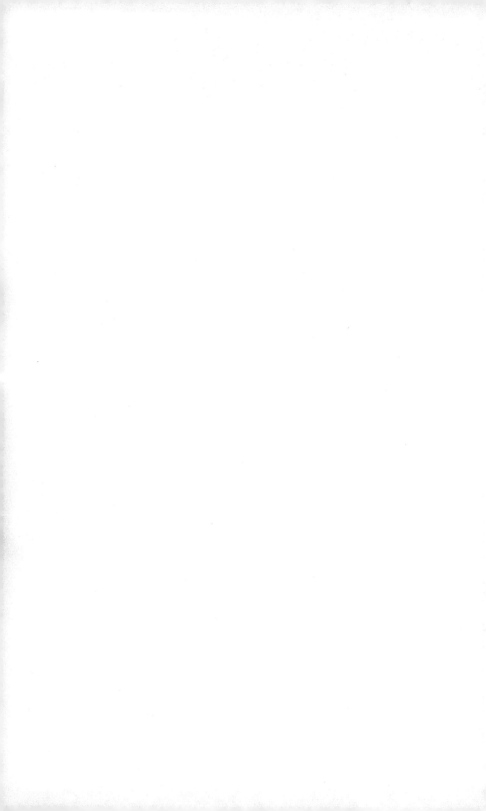

Classics in Psychiatry

Psychological Healing

A Historical and Clinical Study

Pierre [Marie-Felix] Janet

Volume II

ARNO PRESS

A New York Times Company

New York • 1976

Editorial Supervision: EVE NELSON

———◆———

Reprint Edition 1976 by Arno Press Inc.

Reprinted from a copy in
   The University of Illinois Library

CLASSICS IN PSYCHIATRY
ISBN for complete set: 0-405-07410-7
See last pages of this volume for titles.

Manufactured in the United States of America

———◆———

Library of Congress Cataloging in Publication Data

Janet, Pierre, 1859-1947.
   Psychological healing.

   (Classics in psychiatry)
   Translation of Les médications psychologiques.
   Reprint of the 1925 ed. published by Macmillan,
New York.
   Bibliography: p.
   1. Psychotherapy. I. Title. II. Series.
   [DNLM: WM420 J33me 1925a]
   RC480.J3613 1975   616.8'914   75-16710
   ISBN 0-405-07437-9

PSYCHOLOGICAL
HEALING   II

Psychological Healing

A Historical and Clinical Study

By
Pierre Janet

Member of the Institute
Professor of Psychology at the College of France

Translated from the French by
Eden and Cedar Paul

IN TWO VOLUMES.—VOL. II

NEW YORK
THE MACMILLAN COMPANY
1925

Printed in Great Britain by
UNWIN BROTHERS, LIMITED, LONDON AND WOKING

Table of Contents

VOLUME TWO

PART IV

PSYCHOLOGICAL ACQUISITIONS

PART FOUR

PSYCHOLOGICAL ACQUISITIONS

INTRODUCTION

AFTER the methods of psychological treatment which are concerned only with guiding and utilising the existing automatisms, after the methods of treatment which aim at saving the energies while practising the strictest economy, we come to the more ambitious methods of treatment which aim not only at using and saving what a patient already possesses but also at enabling the patient to acquire further tendencies or to recuperate those which he has lost. These methods of treatment are far less precise than the foregoing, and the psychological notions upon which they depend are far less definite. We shall endeavour to study them under three chief heads : education, excitation, and guidance.

CHAPTER TWELVE

EDUCATION AND REEDUCATION

YOUNG children seem to gain fresh tendencies and to increase their energies by daily practice under the guidance of adults. This is the simplest, or certainly the most obvious, process of psychological acquisition, and it is well known under the various names of education, gymnastics, and training. When we try to enable the patient to regain lost functional powers, or to gain new powers, we merely have recourse to the methods which did such good service during youth. Thus the methods of treatment which aim at bringing about the acquirement of really new psychological powers are often described as methods of education and reeducation.

1. HISTORY OF THE REEDUCATION OF NEUROPATHS.

The idea of utilising educational methods for the relief of morbid conditions seems to have first assumed importance in connexion with the work of Seguin (1837–1846) and others interested in the treatment of idiots and defectives. The education of abnormal individuals having given very interesting results, it seemed that it might be useful to apply similar methods to other patients, whose troubles, though less severe, were likewise psychological.

Yet we must not forget that attempts of this character had been made before. Thijssen, in his book, *L'hystérie traumatique* (1888), p. 11, tells us that in the seventeenth century, in the days of Rembrandt, a patient was cured of paralysis by gymnastic exercises. Kouindjy quotes from Amyot an account of the methods used in China to teach those who have been affected with paralysis the re-use of the limbs. Among the French magnetisers I find numerous instances of such methods of treatment.[1] Doctors such as Laisné (1854), Blache (1864), and others, also speak of the use of rhythmical movements in the treatment of chorea. Among the forerunners in the educational treatment of neuropathic disease we must count a number of doctors and pedagogues who have been interested in the education of children with errors of speech, and particularly the education of stammerers. At first the remarkable affection known as stammering was considered quite in isolation, as a mere trouble of speech ; and in early days attempts were made to teach stammerers to speak correctly. As long ago as 1825, Mrs. Leigh of New York advised stammerers to follow certain rules. In especial, she advised them, when speaking, to keep the tongue in contact with the palate as long as possible. But the first application of a carefully thought out and efficacious treatment was made by the French educationist Claudius Chervin, known as Chervin senior, who, after having been interested in the education of deaf-mutes, turned to consider that of stammerers, and who in 1867 founded in Paris a special institution for the relief of stammerers (L'Institution des Bègues). In 1870, his brother, Amédée Chervin, came to help Claudius in the work ; and Claudius' son Arthur Chervin is now the head of the institution. In his book *Du bégaiement considéré comme vice de prononciation* (1867), Claudius Chervin explains that in the treatment of stammering we must induce a psychological discipline of will attention, and emotion. But he does not define this discipline very clearly. It seems to take the form only of trying to give the patient confidence in his own powers. Above all, an attempt is made to restore emotional calm by a silence cure, which the stammerer has to practise during the first week of treatment, The patient, says Chervin, must only communicate with others in writing. Owing to his infirmity, speech is to the stammerer both difficult and disturbing ; the prohibition of speech for a time ensures rest and calm. The second part of the treatment, the only one that is really important, is the motor disciplining of the organs of speech, the organs of respiration, the diaphragm, the thoracic muscles, the alae nasi, the organs of phonation, the larynx, the soft palate, the tongue, and the lips. " The patient is taught to breathe,

---

[1] Lafontaine, L'art de magnétiser, etc., Alcan, Paris, 1860, p. 296.

to control his breathing while he speaks, to speak slowly, to articulate clearly, to scan out syllables, etc. [1]

The course of education by the Chervin method lasted only a few weeks, but the subject had subsequently to continue the exercises for months and years in order to secure permanent results. Chervin's method was thus the educational treatment of a patient suffering from neuropathic disorder.

I think, however, that we have to turn to Charcot, if we wish to find the first interesting systematisation of these educational methods for the treatment of neuropathic disorder. Charcot introduced an orderly treatment of patients suffering from hysterical paralysis by this method of the reeducation of movements. He maintained (the statement is not perfectly correct) that these patients could easily be reeducated, since they had no gross lesions of the nervous system. A remarkable feature was Charcot's demonstration that, in order to render the treatment efficacious, the subject's attention must be concentrated upon the movement he was to perform and upon the sensations of this movement.

Here are the details of Charcot's method. The diagnosis of hysterical paralysis having been made, a distinction was drawn between the cases in which the patient was absolutely unable to move the affected [limb, and the cases in which a certain amount of voluntary movement was still possible. In the former class of cases, the doctor himself moved the patient's paralysed limb, while the patient concentrated attention on what was being done. All that the patient had to do was to attend, to appreciate the movement with all the senses, looking at the movement first of all, and then feeling it when the eyes were closed. To show that he had fully grasped the nature of the movement impressed upon the paralysed limb, the patient had to describe it in words, and to reproduce it voluntarily with the unaffected arm or leg as the case might be. The essential point was to compel the patient to direct his attention consciously towards the lost movements, so that he could learn to repeat them accurately in his mind. After a little time, thanks to the repetition of these exercises, the patient gained the power of making slight movements of

[1] Cf. Arthur Chervin, Du bégaiement et de son traitement, 1879 ; Comment ou guérit les bègues, 1882.

the paralysed limb, and this brought his case into the second category.

Then, by all possible means, it was necessary to increase the consciousness of the movements of the affected limb. Charcot liked to attach an indicator to the end of the finger, so that the patient could appreciate its movements better; and in the patient's hand there was a delicate dynamometer by which the slightest variations in pressure were indicated on a scale. The patient, keeping watch on all these signs of voluntary movement, noticing likewise with careful attention the movements impressed on the limb by others, and also never failing to reproduce the movements with the healthy limb, was enabled by degrees to regain the power of moving the paralysed limb. Continually aware of the advances that were being made, he recovered control, in time, over the dissociated function.

All Charcot's pupils at this epoch emphasised the importance of the method I have been describing, so that it soon became famous. Paul Richer and Gilles de la Tourette recorded cures obtained in this way. Séglas speaks of several cures of hysterical paralysis.[1] Féré, studying twenty-three cases successfully treated by the method, attempted to formulate a theory of the treatment. He considered that the beneficial results were to be explained by the stimulation of the brain centres corresponding to the paralysed areas.[2] This phraseology, half psychological and half anatomical, conveyed no precise significance, and was indeed somewhat absurd; still, it presented an image which had its uses for the moment, since it enabled doctors to understand the psychological facts which they had to translate into their customary speech. Féré's phrase has been a good deal used. Quite recently Lagrange has employed almost identical terms to describe Charcot's method for the reeducation of the limbs in persons suffering from hysterical paralysis, and he gives interesting examples of the success of the method.[3]

At the same period, similar methods came into vogue for the treatment of mutism and of hysterical aphonia. Ernoul,

---

[1] Traitement des paralysies par l'exercice musculaire, " Annales Médico-Psychologiques," March 1887.

[2] Sensation et mouvement, 1887.

[3] Les mouvements méthodiques et la mécanothérapie, 1899, pp. 309 and 312.

in his thesis on hysterical mutism penned in 1898, enumerates the various methods of treatment which have been employed ; they are some of them strange enough. In certain instances, emetics were given, or the mouth was suddenly forced open ; such plans would seem to act by a sort of suggestion. Other methods, such as massage of the larynx, the induction of coughing, respiratory gymnastics (especially advised by Fournier and Garel), efforts to make sounds—are educational exercises. In Charcot's clinic the patient had to listen attentively to simple sounds uttered in his presence. Like deaf-mutes who are being taught to speak, the patient had to touch the doctor's chest and larynx, and thus to become aware of the movements and the vibrations from the sense of touch. By degrees he had to learn how to breathe correctly ; how to make all the voluntary changes in respiration, produce accelerations, pauses, sighs, coughs, yawns, etc. Then he had to try earnestly to make sounds, while attending carefully to the sensations which these sounds aroused in himself. Finally he had to exercise himself in the repetition of syllables and words.

We shall find that an analogous system of reeducation has been applied in patients suffering from various disorders of movement such as astasia-abasia, different forms of chorea, and contractures. Charcot laid especial stress upon the treatment of contracture, which was to begin as early as possible after the onset of the trouble. " We must never let hysterical contracture drag on," he said. The treatment of this peculiar and important affection was to begin by the massage of the muscles affected with contracture.[1] Gilles de la Tourette added : " Such massage acts in virtue of a mechanism which we are unable to understand."[2] Féré, however, said that the massage, just like the mechanical movement of a paralysed limb, stimulated the cortical centres corresponding to the limb.[3] Binet was well aware that in hysterical contracture, just as in hysterical paralysis, the individual has lost consciousness of the sensations of the affected part, and that restoration must be brought about by a method of treatment analogous to that just described.[4] As soon as the patient,

[1] Charcot, Oeuvres, vol. iii, p. 395 ; vol. ix, p. 462.
[2] Traité de l'hystérie, vol. iii, p. 441.   [3] Op. cit., p. 223.
[4] " Revue Philosophique," 1889, vol. i., p. 167.

thanks to the massage, has recovered to some extent the power of moving the limbs, the treatment by passive movement will be the same as that of a case of paralysis. Finally we come to the treatment of hysterical anorexia, which, at the Salpêtrière, was treated by reeducation of the function of taking food. The first part of the treatment was the isolation of the patient. The next stage, and a more important one, was the administering of a graduated diet which reeducated the appetite and the alimentary functions. I myself wrote in 1892 : " It is necessary to put the patients upon a normal diet as soon as possible, for this will speedily reawaken the sensation of normal needs." [1]

The second epoch in the history of treatment by reeducation begins with the application of similar methods to paralyses and other disorders of movement consequent upon organic lesions. I think especially of the disorders of movement that occur in locomotor ataxia. Leyden and Fraenkel were the first to apply such methods in these diseases. They attempted to enable the ataxic to walk better by teaching him how to guide his movements in a way different from that to which he had been accustomed. Owing to the lesions of the spinal cord, the patient, they said, had lost the tactile and kinaesthetic sensations guiding the movements of the lower limbs, and must make the loss good through the aid of purely visual sensations. He must be taught to guide the actions of walking by sight, must be taught to perform purposive movements with the aid of visual impressions just as before he became ill he had performed purposive movements with the aid of tactile impressions. The patient had to learn some specified way of walking, just as anyone else is accustomed to learn an exercise which is regulated by vision—such an exercise as shooting at a target, for instance. The desired gait was analysed into a series of elementary movements, each of which the patients had to watch attentively in others and in himself. At first he performed the simplest movements while he was lying down, passing on from this to the performance of more complicated movements while sitting up

[1] Traitement psychologique de l'hystérie, in Robin's Traité de thérapeutique appliquée ; Etat mental des hystériques, second edition, 1911, p. 687.

and finally while standing. He had to be assisted by very simple mechanical apparatus. For example, he had to place his feet in regular succession upon lines or figures drawn upon the floor ; he had to practice going up and down stairs; and so on. Fraenkel's methods were completed and systematised by Goldscheider and Jacob.[1] They were adopted by Raymond, who introduced them into the Salpêtrière clinic, where they gave excellent results.[2] In the United States, E. W. Taylor and E. A. Lindström have published an account of thirty cases of well-marked locomotor ataxia in which the power of walking was satisfactorily restored by such means.[3] Exercises of the kind have also been carefully described in a book by Lagrange ; [4] and they have been recently expounded with a good deal of detail by Kouindjy,[5] who makes an interesting study of the conditions essential to the success of this therapeutic method.

The methods originally applied to the relief of locomotor ataxia have gradually secured a wider application. J. Madison Taylor tried them in paralysis agitans, a very intractable disease.[6]

We learn also from Maurice Faure's essay that they have been successful in cases of organic hemiplegia, and that they have promoted the restoration of the power of movement.[7] Stephen Ivory Franz records interesting endeavours to bring about the reeducation of speech in patients suffering from aphasia consequent upon organic disease.[8]

In a third phase of development, these educational methods of treatment have been applied in various disorders of movement affecting neuropaths who are not suffering from hysteria in the strict sense of the term ; most of these were cases of motor disorder in persons suffering from psychasthenia, and especially psychasthenics suffering from tics of various

[1] Handbuch der physikalischen Therapie, p. 256.
[2] Leçons sur les maladies du système nerveux, 1897, p. 581.
[3] Experiences in the Treatment of Tabes by Coordinate Exercises, " Boston Medical and Surgical Journal," December 13, 1906.
[4] Op. cit., p. 330.   [5] " Journal de Physiothérapie," March 15, 1910.
[6] The Amelioration of Paralysis Agitans and other Forms of Tremor by systematic Exercises, " Journal of Nervous and Mental Diseases," 1901, pp. 28 and 133.
[7] La rééducation motrice, " Revue Scientifique," 1902, vol. ii, p. 73.
[8] " The Journal of Philosophy, Psychology, and Scientific Methods," October 1905, pp. 589–597.

kinds. In 1889 I myself pointed out the part played by automatism in the tics so common in these patients, and I referred to the educational procedures by which the abnormal motor tendencies might be modified. Morton Prince laid stress, as concerned these association neuroses, upon the abnormal grouping of movements which he termed neurograms. Subsequently he compared them to the artificial associations produced in the dogs experimented on by Pavloff. According to Prince, the essence of the treatment lay in effecting the dissolution of these artificial associations by an education the reverse of that which produced them.[1]

Other psychologists, such as Payot, have insisted upon the law of memory in accordance with which every memory which is not refreshed from time to time has a tendency to become less distinct and to disappear. Now, to a certain degree, it is within our power to favour or to hinder the reproduction of movements and thoughts, and we can thus condemn a memory or a motor tendency to death by refusing to exercise it. An interesting method for the treatment of tics has been organised out of these various elements.

In former days, doctors made almost no attempt to cure tics and habit-spasms, regarding them as of trifling importance or as incurable. Charcot and Georges Guinon did not take an encouraging view with regard to the curability of tics, and, like Trousseau, they were extremely reserved upon the subject. Treatment by reeducation began with Jolly in 1830 and with Blache in 1854. The methods were studied and rendered more precise by Brissaud, and by his pupils Meige and Feindel.[2] According to the last-named authors, we are concerned with a method of treatment by a prescribed immobility; the main principle of " Brissaud's method " is the disciplining of motionlessness and of movement. The first procedure is to preserve absolute immobility, the motionlessness that is needed for the taking of a photograph, maintained by a limb or by the face, at first for a very short period, but for a period which progressively increases. The subject, to begin with, must remain motionless, controlling the tic, for a moment merely, while we count " one, two, three," for

[1] Morton Prince, The Mechanism of Recurrent Psychopathic States, " Journal of Abnormal Psychology," July 1911, p. 135.
[2] Meige and Feindel, Les tics et leur traitement, 1902 ; Meige, Histoire d'un tiqueur, " Journal de médecine et de chirurgie," Aug. 25, 1901.

instance. He will be able to do this quite easily, and we gradually increase the duration of the motionlessness by two or three seconds at a time, up to several minutes; until, at length, the patient becomes able to remain in various postures for a whole hour without giving way to the tic.

When immobility is thus secured for a sufficiently long time, we must teach the patient to perform voluntary movements without the tic or habit-spasm. If we are concerned with a twitching of the head or with a spasmodic wry-neck, we shall first make the patient perform movements of the arms or legs without disturbing the immobility of the head. Then we shall try to induce the patient to make voluntary movements of the head itself, of the eyes, of the mouth, without the reappearance of the twitching of the head or of the spasmodic wry-neck. These exercises must be repeated in the presence of persons who are able to watch their carrying out with attention, and to point out the failures as well as the advances. When the patient has made considerable improvement, he will be able to repeat them when he is by himself, watching the performance in a mirror. The essential point is that the patient shall be interested in his own treatment and shall practise it with close attention for a long time, for several months in succession as a rule; and he must persist long after the apparent cure of the spasm, for these troubles are extremely liable to relapse.

The close kinship between the various kinds of habit-spasm and stammering has led to the application of the same methods of reeducation for the relief of stammering. Pitres has proposed for the treatment of habit-spasm, a method based upon the regulation of the breathing.[1] During a sitting of ten minutes, daily or twice a day, the patient must practise deep breathing, must breathe as slowly as possible and as deeply as possible, raising the arms while breathing in and lowering them while breathing out. Writing of Pitres' method, Meige and Feindel say : " It seems to us that the efforts of attention made by the subject to carry out the respiratory exercises must have a salutary effect. No matter whether we are concerned with a deliberate respiratory movement or with a voluntary movement of the limbs to which the per-

---

[1] Tcis convulsifs généralisés, traités par la gymnastique respiratoire, " Journal de Médecine de Bordeaux," Feb. 17, 1901.

former carefully attends, what we ask of a patient suffering from habit-spasm is that, for a moment, he should discipline his capricious will, should master the inappropriate motor reaction which is inclined to distort the deliberate gesture." [1] Such reeducative procedures have effected remarkable cures, and the before-mentioned authors have published accounts of them.

An interesting application of the same methods has been made in the case of the occupational cramps which are often varieties of psychasthenic habit-spasm. Happily, doctors no longer prescribe in such cases more or less absurd surgical methods of treatment ; and they have abandoned, for the most part, the immobilisation of function which Charcot used to advise when he would forbid patients suffering from writer's cramp to use the pen for many months. Nowadays, such patients are promptly subjected to educational treatment. Thiol, of Riga, and Montarani have pointed out various rules which must be observed in the treatment of these affections ; their remarks apply especially to writer's cramp.[2] Kouindjy in a series of interesting studies has summarised the work of the before-mentioned writers, adding useful observations of his own, and thus formulating a gymnastic system for such patients.[3] He tells us that in cases of writer's cramp there is almost always a hypertony of the flexor muscles and a hypotony of the extensor muscles, and he begins the reeducation by a series of exercises which provide work for the extensor muscles. For the same reason, he has the patient taught to write with the hand supinated, writing with the aid of the flexor muscles being thus transformed into writing with the aid of the extensor muscles. Then he makes the patient learn to write slowly ; " Gilbert Ballet used to say that it was often enough for the patient to learn to write slowly, and then the condition of cramp would be much mitigated." There must be a continued practice of all the exercises which develop accurate movements of the hand, such as those of the pigeon-holes, the planchette, the triangular prisms, the keyboard, etc. According to this author, we

---

[1] Meige and Feindel, op. cit., p. 574.
[2] Montarani [A Case of painful Writer's Cramp cured by rational Psychotherapy], " Rivista Sperimentale di Freniatria," December 1909.
[3] La crampe professionnelle et son traitement par le massage méthodique et la rééducation, " Nouvelle Iconographie de la Salpêtrière," July 1906.

shall usually secure good results by such exercises after the lapse of from two to four months.

Akin to such methods of treatment are those which aim at the restoration of the power of satisfactory speech in stammerers, methods which were advocated long ago by Chervin. Nowadays, for this purpose, we have more generalised methods ; and we also have methods of gymnastics which aim at modifying the neuropathic motor disorders. Claudius Chervin's methods are still applied by his son Arthur Chervin. In Belgium, Romma uses similar methods ; and he also advises prolonged expiration during the pronunciation of the vowels, and strong inspiration at the beginning of phrases, with efforts to breathe and phonate rhythmically. He likewise recommends the subject to make sweeping gestures with the arms while speaking. This would seem to be a practical application of the results of certain experiments made by Féré, who had demonstrated (so he believed) that the speech function excited the activity of the right arm ; and, conversely, that movements of the arm had a stimulating effect upon the speech, owing to the irradiation of energy from one nerve centre to another adjoining it.

Other authors, such as Liebmann of Berlin (1898), and Netkacheff of Moscow (1900), protest against these exercises of breathing and speech, which, they say, serve only to concentrate the patient's attention upon his malady. They want to restrict the treatment to the control of emotionality, by aiding the patient to overcome the difficulties he finds in speaking in the presence of others. They practise him in telling stories, and in longer and longer conversations, at first in the presence of the teacher only, then in the presence of relatives and friends, and finally in the presence of strangers.

Robert Foy, in an interesting essay on stammering,[1] takes up an intermediate position. His contention is that stammering is akin to occupational cramps, to emotional disturbances, to verbal phobias, and to social obsessions. Stammering is merely a specialisation and localisation of the natural emotionality (exaggerated or perverted)—a localisation in the organs of speech. He writes : " The primary disorder is a disorder

---

[1] Le bégaiement, nouveaux essais pathogéniques et thérapeutiques, " Bulletins et Mémoires de la Société Française d'Oto-Rhino-Laryngologie, Congrès de 1913."

of the coordination of the muscles of respiration and of those of phonation, a disorder which is in rapport with the emotional state. The twitching mouth and the modifications of pronunciation are no more than secondary phenomena, no more than compensatory movements superadded to the primary trouble. The dread of speaking, the fixed ideas, and the intellectual timidity, are likewise superadded phenomena, superadded at a later stage. . . . These emotional troubles are to be dealt with by a psychomotor treatment, which must demand from the patient considerable efforts of attention, will, and reasoning." But only those who are approaching years of discretion can, he says, make such efforts ; and the treatment of stammering by this method could not begin until a child is twelve or fifteen years old, whereas stammering makes its first appearance at three or five years old. What we want is a method of treatment applicable in those early years, when the child, if capable of acquiring a bad habit, is also readily able to rid himself of it. Furthermore the methods under discussion, tend to fix the attention upon articulation, and nothing makes us more likely to perform a movement badly than being afraid that we are going to perform it badly. Finally, these efforts of attention and will tend to exhaust one who is already prone to exhaustion. " What we want is to enable the patient to use a natural, reflex, and automatic speech ; and not a conscious deliberate, and artificial speech."

This author, then, is inclined to pay little attention to the disorders of articulation, which he regards as secondary and compensatory phenomena, and to aim merely at the reestablishment of coordination between breathing and phonation. He hopes to achieve this by a few simple exercises repeated every morning and every evening. The reeducation of the breathing is essential, for stammering is attended by spasms of the diaphragm and by all kinds of respiratory incoordination. Nose breathing, slow, deep, and silent, while the alae nasi are kept dilated ; expirations that are still slower and still more complete while the alae nasi are allowed to collapse ; various kinds of pressure exercised by the hands on the epigastrium, the abdomen, and the base of the thorax— these will help to dilate the epigastric region during inspiration and to compress it during expiration. The stammerer must learn to sing in order that he may consolidate the coordination between the phonetic functions and the auditory functions, for this coordination is the basis of the treatment. If he stops his ears, he will be better able to hear and supervise his own laryngeal vibrations. A respiratory girdle, which the author calls the "ductophone," is so arranged as to ring an electric bell when the chest is empty. The subject acquires the habit of beginning to inspire when this signal sounds, and of keeping his chest expanded during the exercises of phonation. Such exercises counteract the principal cause of stammering, which is respiratory incoordination. Finally, the use of a phonograph enables the patient to control and correct himself. All these methods of treatment, which are interesting, and perhaps less different from Chervin's methods than the author imagines, facilitate the reeducation of speech in neuropaths who stammer.

To a larger extent than is commonly supposed, disorders of sensation (or of perception) are related to disorders of movement. It is not surprising, therefore, that a great many authors have attempted to restore the perceptive functions to health by the reeducation of the movements which accompany and constitute perception. Nattier, Marage, and various other otologists, have tried to reestablish the hearing of the deaf by teaching the patients to react correctly on hearing certain definite sounds. The treatment of various troubles of sight has been found more successful. Parinaud, Javal, Rémy of Dijon, and Cantonnet, have worked at the cure of strabismus by the reeducation of binocular vision. Javal's stereoscope has been variously modified and improved, and a course of gymnastics for the eyes has come to play a considerable part in such treatment.[1]

As we have just seen, the reeducation of speech must be essentially based upon the reeducation of breathing; and we have already learned that the reeducation of breathing is of great importance in cases of hysterical mutism. No doubt this form of reeducation concerns a visceral function, but this visceral function is not completely independent of the will. Such respiratory exercises have speedily become independent of the treatment of disorders of speech, and have

[1] Cf. Cantonnet, La rééducation de la vision dans le strabisme, ' Presse Médicale," May 15, 1919.

shown themselves to be essential for their own sake.   The teachers of Swedish gymnastics, and especially Ling, have shown the importance of methodical respiratory gymnastics, and have formulated the rules of the practice.   Deep-breathing exercises ventilate the lungs more fully, and sweep out the residual air.   They have great influence upon the general health, and perhaps also upon mental activity.   They ought to form, more often than they do, a regular element in the general treatment of neuroses.   Breathing exercises are often more important when the neuropathic troubles affect the respiratory functions.   I have already shown more than once [1] that respiratory gymnastics are not only useful in hysterical mutism but are also useful in the paroxysms of coughing, yawning, sniffing, sighing, and hiccough which are so common among neuropaths.   Lagrange also lays stress on the importance of these breathing exercises.[2]   He appears to consider that such gymnastic exercises must sometimes be carried out mechanically with the aid of apparatus which bring about movements of the limbs and the thorax while the subject remains passive.   It is quite possible that exercises of the kind may be useful in organic diseases ; but where we have to do with neuroses, it will always be well, if I mistake not, that the exercises should be performed with the aid of will, effort, and attention.   More recently, Georges Rosenthal has shown how common and how serious respiratory insufficiency is, and has given an excellent formulation of the rules for such special respiratory gymnastics.[3]

At first, treatment by the education of the function of feeding had only been applied in cases of hysterical anorexia, but at about this time its use became more generalised.   Paul Dubois, recalling the work of Barras, *Traité sur les gastralgies et les entéralgies ou maladies nerveuses de l'estomac et des intestins* (1823), maintained that a large number of gastric disorders were connected with bad habits, emotional troubles, and the various neuroses ; and he insisted upon the importance of an alimentary education which disregarded the fears, the prejudices, and the bad habits of the patient. In Parker's *Psychotherapy*, R. C. Cabot ingeniously classes this treatment among " Work Cures " : " A young college

---

[1] Névroses et idées fixes, 1898.   [2] Op. cit., pp. 132–180.
[3] " La Revue des Hôpitaux," 1905.

student . . . was under my care for what he thought was a serious disease of the stomach." Taking food gave him pain, so that he nearly starved himself to death. Cabot " told him that he must eat whether his stomach hurt him or not, . . . assured him again and again, like a phonograph, that he could and must force his stomach to work." The prescription was effective—it was a " work cure." . . . " Work makes people's stomachs, their bowels, their sexual organs, as well as their brains, perform their proper functions and keep their places." [1] The same ideas find interesting expression in an article by A. Blix on the influence of the mind upon the digestion.[2] Dejerine and Gauckler reiterate Dubois' theories on this subject. They see how the appetite is disturbed by various mental causes, how bad habits play their part in producing bulimia or anorexia, and how important alimentation is in practical life. They contend that a great many serious symptoms of the neuroses can be overcome by a judicious training of the function of food-taking. Sollier and de Fleury protest against some exaggerations of this doctrine, showing that those who have applied the method have been inclined to overlook a large number of organic stomach troubles, and, perhaps, to encourage the development of intoxications of a digestive origin. The protesters are right, but the previously mentioned authors are also right. It is always a question of exact and carefully considered diagnosis. Most of the writers who study digestive disorders recognise in their etiology the great importance of all dietetic habits, such as inadequate mastication, unduly rapid deglutition, aerophagia, etc. ; and they insist upon the need for some sort of education of the function of food-taking.[3]

The genital functions and also the functions of sleep have been the objects of attempts aiming at their regulation by educative exercises. In Parker's *Psychotherapy* (III, i, 74) there is an interesting article by the Rev. Samuel Fellows upon " Insomnia, its Nature, Causes, and Cure." The author shows how often bad habits play a part in such troubles, and how education can improve our powers of sleep. Dejerine

[1] Parker's Psychotherapy, III, i, 27–28.
[2] Ibid., iii, 48.
[3] Cf., in especial, J. Guisez, De l'étiologie et de differentes formes des sténoses inflammatoires de la région cardiaque de l'oesophage, " Presse Médicale," June 4, 1917.

and Gauckler also insist upon the need for educating sleep (op. cit., p. 517) ; and the champions of the New Thought method in America give a series of rules as to the position to assume, the words the would-be slumberer is to repeat to himself, the various measures to be taken in order to ensure satisfactory sleep. This rapid review shows us how remarkable an extension was undergone at one time by the method of training the motor and visceral functions liable to be disordered in neurotic patients.

But reeducation has been given a yet wider scope, for it has been applied to the treatment, not only of purely motor troubles, but also of disorders that are more obviously and more strictly mental. At first, disorders of the mind were dealt with only through the intermediation of the disorders of movement.[1] As I have already shown more than once, the patient whose most obvious symptoms seem to be phobias, obsessions, and even delusions, and in whom there is nothing to direct attention to the disorders of the movements of their limbs, nevertheless exhibit many disorders in those movements. I have frequently insisted upon the weakness, the suddenness, the irregularity, and the awkwardness of the movements in such persons. These characteristics of their movements have often been noted since childhood, long before the appearance of the typical mental disorders. The awkwardness of the movements is related to the disorders of activity characteristic of neuropaths—the disorders which are the source of all their subsequent troubles. Does it not seem likely enough that a transformation of these movements by means of a process of education may have an effect upon the totality of the patient's activities, and thus prove competent to prevent or remove the mental troubles ? That is what I suggested already in my book on obsessions in 1903, when I advised that a child predisposed to such disorders should be habituated to movement, which is one of the great antagonists of brooding. " Such a child " I wrote, " must practise a number of physical exercises of all kinds. These exercises must be regulated and skilful, for it is essential to develop in

[1] Cf. Charles K. Mills, The Treatment of Nervous and Mental Diseases by Systematised Active Exercises, The Transactions of the Philadelphia County Medical Society, Jan. 11, 1888.

the child a skill in the performance of bodily movements. Over-scrupulous persons are clumsy, and are afraid to touch or handle anything. We must accustom them from their earliest years to use their hands, to practise manual crafts, to dig, to do work in wood or paper, to cultivate plants, to make various articles, to act upon real objects." Ideas of this sort have been adopted by those who are interested in gymnastic methods of treatment, but with great lack of precision. Lagrange speaks of the importance of continual training in bodily carriage, and of the persistent watchfulness which it is necessary to exercise over certain neuropaths in order to call their attention to their muscles.[1] " The influence of bodily attitudes is very great," write Camus and Pagniez : " a neurasthenic's energies are developed by making him adopt energetic and vigorous attitudes." [2] Dejerine and Gauckler insist upon the need for correcting " disharmonic attitudes," to which they attribute an important role in the production of phobias and obsessions of fatigue. " It is important to make the patients walk slowly, counting their footsteps, and stopping to breathe. We must teach them to stand upright without aiming at absolute immobility. We must safeguard them against all disturbances of balance. In a word, we must teach them how to break up their movements into the component elements, and how to regulate them." [3] Cabot writes : " Why is it that we contract all our muscles when the need is to contract a few and leave the rest slack ? How comes it that when we sit down to write a letter, we write not with the fingers of one hand but with all the muscles of the right arm and shoulder, and not infrequently with our faces, our tongues, and our legs ? " We must learn to guide our motor energies intelligently, and to correct these bad habits.[4]

It seems to me that the growth of this idea has been one of the most important characteristics of the therapeutic movement which has developed in America, in opposition to Christian Science, under the name of New Thought. Most of these authors endeavour to modify the mental state of neuro-

[1] Lagrange, op. cit., p. 361.   [2] Camus and Pagniez, op. cit., p. 550.
[3] Dejerine and Gauckler, op. cit., p. 150.
[4] The Use and Abuse of Rest in the Treatment of Disease, Parker's Psychotherapy, II, ii, p. 25.

paths by the education of the movements of the limbs and by the suppression of all the minor disorders by which these patients are characterised. Walker Atkinson recommends that the following exercises should be made several times a day : " Walk up and down holding a glass full of water stretched out in front of you, being careful not to spill a drop. This will teach you to keep watch over tremors and involuntary movements. You must learn to read without allowing your lips or your tongue to move while you are reading. You must practise opening the fingers slowly one by one, and then practise closing them slowly, doing this exercise for ten minutes, watching all the while with great care the opening and closing of the fingers." Turnbull recommends exercises of the same character, and insists upon regular breathing while the exercises are in progress. " The accomplishment of these apparently trivial tasks is important, for it strengthens the will. Do these things simply as a task." The same author emphasises the importance of exercising the powers of sight : " We must practise ourselves in fixing the gaze with great intensity upon a black point on a sheet of white paper. Begin by fixing the gaze in this way for a minute, but practise it until you can maintain it for a quarter of an hour ; then change the direction of fixity and maintain the new direction for a time. . . . Look at yourself fixedly in a mirror in order to accustom yourself to endure another's glance ; look others firmly in the eyes, or if you cannot at first bear to look them in the eyes, fix your gaze on an imaginary point at the root of their nose. . . . Do not forget that an energetic man always gives us the impression of being at rest. He is not nervous ; there is no agitation about him ; he is confident of his own reserves of strength."[1] It is needless to enumerate all these exercises, which are always of the same kind, which have the same general characteristics. They show the same therapeutic trend. The invariable object is to train the attitude towards things, in order thereby, in the end, to modify the morale. There has been a great spread of this notion of late, and it has even made its way into ordinary literature. In Pierre de Coulevain's novel *Sur la branche*, we find the following description of a nursery in which the children were being trained : " When I went into

[1] W. Turnbull, Course of Personal Magnetism.

the nursery the other day, I saw Francis sitting gloomily in the middle of the room. He had no toys, and his hands were resting on the arms of his chair. ' What are you doing there ? ' I asked. ' What is he doing ? ' answered Sarah, surprised at my question. ' He is learning how to keep perfectly still. He does it for ten minutes every morning and every afternoon. He practises repose, and so do I.' " This practice of repose may certainly be recommended as likely to do a great deal of good to unstable neuropaths. All these gymnastics for the training in rhythmical movement and for the training of bodily carriage which are so popular to-day give expression to the same therapeutic idea.

Quite a number of therapeutists, bolder than those hitherto mentioned and more logical, must now be considered. Since mental disorders have to be modified by education, the troubles, say these, must be attacked directly. What we have to amend are not the movements of the body but the movements of the mind. We should exercise the mind itself, and by mental gymnastics should encourage the development of the faculties which seem to be lacking in the patient, the faculties which will enable him to make headway against his malady. Morton Prince was one of the first to lay stress upon education in these things as a means for the treatment of neuropathic disorder. He has written on *The Educational Treatment of Neurasthenia and Certain Hysterical States.*[1] In this essay he justly criticises Weir Mitchell's rest cure when applied in an exaggerated manner and in the absence of moral influences. To improve a patient's nutrition, and even to enable a patient to put on fat, does not necessarily lead to the cure of mental disorders. An improvement in nutrition is more apt to be the effect than the cause of the reestablishment of nervous health. Besides, the Weir Mitchell treatment has its inconveniences and even its dangers. Prince prefers to attempt the reeducation of the patient's character. What he advises is, not to isolate the patient, but to separate him from his customary environment, and to teach him how to live more wisely in a new environment. " The most difficult and the most interesting thing is what I call the education of the patient. It is to this that I look when I want to give the

[1] " Boston Medical and Surgical Journal," October 6, 1898.

of controlling emotions and passions.[1] We must learn to check at the outset sudden attacks of anger, fi\ obstinacy; we must not allow children to fly into a 1 to weep, to wring their hands in despair. Sick people, \ children, must be habituated to have always present in t. mind ideas which can antagonise anger, and speedily overcom it by a vigorous act of will which gives a fresh direction to the sentiments. Nay more, we must accustom children to bear sudden shocks upon the senses, to hear loud and unexpected noises without being startled; we must expose patients to conditions which will arouse little causes of emotion so that they may be accustomed to exercise their powers of inhibition. They will thus become less and less emotional, and this will greatly diminish anxiety and various other neurotic troubles. The same conception inspires the work of J. E. Donley,[2] who shares Oppenheim's views as to the aim of psychotherapeutics. "Above all," he says, "we must get rid of the habit of fear, which is the main factor of most neuroses."

The same idea, I think, forms the essential part of the writings of Paul Emile Lévy, a French physician. This author shows that many troubles which appear to be of organic origin are really the outcome of unrecognised neuroses, and that in these cases excess of physical care is harmful rather than helpful.[3] The preferable psychotherapeutic method, the great aim, is neither suggestion nor persuasion, for these furnish no more than an insufficient formula. What he advocates is the education or the reeducation of the neurotic patient. By this term "education" he wishes to imply, not only that psychotherapy must be rational, must address itself preeminently to the reason; but also, and above all, his theory is based upon a fundamentally important pathogenic datum. He holds that the hysterical or neurasthenic neuroses are, primarily, the consequence, the inevitable result, of an initial lack of ·education, or of an erroneous education. "The neurasthenic, the nervous person, is, more than anything

[1] Cf. Oppenheim, Psychotherapy in Child Training, in Parker's Psychotherapy, I, ii, 51.
[2] Psychotherapy and Reeducation, "Journal of Abnormal Psychology," April 1911.
[3] Lévy, Les névroses méconnues. Pathogénie psychique et psychothérapie. "Journal des Practiciens," 1906, No. 32.

patient health of body and mind, so as to enable him to p
his own part in the battle of life. . . . To this end we n
modify our patients' beliefs, must relieve them of their fe
and must help them to get the better of their disast
inclination to regard every disagreeable sensation as the
of some grave and incurable lesion. We must accu:
them to control and suppress emotional states, and her
doctor's tact and personal character are of pri
importance." Finally we must teach the patient to u
take as many actions as possible—when they can be u
taken without doing him any harm.

Lewellys F. Barker lays stress upon similar condit
For him the treatment of neuroses consists chiefly of iso
and psychotherapy. By the latter treatment he understan
reeducation of emotion, attention, and will. The docto
inspire confidence in his patient, must teach him firmn
will, and must enable him to pass by degrees from at
reliance upon the medical adviser to self-guidance. W. S
Thayer [2] also insists upon the importance of the
reeducation of the mental and voluntary functions, ar
wise of the digestive functions. T. A. Williams adds
is the doctor's business to cure the patient of bad ha
developing good habits to counteract them.[3]

Most of these studies concerning reeducation are
and seem to bear upon all the functions of the mind
distinction. A few, however, are more precise, sing
special faculties by preference. A good many aut
instance, are occupied with the tendency of the mind
exaggerated emotion, towards what is known as e
which plays a great part in many disorders; a
consider the resistance to emotion to be a function v
be developed by gymnastics. Oppenheim, in his /
Psychotherapeutics (1907), and in more recent article
us to begin in early childhood the cultivation of t

[1] On the Psychic Treatment of some of the Functional Neu
also, Some Experiences with the simple Methods of Psychother
education, " American Journal of the Medical Sciences," Octobe
[2] On the Importance of simple physical and psychical Meth
ment, " The Johns Hopkins Hospital Bulletin," November 1907.
[3] A few Hints from personal Experience in Psychotherapy i
physiological Analogies, " Monthly Cyclopaedia and Medic
July 1908.

else, one who has been badly or insufficiently educated. Education, therefore, is the most essential point in the treatment of neuroses. Education alone, if conducted on the right lines and pushed far enough, can not only restore health, but can (I wish to emphasise this point) maintain health definitely." [1]

This education must fight against the patient's prepossessions. The patient must be shown how important it is for him to regulate his emotivity ; he must be made to understand how large a part this emotivity plays in giving rise to his symptoms. In order to stop emotional crises, Lévy advises the patient to breathe more gently ; not to cry out, not to weep, not to complain. " In a word, I teach him to calm his impressionability, not· contenting himself with a general and commonplace suggestion ; but trying to establish this calm in every detail, in all its diverse manifestations, which are the outward and visible sign of the impressionability." [2]

Whereas the before-mentioned authors are mainly concerned with the education of emotion, others have aimed chiefly at the education of attention. I myself studied this question in 1892, when I described the difficulties I had found in treating a patient named Justine, suffering from a remarkable form of hysterical obsession, and when I recounted the results secured.[3] I showed how making the patient do mental work—a very difficult task at the outset—seemed to facilitate greatly the restoration of mental activity. I shall return to the consideration of this case when I come to deal with stimulant methods of treatment. De Fleury, who likewise insists upon the importance of mental work, details the ways in which we can make it comparatively easy for our patients to undertake it. He shows that in the case of mental work, as in the case of other kinds of work, there is a considerable element of habit, which has to be developed, and upon which we must mainly depend. Routine, in fact, enables us to begin work without effort, and economises energy in various ways. De Fleury insists that the work must be done daily,

[1] Lévy, Les principes de la psychothérapie, la rééducation, " Bulletin de la Société de l'Internat," November 1904.
[2] Lévy, Traitement psychique de l'hystérie, " Presse Médicale," April 29, 1903.
[3] Histoire d'une idée fixe, " Revue Philosophique," February 1894, p. 121 ; Névroses et idées fixes, 1898, vol. i, p. 156.

at a fixed hour, without fail ; and he says that all the most
noted writers have been able to secure splendid results by this
methodical way of working. " Make the habit of daily work
second nature, make it something approaching a mania."
This is what will do most good to inattentive and idle patients.
R. C. Cabot, in his interesting essay on the *Work Cure*, insists
that the patient must use mental work as a means of cure.
Let the patient learn to work, to throw off worries while he
is working ; let him learn how to give full attention, after a
period of complete relaxation ; and let him also learn how
to stop work. " He must know how to shut up his mind as
if he were turning off a gas tap after a certain period of work." [1]
Finally I may recall that Dejerine and Gauckler have
developed the same ideas of the importance of mental work
in the education of the attention in neuropaths.[2]

This historical summary, though cursory and incomplete,
is an attempt to display the remarkable evolution of the
methods of treatment by gymnastics and education. At the
outset, the endeavour was to treat by these means various
elementary and circumscribed disorders affecting well-known
motor-functions. Then the claims of gymnastics were enlarged,
and they were applied as remedial measures to functions
of a more lofty and complicated character. The aim was
to practise the gymnastics of emotion and attention just as
at an earlier stage there had been practised the gymnastics
of walking and speech. We are entitled to ask whether, in
this ambitious extension of the scope of education, education
has preserved its characteristics, and whether we have a
warrant for expecting from these later forms of education
the same effects that were secured from the former.

2. THE CONCEPT OF EDUCATION.

The treatments we have just been discussing were considered under the caption " Education and Reeducation."
But now we have to come to an understanding as to the
psychological significance which ought to be attached to
these words, for this will enable us to appraise more accurately
the worth and opportuneness of the methods.

[1] Cabot, Work Cure, in Parker's Psychotherapy, III, ii, 24-25.
[2] Op. cit., p. 523.

There can be no doubt that in a great many contemporary works these words are understood in an extremely general sense. For the successful transformation of a morbid form of behaviour, when the transformation occurs slowly and gradually, and when it seems to be due to the influence of some one who acts upon the patient at regular intervals, the term "education" is used. Many authors, especially in books on psychotherapy published in the United States of America, also employ the term "education" to denote any kind of psychological treatment, much as, a few years ago, people used the word "suggestion" in the same sense. Without recapitulating what has already been said regarding this word suggestion, I shall be content to point out that so general an application can only introduce numberless confusions, that it annihilates diagnosis, and renders accurate treatment impossible.

We cannot enter here into all the problems of pedagogy, nor enquire what we are to understand when we speak of the education of children or education of supposedly normal persons. We have only to ask what we mean by education when we are thinking of neuropathic patients ; and when, under the head of educational treatment, we are searching for a definite method applicable to such patients, and distinct from other methods of treatment. In our search for a definition of education, understood in this restricted sense, we must first make certain psychological observations.

Life does not consist only of the exercise of tendencies which exist in a latent state in living beings ; it consists also of *the acquirement and fixation of new tendencies.* Every living being transferred to a new environment, adapts itself thereto in the first place by new combinations of movements, which achieve an appropriate reaction to the new environmental stimuli. In due course, these combinations of movements become fixed, through the formation of corresponding tendencies. That is to say, there arise dispositions to produce the desired reaction correctly, rapidly, easily, and automatically.

When the individual is alone in the new environment, he acquires these new tendencies by the method of trial and error, and he fixes them by numerous repetitions. At first a protective agitation drives him to make all sorts of movements, good, bad, and indifferent. Little by little, he learns to discontinue the unsuccessful movements, and to repeat only the successful movements. The experiments made by psychologists upon the behaviour of animals have proved the existence of this mechanism of acquirement. I think especially of the experiments of Thorndike.[1] A cat is confined in a specially constructed cage usually termed a " puzzle-box." The door of exit can only be opened when the cat presses a knob, and pulls a string with the teeth ; and the animal's food is placed outside the cage. Wanting to get to the food, the cat turns restlessly round and round in the cage, pushing against the walls, pawing them, biting everything it can reach. After a number of futile efforts, and after a time which may be considerable, the animal comes across the knob and the string, and thus succeeds in opening the door. Put back into the same cage next day, the beast begins the same disorderly movements and makes the same attempts, but reaches the correct series of movements earlier than before. After repeated experiences of the kind, the cat learns how to open the cage immediately, without any agitation, and without fruitless trials. It finds its way out as soon as it sees the food outside the cage. This mode of acquiring tendencies is, then, real and useful ; but it is inconvenient, for it is very slow, and necessitates a great expenditure of energy, demands the maintenance of extreme attention during a long series of efforts.

If another individual has already acquired the new tendency, the mere presence and example of this skilled individual will greatly facilitate the acquirement of the movements by an animal which has not learned them. If the cat is shut up in the cage in the company of another cat which has already become acquainted with the mechanism and knows how to get out quickly, the new cat will learn the trick sooner. If the skilled companion is a human being, is a person capable of watching and understanding, he will instruct the animal far more quickly, for he will have discovered methods of instruction which will lighten the labour of learning. In Pavloff's experiments, a dog is taught to water at the mouth on hearing a whistle blown or on seeing a flash of light. This peculiar reaction would have taken a very long time to acquire, and would perhaps never have been

---

[1] Animal Intelligence, 1898 and 1911 ; see also Woodworth, Dynamic Psychology, 1918, p. 90.

acquired, had it not been possible to make use of an association between a conditional and an unconditional stimulus of the salivary reflex. The operator, to begin with, had accompanied the blowing of the whistle or the flashing of the light with the ordinary stimulus of the salivary reflex, namely with the smell of food. In other cases, when concerned with a series of complex movements, the operator decomposes into its elements the movement he wishes to teach the animal, introducing at a suitable moment by associated stimuli the movements which the animal already knows how to perform, gradually following them up by appropriate stimuli (rendered more complex by degrees), and having the movements reproduced in a definite order. He supervises the performance of the act in its totality, checking at the very start the useless movements and encouraging the useful movements. In this way he obtains remarkable results, and is able to shorten very considerably the period of apprenticeship.

Finally, if the pupil, likewise, be a human being, and therefore one capable, in virtue of antecedent tendencies, of reacting to speech and of obeying spoken orders, the association of the stimuli, the repetition of previously acquired movements, the checking of useless movements, the encouragement of useful movements, will be vastly facilitated, and the process of education will be still more rapid. Numerous researches, summarised by Woodworth and others, have shown that by such educative methods a normal human being can greatly modify even the most elementary amongst his actions ; that he can gain control over his reflexes ; can modify the functions of urination, defaecation, and even respiration. In my course of lectures on psychotherapeutics, delivered in Boston, U.S.A., during the year 1906, I recalled in this connexion a remarkable experiment made by J. H. Bair upon the voluntary movements of the ears.[1] Most normal human beings are unable to move the external ears, but by suitable education, by the association of the desired movement with voluntary movements of the forehead, they can easily learn to do so. A fortiori, a carefully considered education can modify the movements of the limbs, over which we already possess so large a measure of control. We note that human beings are

[1] The Development of Voluntary Control, " Psychological Review," 1901, p. 474.

capable of learning numberless actions, and that, thanks to education and instruction, they become capable of the most difficult mental operations. At first these operations demand intense conscious effort ; but, through repetition, in virtue of the mechanism of habit, they are performed with increasing ease and quickness ; so that, at long last, they can be executed correctly without attention and almost unawares. Education thus consists of the production and repetition of a new action performed in the presence of a competent witness, who supervises it, corrects it, and has it repeated until the action becomes, not merely correct, but automatic.

In these circumstances it is natural that the attempt should have been made to apply these educational methods to the treatment of certain patients whose trouble seemed to consist principally in their inability to perform a certain action. It would suffice to teach them how to perform this action ; and it would be all the more easy to do so seeing that, in most instances, they had formerly known how to perform the action correctly. Presumably their organism would have preserved traces of the tendency which had once been complete. These persistent traces would facilitate the education, seeing that, as a rule, it would be a reeducation.

This method of treatment by education must be distinguished from the treatments by suggestion which we have previously studied. What characterises suggestion, properly so called, is that it does not create new tendencies. It merely awakens, brings into active functioning, preexistent tendencies, by inducing conditions in which the activation of these tendencies is easier, thanks to the phenomena of automatism, and in particular, thanks to the automatism of assent. If I do not know how to ride a bicycle, no suggestion would enable me to keep upright upon this machine. In spite of my assent to the words of the hypnotiser I should promptly fall. A special kind of education would be needed to enable me to learn the combination of movements that are necessary ; then, perhaps, a suggestion will enable this tendency, once it has been acquired, to be activated more easily. It follows from this fundamental distinction that education can be successfully applied in cases where suggestion would have been quite without effect.

From one outlook, education is akin to treatments by repose and by economy. The possession of a tendency which is well adapted and has become automatic, will obviously be the starting-point of notable economies of energy when the subject is placed in circumstances to which the education will have adapted him. He will then make correct and automatic reactions which will spare him the loss that would be caused by failure, as well as the cost of agitation and emotion. Neuropaths are apt to complain of not having secured a sufficiency of good habits which would help them when the circumstances are difficult. For instance, a neuropath will say : " Other men walk along rails ; between shafts, which support them and push them forward. For my part, I always have to walk along an unmarked road. That is what tires me out. It is a great exertion to have to discover one's life from moment to moment." A good education, creating in the individual a large number of useful automatisms, would put the patient on rails, between shafts, and would greatly facilitate the journey. We may say, then, that education paves the way for economy and repose. Nevertheless, we must not confound education with repose, for in actual fact, when the tendency has not been formed, and must be brought into being, the subject is obliged to make with effort a large number of new movements, many of which are useless ; he must arrest and suppress these, he must begin the action again at the word of the educator. Now, all these things involve a great waste of energy. In such cases, the action is a costly one, and cannot be likened to repose, to economy. Here another therapeutic method will obviously be in place. We must not immediately try to increase our income by an economy of expenditure ; we must aim at a prospective augmentation of income that will ensue upon an increase of capital. From this outlook it may be said that educational methods are intermediate between the methods of pure economy, which make use of repose and isolation, and the methods of pure acquisition, which make use of excitation. This last will be considered subsequently.

3. DIFFICULTIES OF EDUCATION.

These reflections enable us to understand the difficulties of applying such educational methods in neuropathic disorders.

It is easy to ascertain that the patient, if left to himself, will not be able to educate himself. He remains just as awkward when the circumstances recur as he was at first. He does not acquire the tendencies which ought to enable him to respond correctly and automatically. He does not even succeed in reeducating himself when he has lost a tendency which he used to possess more or less perfectly. He does not know how to rediscover it, and how to refix it in a more stable manner. Why is this? For two reasons. First of all, the patient does not fully understand the nature of his troubles and the nature of the action he is unable to perform. It is difficult to grasp the fact that all neuropathic disorders are due to the insufficiency of some action, and to find out precisely what action is lacking. The patient, unaided, will certainly never make these discoveries. Even if he were able to become aware of this difficulty in himself, he would not know what steps to take in order to remedy it. He is not familiar with the mechanism of the action which he is trying to learn. He would not know how to decompose it into its elements; he would not be able to repeat the useful elements of the movement one by one or to eliminate the futile elements; and he would not be able to perform the action with that peculiar attention whereby a tendency becomes fixed. He is reduced to the method of acquirement by incoordinated agitation, which can only culminate in a result after a very long period of time, enormous expenditure of energy, and vigorous efforts of attention to seize and to stop on the wing the most trifling and useful acquirements and to preserve them. Secondly, this work would require a great expenditure of energy and great perseverance. He is incapable of such efforts, which demand keen psychological attention; and above all he is incapable of prolonging such efforts for a considerable time. As a rule, therefore, he confines himself to temporary efforts of agitation, which exhaust him yet further without producing any useful result.

This education is only possible with the aid of a teacher who demonstrates in detail the action which is to be acquired, and, by guiding the apprenticeship, reduces the inevitable expenditure. Now, can the teacher, who in this case is the doctor, completely overcome the difficulties I have enumerated? This seems to me very doubtful. The two before-mentioned difficulties can perhaps be lessened, but in large measure they will persist. To begin with, let us consider the first difficulty. Can a doctor who is playing the part of teacher ascertain precisely what action is lacking to the neuropath, and is he in a position to teach the subject how to perform this action correctly? We have only just begun to realise that neuropathic disorders are an indirect consequence of inadequacies of action, and that the emotion from which neuropaths suffer is no more than an agitation by derivation which replaces an inadequate mode of adaptation. In most cases it is very difficult to ascertain with certainty what action is lacking, and our capacity for analysing this action is still rudimentary. The educational process does not thrive unless we have to do with artificial actions which human beings have invented for themselves, and whose mechanism is perfectly known to them. A teacher of dancing, who has made a new dance by grouping elements drawn from old dances, will be able to teach it quite easily. The things taught to normal children are little else than things of this sort, sciences and arts invented by human beings and well understood by human beings. But it is risky to compare, as people often do, the education of neuropaths to the education of children in the schools, for education is very different in the two cases. What we have to teach neuropathic patients is not an art deliberately invented by human beings ; but one or more natural actions unconsciously invented by living beings in ages long past, and constructed out of elements which are unknown to us and combinations which we do not understand. We cannot dream of being able to teach these things as we teach dancing or mathematics. We can only teach satisfactorily what we know well ourselves; and since we know very little about the psychology of behaviour, we shall teach it badly. Our pupils will have to make good the defects of this teaching by a greater psychological attention and a larger expenditure of energy.

Let me give an example in illustration of this first difficulty in the education of neuropaths. The case I am about to consider is one of those illnesses which people have proposed to treat by an education which is apparently very precise. Gb. (f., 39) appears to be affected with nothing more than writer's cramp. As soon as she tries to write, her fingers close spasmodically on the pen ; they ride one upon the other ; her whole arm becomes contracted. As a result of this, her hand rests too heavily on the pen, digs it into the paper, so that she becomes unable to write legibly after the first two or three words. To begin with, we may fancy that we are concerned with a trouble of the function of writing, and that it will suffice to reeducate the tendencies bearing on the act of writing. In accordance with the foregoing rules, we shall set to work upon the education of the muscles of the hand, shall develop the strength of the extensor muscles, reduce that of the flexor muscles, and so on. But the patient has performed the exercises conscientiously for several months without any good result. She is simply more exhausted, more depressed than ever. She now suffers, in addition to the original trouble, from all sorts of nervous crises, with doubts and attacks of anxiety, as soon as she tries to touch a pen. In view of this failure, let us examine the malady more closely, and study its development with greater care.

From early youth, this young woman seemed different from other children. She was extremely well behaved and over-scrupulous, tried to be absolutely blameless in her conduct, with an overwhelming desire for orderliness and neatness. Her parents were inclined to make fun of her, regarding her as ridiculously finical. They wanted to check her tendency to rise at four in the morning, that for hours together she might dust, arrange, and rearrange the few articles in her little room. This over-scrupulousness, this aspiration towards perfection, became localised (if I may use the term) towards the age of twenty upon one particular action, that of writing. Though she had not had much education, so that writing had never become for her a habitual and cursive matter, she was seized with a passion to write clearly and well. If she had to write a short letter, or to write down the accounts of the housekeeping, she wanted the result to look pretty, to be irreproachably neat, and she would work at this for an indefinite time with a sort of vanity and pleasure. What made her rather unhappy was that her handwriting, though pretty enough, was not sufficiently regular to please her. She said that always some of the letters were a little above the line and some a little below the line, and that the upstrokes varied in fineness. That is why she took such a lot of trouble, trying all sorts of ways of holding her pen. In short, by the time she was twenty-five she had a perfect mania of scrupulousness and desire for perfection localised upon her handwriting. In accordance with a law which we have often had occasion to formulate, an action which is performed in this way becomes more and more difficult and untrustworthy. Then, a few years ago, a trifling incident occurred which, on the one hand, caused her a considerable amount of emotion and lowered her tension largely ; and, on the other hand, concentrated her attention yet more upon her handwriting, and made it more and more difficult for her to write. She was promoted at the works, and became one of the leading hands. Her duty now was to write up in a book the time of her fellow workers' arrival and to record the amount of work they did. How important was the keeping of this official record ! She trembled when she thought of it. Looking at her unfortunate handwriting, she was terrified at the thought that she would now have to write in public. And thenceforward her powers of writing were hopelessly impaired. It was no longer an irregularity in the handwriting of which she had to complain, her writing had become absolutely illegible.

When we had studied this history, the case seemed much less simple than it had done at first. We were really concerned with a trouble of the handwriting function, and should we be able to cure the patient merely by teaching her how to write ? Though our attempts to teach her to write had had nothing but bad results, this might have been because the education did not bear upon the essential factor. The trouble with the writing was merely an external localisation of a disorder of action having far deeper roots. If we are to transform the patient by education, we shall obviously have to educate something more than the powers of extending the hand ; and unfortunately it is not easy to ascertain with precision the nature of the tendency which has to be reeducated, and the technique of the required education.

Difficulties of this character recur at every moment. Can we say with certainty that a woman suffering from hysterical paraplegia has lost the function of walking ; and will it suffice to teach her once again the series of movements required in walking ? Numerous observations, many of them dating from a long time back, have shown that this is not the case. One who suffers from hysterical paraplegia is, in truth, sufficiently well equipped as regards the function of walking ; just as the hysterical mute is sufficiently well equipped as regards the function of speech : and in both cases it is hard to say precisely in what the trouble consists. When speaking of the treatment of tics and habit-spasms, I described under the name of " Brissaud's method " a treatment which mainly consists in teaching the subject to maintain voluntary immobility. This seems to imply that what is lacking in the person suffering from habit-spasm is the function of voluntary immobility. But is that the fact ? Has it been clearly proved that every normal individual who is free from tics is endowed with extensive powers of voluntary immobility ? I have seen plenty of children, and even adults, who were absolutely unable to remain perfectly still in order to have their photographs taken ; and yet they were quite free from habit-spasm. A man who is incapable, when subjected to military drill, of presenting arms, is not necessarily a sufferer from habit-spasm. The sufferer from habit-spasm may have a great many other troubles quite apart from the lack of the power of voluntary immobility. Consequently, while the treatment of habit-spasm by education in the practice of voluntary immobility may sometimes be successful without our knowing very well why, it will fail in other instances, probably because we have not really succeeded in " touching the spot " with our reeducation.

Far too often do we find that tics persist in spite of efforts at education which may at first seem to have been adequate as well as earnest.—Ay. (f., 43) suffered from typical spasmodic wry-neck as a sequel to anxieties concerning draughts. She was a restless woman, obviously hypochondriacal, but she made sincere attempts in the way of reeducation, without achieving any definite result after four months.—Ic. (f., 45) had her first crisis of spasmodic wry-neck when she was twenty-seven years old, after undue fatigue, and the spasms persisted for eight years in spite of treatment. Gradually a cure ensued ; she was quite well for seven years. Then, about three years ago, maybe in connexion with the menopause, the spasm recurred. Elaborate attempts in the way of gymnastics and reeducation, sedulously and conscientiously carried out for two months and a half, seem to have reduced the spasm a little ; but they certainly have not cured it.

Let us pass on from these tics and occupational cramps to study cases of agoraphobia, all sorts of phobias, genital perversions, obsessions, delusions. Can we suppose that we know exactly, in each case, what tendency is disordered; and can we initiate a reeducation? Can we seriously contend that it is the function of speech which is troubled in a shy person; or that it is the function of walking which has gone wrong in a sufferer from agoraphobia? When we have to do with a sufferer from delusions, does it suffice to say that there is a disorder of attention? Our contemporary psychologists are no longer quite certain whether attention is a special function, and whether there actually exists an operation corresponding to the totality of factors roughly classed under the name of attention. Some psychologists would even like to erase the word "attention" from the psychological vocabulary. Since we know so little about attention, are doctors competent to reeducate this faculty in their patients? We need hardly be surprised if our treatment often fails.

Nevertheless, we need not be wholly discouraged by these reflections. They show us that the failure of our educational methods is not due to the weakness of the procedure, but to the ignorance of the operator. A deeper knowledge of the physiology of walking has enabled us to be more successful in reeducating the gait in tabetics. Advances in psychological science providing us with fuller information regarding the tendencies involved in the various forms of behaviour, and regarding the mechanism of those tendencies, will, some day, make the education of neuropaths easier and more effective.

Unfortunately, our earlier studies concerning the nature of education have enabled us to foresee another and still more serious difficulty. Even though we may suppose that we know precisely what it is we wish to teach the patient, the question arises whether he will be able to obey us and understand us. The understanding of a new thing presupposes a superfluity of energy able to create new combinations of movements, to make trials, to choose, and to fix an acquisition. This is the capacity which is possessed by natures rich in psychological tension, as we see in normal children. One of the great characteristics of a lowering of psychological tension such as we may witness in our patients, is the reduction and the disappearance of this power of acquisition, an insufficiency of adaptations and of new acquirements. The phenomenon is observed in the persistent amnesia of these patients, in their incapacity to adapt themselves to new situations. "I am just as incapable of learning a new piece of poetry as I am of accustoming myself to my rooms or my wife." When they try to acclimatise themselves, to adapt themselves to these changes of situation, they display insufficiencies, signs of fatigue, anxiety, or obsession. If you ask them to make a particularly difficult kind of adaptation, however you may simplify it, you will merely exhaust them by inducing them to make fruitless efforts ; you will increase their depression and their agitation.

In many instances, experience justifies these fears. If we consider matters without prejudice, we are forced to admit that, only too often, attempts at reeducation, however reasonable they may appear, do the patient more harm than good. In this connexion I have already referred to the risk of trying to educate persons suffering from habit-spasm. It is often unwise to make patients whose mental state is not very well known to us, engage in detailed practices of this kind for a long time. Hypochondriacs, and persons suffering from over-scrupulousness, will readily transform the exercises we prescribe to them into tics and obsessions ; I have seen this again and again. Hn. (m., 43) began to practise Javal's treatment and stereoscopic exercises for the cure of a congenital squint, for which he sought advice rather late in life. His doctor recommended him to avoid monocular vision and to keep the left eye closed for some time, only opening it when practising stereoscopic exercises, and when this left eye could participate in binocular vision. For three years, Hn. wore a huge leathern bandage of his own manufacture over the left eye, and took incredible precautions to prevent the least ray of light from making its way into his left eye ; he was terribly distressed when he fancied that this was happening. When he took off the bandage, he practised complicated gymnastic exercises with the eye, and then covered it up again instantly. In a word, in his attempts at reeducation he created morbid impulses and even delusions. Obviously the same kind of thing can happen in the case of any treatment, especially if it is not carefully supervised by the doctor ; but we shall do well to note that gymnastic treatment is not exempt from such dangers.

It must also be remembered that gymnastic treatment demands serious efforts, and may make the patient excessively tired. The exercises that are prescribed are not always so simple and natural as they seem. It is not true that a normal person will invariably find it easy to maintain deliberate motionlessness for a long time together, or that he will find it easy to perform movements very slowly while watching constantly what he is doing. This is not the way in which we commonly act. It is often difficult to teach recruits to stand perfectly still when they are presenting arms, and this is a fatiguing exercise. No doubt the practice of immobility will be useful to the sufferer from habit-spasm, and will help him to check his abnormal movements ; but to gain this advantage he must put himself into very artificial conditions, he must make strong efforts, and must endure considerable psychological tension. It is not surprising, therefore, that weakly persons become exhausted thereby. I have previously referred to the interesting case of Emile, a lad of fifteen, scrupulous, and suffering from phobia, with spasmodic affection of the eyes, the face, and the hand—all related to his obsessions. The attempt was made to treat him by the simple reeducation of his movements without sufficient regard being paid to his mental state, and he conscientiously tried to do as he was told. The result was deplorable. Becoming completely exhausted, he now suffered from digestive disorders, from attacks of muco-enteritis with fever (to which he was always subject when greatly fatigued). In the end, his mental depression became greater than ever, and his obsessions were transformed into delusions.

While results so unfortunate are rare, failure is quite common. One of the most frequent results of this method of treatment is a change in the symptoms of the illness. The tic which we are treating may undergo improvement ; but when that particular symptom is relieved, we shall find that, either in the same part of the body or another, there now develops a new tic more troublesome than the first.—In Co., spasms of respiration and an inclination to unmeaning exclamations replaced spasms of the eyes and face.—Sometimes, during treatment, other psychasthenic symptoms appear, symptoms of mental mania or obsessions.—Kd. (m., 15) was relieved of the spasms which affected him when walking, but, instead, he became tormented by phobias and obsessions relating to little creatures, to imaginary insects, which he crushed in fancy when he was walking—though his gait now seemed more normal to his relatives.—Dc. (f., 48) had for years been suffering from polypnoea associated with a tendency to sniff. Respiratory exercises relieved this trouble, but instead the patient now became affected with paresis of the legs and with delusions.—Hq. (f., 17), suffering from anorexia, had for a year obstinately refused food. By degrees she was reeducated as regard the function of food-taking, but then became affected with somnambulist states attended by attacks of delirium. Hers was the fifth case in which I had noted this remarkable substitution of a garrulous delirium for anorexia.— Xof. (f., 21), who had been cured of spasms of the throat and of spasms and contractures of the feet, was affected thereupon by various other forms of spasms.

A great many patients are not troubled by these changes of symptoms, because they are not capable of carrying on a reeducative treatment for any considerable time. They seem to grasp the nature of what is asked of them, and give a sort of voluntary consent ; but they do not perform the exercises with a sufficient amount of attention, and they become discouraged before having secured any notable results. A woman of forty-one, always timid and scrupulous, had a terrible fright because she had nearly fallen from a verandah, and had looked down into the abyss into which she was about to fall. Since then she had been subject to a peculiar spasm of the eyelids. From terror of looking down into the abyss, she had formed the habit of half closing her eyes. By degrees, the spasm of the eyelids became so severe that she was no longer capable of keeping her eyes sufficiently open to see her way in the street, so that for practical purposes she was blind. At first, the treatment by reeducation seemed to go smoothly enough. She could easily keep her eyes open for thirty seconds when the doctor was close at hand ; and to all appearance nothing more was needed than perseverance. But after a few days, although there was obvious improvement, the patient refused to continue the exercises. " I can't make such efforts any longer, for they upset me and worry me. I would rather remain blind for the rest of my life than have to fight against myself in this way."

I now come to a remarkable instance, to a case which at first seemed to present very favourable possibilities for educative treatment. A man of forty-one was affected with a phobia of staircases and of rising slopes. When he tried to go up such a slope or to go up a few steps, his stomach became greatly distended and he was affected with palpitations and with intense anxiety. The symptoms were due to the swallowing of large quantities of air, which took place involuntarily and unawares as soon as he saw the slope or the staircase. To escape these distressing symptoms, he made a practice of walking upstairs backwards; and when he had to cross the street, he would walk backwards until he reached the middle and had got to the top of the camber—for he had no trouble so long as he did not see the ascent. It is easy to understand that the original disorder had been a habit-spasm taking the form of aerophagia. Whenever the patient had had an emotional disturbance, he had swallowed a quantity of air, thus distending the stomach; then he became alarmed at the distension, and at the respiratory discomfort which ensued. The tic was localised, and was associated with a special form of agoraphobia, and thus there came into existence the remarkable disorder from which this patient suffered as soon as he saw an upward slope. Since the man seemed intelligent enough, and fairly active, might we not have expected to do him good by respiratory exercises, by the reeducation of the function of swallowing (since this is found successful in relieving aerophagia), and by reeducation in walking? The patient seemed to understand, but he lacked courage and perseverance, and gave up trying to follow the doctor's directions before any improvement had resulted.

A good many patients will not even begin the treatment. They may seem to accept our advice in theory, but they cannot begin the practice. They argue, hesitate, spend hour after hour in contortions without having made a hundredth part of the movements we describe to them. Aj. (f., 37) has since girlhood been affected with all sorts of disorders of will, absence of mind, tardiness, a mania for doing things over and over again, obstinacy, etc. She recognised the error of her ways, was greatly distressed, and wanted to amend. With the aid of her husband, who undertook her education, she made persevering efforts. But the husband gave up the attempt in despair when he found, after three years, that not the least progress had been made. The patient admitted that the trouble lay with herself. " As soon as my husband speaks to me, I think of something else. While he is explaining things to me, I turn over in my mind the nice dishes I can cook. I cannot follow what he says to me."

When we turn to consider the various disorders classed under the names of abulia, obsessions of scruple or sacrilege, phobia of contact, etc., we shall readily understand that we have to do with disorders of action, and that we must try to educate the patients, by degrees, to perform more correctly the actions which they dread and which induce anxiety. They seem to accept our advice, but they understand perfectly well that our aim is to make them handle the objects of which they are afraid ; and although they pretend to recognise the absurdity of their fears, they lack the courage to make the attempt. We may spend hours in trying to make them begin the desired action, and they will always stop at the critical moment under some absurd pretext—declaring, like Clarisse, that they will disinter their father's dead body if they are compelled to remain alone for a moment or to dress suitably. In serious cases of asthenic delirium or mental confusion, the question of education does not even arise, for the doctor perceives at once that there is no possibility of inducing these patients to perform any definite action or to repeat any kind of effort.

In these circumstances, how can we watch, correct, perfect an action which is never performed when we order it ? How can we hope that this action can be perfected, and can be fixed by repetition, when there is neither action nor repetition ? Education has no place in diseases where action is entirely annulled. This is the great argument voiced by many of the doctors in charge of lunatic asylums, who are accustomed to watch the development of these neuroses, and who laugh at psychotherapeutics. As far as neuropaths are concerned, they say and reiterate, education and reeducation are no more than philosophical speculations. Such practices will only be successful in very slight cases of illness, or when the patient is already more than half cured. When we have to do with those who are seriously ill, no real psychotherapeutic action is possible. That is what Deschamps means when he declares that asthenics are incapable of being trained or educated. " These patients," he says, " are suffering from aphoria. They are incapable of modifying themselves by repeated efforts ; and after a year of effort they are just where they were when they began." Deschamps' conclusion is that it is futile to try to compel them to make such sterile efforts, and the only treatment he recognises as useful is treatment by the economising of energy and by repose.

4. Attempts at Education in Motor Disorders.

Still, we should go too far were we to draw wholly pessimistic conclusions. No one can doubt, after all, that education has a certain effect upon neuropaths, and that the consequences of bad education play a considerable part in aggravating the symptoms.

Here is one example among a thousand. A woman of fifty years of age is affected with a very remarkable degree of depression and is suffering from a most painful obsession. For the last two years she has been able to think of nothing but her stools, and of the faeces she passes. Incessantly, all day and even all night, she speaks of the last motions she has had, how they have been too small or too large ; she talks of the constipation or of the diarrhœa, real or imaginary, with which she is affected ; she speaks of the way in which she has been to stool or in which she is going to stool ; of the hour that she will choose for this purpose the next day ; of the examination of the stools, which she cannot bear to undertake herself and which must be done for her by some one else ; of the movements of her anus, of her digestive organs, and so on. She is intensely distressed because she is constantly thinking of these improprieties ; she groans at her own intellectual decadence, and yet in spite of her self-contempt she begins the whole story afresh, and clamours for astringent or laxative medicines. It is interesting to go into her history, and to find out how this mental condition came into being. We evidently have to do with one who is markedly psychasthenic. Since early youth she has been affected with all kinds of disorder of action and attention, and has suffered from every variety of the sentiment of incompleteness ; but we find, furthermore, that her mind has developed under very peculiar circumstances. All the members of her family were hypochondriacal ; she lived in an environment where there was constant talk about digestion, dietetic regimen, and drugs. Affected with a morbid desire to attract attention to herself, and by a wish that every one should sympathise with her, she followed the example of the other members of her family, was continually thinking of her health, and spent all her life studying her own internal sensations. " I am like a broken doll whose eyes have fallen inside it." That often happens in the case of neuropaths. She really suffered for years from constipation and from muco-membranous colitis. Doctors held consultations over her case ; she stayed in spas ; underwent numberless curative treatments ; and innumerable enemata filled up the measure of her days. For many years all her thoughts directed her hypochondriacal impulses towards the intestinal functions. Now comes a very curious fact, to which we shall have to return. The real intestinal troubles, including the genuine muco-membranous colitis, underwent a complete cure ; they disappeared as soon as the mental depression ensued. But it was now that the obsession became fixed, became concentrated upon the antecedent intestinal troubles, so that the real colitis was replaced by an obsession of colitis. May we not say that the actual mental condition is the outcome of a prolonged education on the part of her family and her doctors ; that it was this education which gave the neurosis its specific trend ?

Here is an equally striking example. Clarisse (f., 35) had been ailing since childhood, but the first severe morbid symptoms were manifested towards the age of fifteen or sixteen. At this epoch she began to suffer from scrupulous obsessions, such as are often seen in young girls, taking the form in her case of dread of action. " I am afraid of behaving badly, afraid of being immodest, afraid of doing injury to others, afraid that I shall put fragments of broken glass into the water-bottle and give this water to my father to drink," and so on. By a great effort, she succeeded in refraining from such actions, she repressed these imaginary desires. Then came a second phase, towards the age of nineteen, when she passed to the second degree. The desire for action, which had been incessantly repressed and had been thought so dreadful, grew stronger and took the form of an impulse. " I was no longer afraid of behaving badly, for I now had a terrible longing to behave badly ; I was no longer afraid of poisoning people, but felt a strong inclination to poison them." In this phase of the disease, the patients are not content with merely repressing the desire in thought, but they take precautions against themselves ; they refuse to touch the dangerous objects ; they ask people to watch them ; they do not wish to be left alone. Belonging to a family of scrupulous persons with religious inclinations, persons who had little knowledge of mental disorders and little strength of character, Clarisse was able to indulge in all her caprices. If she was afraid that some object had been soiled, it would be washed in front of her as she wished. If she fancied that she was harbouring dangerous microbes, whatever antiseptic practice she demanded would be carried out. When she believed herself to be contaminated and dangerous, the other members of her family avoided touching her ; they would only go to her when they were wearing aseptic blouses and amid fumigations. In a word, all the symptoms of the disease were sedulously fostered. After ten years of this sort of education, the patient was afflicted with the most typical psychasthenic delusion that can possibly be imagined. She spent most of the day in a bathroom, having all parts of her body washed by two women whose whole business it was to drench her with antiseptics. At night she would have herself tied firmly down in the bed, with cords which made deep furrows in her skin, this being done to prevent her from walking in her sleep and committing nameless crimes. One concession after another had ended by developing the disease to an almost incredible degree, and by making the poor young woman's life utterly wretched.

The way in which symptoms become aggravated in the case of " a delusion affecting two persons at once " has been often described by alienists. Two persons in one family suffering from the same type of mental disorder will lead one another on, stimulating one another, watching over one another, and thus fostering and perfecting one another's delusion. In such instances we cannot doubt the power of pathological education. But if this power be real, we have to agree that the mechanism of education exercises a certain influence over neuroses and psychoses. Why then should we deny that the same forces, under better guidance, can exercise a remedial influence ?

It is true that a little while ago I had to point out that education, in the strict sense of the term, is not all-powerful, and that attempts to apply it therapeutically often culminate in failure. This is perfectly true, but we must not forget the cases in which the results of such treatment are favourable. In many instances, patients have got better, and have even been cured, thanks to therapeutic procedures which perfectly correspond to our definition of education.

In the first place I wish to record (I do not wish to stress the point unduly, since I have not devoted special attention to the study of this particular technique) the reeducation of walking in two tabetics suffering from ataxia so extreme that at the beginning of the treatment they could hardly rise from their chairs and walk two or three steps without being supported. One of them within four months, and the other within six months, was able to take long walks in the streets with no more support than that of a stick ; but they had to continue their exercises indefinitely and to keep a close watch upon themselves. The results were less fortunate in a case of spasmodic hemiplegia ; but even in this case reeducation restored the powers of walking, though slowly, whereas for some time the patient had been completely unable to walk. Finally, in the case of a young man suffering from remarkable symptoms of disorders of the cerebellum, prolonged efforts, aided by the notable energy of the patient, led to no more than a moderate improvement in the gait. Still, the general result of such attempts at treatment was such as to convince me that specialists in the method, better informed than myself regarding the physiology of walking and the mechanism of these various disorders, would easily secure valuable results. As Maurice Faure justly remarks : " The patient must not be allowed to engage unaided in the performance of exercises which may often be futile and even dangerous ; the technique must be accurately adapted to the end we hope to secure and to the nature of the trouble which has to be cured." [1] Here the door is open to therapeutic methods which will become

[1] Faure, " Bulletin de la Société de l'Internat," January 1908.

more potent in proportion as our knowledge of the physiology of movement becomes fuller.

Educational treatment of the various forms of hysterical paralysis, of chorea, and of hysterical spasm, is less simple from the theoretical outlook. Here we are no longer concerned with a disorder of the simply mechanical performance of movement, for the malady affects actions which are, strictly speaking, psychological ; it is related to attention, to the consciousness of individuality, and to fixed ideas. Moreover, the subject's mental condition is less satisfactory, and the illness is attended by typical mental depression. The treatment, therefore, is as a rule more complicated. A moral disinfection, disclosing and influencing the subject's fixed ideas, becomes an essential part of the treatment ; so does an economising of energy by repose ; and so does suggestion. Still, I find in my notes the record of a certain number of cases in which these adjuncts to the treatment could not be applied, or in which they had failed ; and yet the simple reeducation of movement, with a concentration of the patient's attention thereon, sufficed. In seven instances, the patients had for a long time suffered from paraplegia, or from abasia, or from paralysis of one of the limbs, and complete cure ensued after several months of methodical gymnastics. A very remarkable instance was that of Madame X., who at the age of fifty was still suffering from troubles of the function of walking, sequels of severe abasia which had supervened when she was twenty years of age and had never been more than partially cured. Now, thirty years later, six months of graduated exercises relieved her of her troubles. In the case of another patient, Na. (f., 30), twitches and spasms of all kinds had become associated with the abasia, and she had to be taught, not only to walk correctly, but also to check the twitches and her tendency to utter involuntary cries. The process of education was a long one, lasting more than eight months.

In six cases of hysterical mutism, the effect of suggestive treatment and of treatment directed towards removing the fixed ideas seemed to me practically nil, and a cure was only achieved through gymnastics of respiration and speech, continued for a considerable time. I wish to draw special attention to the remarkable case of Oa. (f., 14), who, after a series of emotional stresses, suffered simultaneously from mutism and agraphia, although before the illness began she had spoken perfectly and had been able to write very well. This was one of the cases of association between disorders of speech and of writing in a hysterical patient. They are rare, but I have recorded several instances.[1] Oa. had to be taught anew both to write and to speak, and was not fully restored to health until after three months.

The education of the movements of the limbs also plays a great part in the treatment of the hysterical contractures which so often complicate the maladies previously described. I must point out here that certain practices are absolutely disastrous, and must be carefully avoided. The physician should never directly and forcibly attack a hysterical contracture on the pretext that it is a mere whimsy, and due to the patient's obstinacy. It may seem incredible, but doctors, endeavouring to overcome a hysterical contracture by the direct application of force, have actually dislocated a joint or broken a limb, and we must admit that this is a rather remarkable way of trying to cure ! Even if the doctor is less violent, the use of a minor degree of force will serve only to increase the obstinacy of the patient and to make the contracture worse. Above all, when we are dealing with such troubles, we must be gentle. Another equally unfortunate method of treatment which was formerly in vogue was to confine the contractured limb in some sort of apparatus, the commonest being a plaster of Paris case. By this method, we immobilise a limb which is permanently contractured ; or, if the contracture be remittent, we prevent the patient from moving the limb from time to time. Thus we cannot fail to aggravate the disorder. It may be necessary to put the patient under an anaesthetic in order to make quite sure that there is no organic cause for the contracture—in order to verify our diagnosis of hysteria. But when the patient recovers from the anaesthetic we must leave the affected limb quite free, even if it should resume its abnormal position, and we must have recourse to other methods of treatment. Charcot used to give excellent advice, that we should intervene at the very beginning of the trouble, or at any rate as soon as the existence of a hysterical contracture had been recognised. These troubles undergo evolutionary

[1] Névroses et idées fixes, 1898, vol. ii, pp. 404 and 454.

change ; their psychological nature becomes modified and they grow more obdurate when they are allowed to last for a certain time. Charcot said : "We must never let contractures drag on."

Hysterical contracture is a disorder to which I have paid a great deal of attention. In most cases it is an extremely complicated phenomenon ; at the outset it is often a more or less conscious expression of certain fixed ideas or permanent emotional states. Many of the patients, when they first become ill, exhibit systematised contractures related to definite emotional states which persist almost unconsciously, and it is not until a later phase in the development that the contractures become generalised throughout the limb so as to give rise to the classical type of total contracture. Connected with contracture, moreover, is a very peculiar mental state, a sort of obstinacy, a morbid resistance which modifies the customary abulia of these patients. Some patients exhibit, simultaneously with the contracture, persistent manifestations of freakishness ; and they are no more capable of overcoming these caprices than they are capable of relaxing the contractured muscles. Sometimes there will be a simultaneous intermission of the mental symptoms and of the contracture. But, independently of all these phenomena, there occurs in cases of contracture, just as in cases of hysterical paralysis, a strange forgetfulness of the function of the limb, a sort of detachment from normal functioning which leaves all the muscles at the disposal of automatic tendencies. Various explanations of the origin of this forgetfulness are possible. We may suppose it to be due to suggestion, or to fixed ideas, or to an exhaustion of function in persons suffering from depression and in whom the field of consciousness has been restricted. No matter what the reason may be, we have to take the characteristic into account when we are treating contractures.

The methods of moral disinfection enable us to modify fixed ideas.—In Yz. (f., 17), we were thus enabled to annul a memory of her father's illness, the memory of which, as we saw, led her to simulate her father's malady.—In Pc. (f., 19), we could modify the persistent dread of the omnibus which had induced the position of the shoulder.—In five other patients, we were able by moral disinfection to rid them of the memory of some localised accident, such as a sprain or a fracture, the memory which was responsible for the maintenance of the morbid posture. Treatment by methods which economise mental energy, and by other methods presently to be described, enable us to lessen the abulia and the depression. Here we encounter a problem analogous to that which we have noticed in connexion with the treatment of hysterical paralysis. We have to accustom the subject to resuming possession of the function whose control he has lost ; we have to enable him to regain a knowledge of his limbs and their movements.

We sometimes have to do with patients who are almost incapable of moving their limbs voluntarily and of undertaking methodical gymnastics. In these cases, the only exercises that can be practised to enable the patient to regain a consciousness of movement take the form of passive movement of the contractured limb. When the muscular resistance is too great for passive movements to be possible, we have to fall back upon massage of the contractured muscles. In recent cases, when fixed ideas play a great part, the practice of massage must be superadded to the methods previously described. In long-standing cases, in which the originating ideas have ceased to play an active part, massage alone often suffices to effect a cure. Passive movements and massage may be practised with advantage during hypnotic sleep, but often they can only be practised during the normal state. I have records of about fifty cases in which passive movements and massage were used with good effect. It is impossible to give all the details. In a dozen of them, a few sittings were fully successful. In the others, a larger number of sittings was required ; but in most of these, too, the hysterical contractures were ultimately cured.

The main effect of the massage and of the passive movements is, I think, achieved through the education of the subject. He gradually comes to be consciously aware of the modifications in this limb which he was far too apt to leave in oblivion in its attitude of fixation. In the case of contracture, just as when we are treating paralysis, we must concentrate the patient's attention upon the diseased limb. In many cases for which massage is prescribed, where the malady is of a very different kind, the patient may be permitted to read while the doctor is making the passive movements and is kneading the muscles. That indulgence is impossible in the cases we are now considering. The patient must be compelled to look at what is being done, to feel the movements, to collaborate as far as he is able. Besides, when the massage of the contractured limb is efficacious, it gives rise to a special kind of pain. I have frequently had occasion to note that one who is suffering from contracture and does not complain that the massage hurts, is not making any progress. It is when pain is noticed that we find that the muscles are yielding and are being relaxed. In especial we find that it is apt to be very painful when we massage the rectus muscles of the abdomen, which are so often contractured in neuropaths.[1] There is also a great deal of pain when we massage the temporal muscles, the masseter muscles, and the muscles of the neck, as we often have to do when there are disorders of speaking and deglutition. The subject complains of formication, nervous irritation, and severe pain. Sometimes this culminates in hysterical crises, unless we proceed cautiously. As soon as a certain amount of improvement has been noted (thanks to the massage), we must take advantage of the fact, first in the way of more extensive passive movements of the limb, and then in the way of asking the patient to make voluntary movements of the affected part, even though they may be very slight ones. Thus we pass by degrees to treatment by the reeducation of voluntary movement.

One of the great difficulties arising in the treatment of hysterical contractures is that the symptoms are so apt to recur during the days or the hours that intervene between the spells of treatment. It is certainly important, if we wish to avoid these relapses, to study the patient's fixed ideas, morbid autosuggestions, and depression; but we must also take precautions bearing upon the reeducation of movement. We must be careful not to leave in the affected limb partial contractures of this or that muscle, which may cause fixation in various postures, and may form the starting-point of general contractures. In Qa. (m., 25), even after the affected leg had been subjected to passive movements which were apparently complete, it remained affected by slight contractures of the short extensor of the toes, which caused a false position of the

---

[1] Notes sur quelques spasmes des muscles du tronc chez les hystériques et sur leur traitement, " La France Médicale," December 6, 1895 ; Névroses et idées fixes, 1898, vol. i, p. 347.

foot. When he had walked for a few minutes, this erroneous position, which immediately after the sitting had been hardly noticeable, became exaggerated, and the contracture of the leg reappeared. The treatment, and the overcoming of these slight residual contractures, together with precautions to avoid a faulty position, will stabilise the cure. Furthermore, during the hours that follow a decontracture, the patient must shun sudden movements, uncomfortable attitudes, and needless fatigue. We shall, therefore, have to keep watch upon the patient for some time, to ensure that his movements are correct and prudent. The education of movement will continue to play a great part, if we are to prevent the incessant reappearance of contractures, which is so grave a trouble in many of these patients.

It is hardly possible to lay too much stress upon the importance of the treatment of contractures in neuropaths. Ordinarily, doctors do not trouble much unless they have to do with typical contractures of the arms or of the legs, which are in fact comparatively rare. They do not attach enough importance to contractures of the muscles of the neck. Contractures of the muscles of the jaw, the laryngeal muscles, and the muscles of the tongue and of the neck, play a part in causing disturbances of mastication, deglutition, and phonation. Contractures of the neck, of the trapezius muscles, the intercostal muscles, the various sphincters, etc., give rise to disturbances of respiration, digestion, and defaecation, and cause various pains, alimentary phobias, pain during digestion, vaginismus, etc. The aim of the treatment must be to effect reeducation of these different functions; but a careful examination of the state of the muscles must always precede an attempt at reeducation.

Analogous methods of reeducation are certainly competent to relieve various disorders of movement characterised by agitation, and taking the form of chorea, habit-spasm, or some other tic. Brissaud's method consists, as we have seen, in making the subject practise the maintenance of immobility for considerable periods, and in making him perform slow movements under the control of voluntary attention. This method is obviously founded upon the hypothesis that the disorder of movement is related to an insufficiency of the motor tendency

which presides over the prolonged maintenance of motionlessness, and of the other tendency which presides over accurate
voluntary movements performed under the control of voluntary
attention. I doubt whether the accuracy of these hypotheses
from the psychological point of view has been directly proved
by the psychological analysis of the mental state of sufferers
from habit-spasm ; but that it is presumably correct is
proved by the therapeutic results of the method of muscular
reeducation.

Additional observations could easily be quoted to confirm
the fortunate results reported by the before-mentioned authors.
I have myself published two records of the cure of habit-spasms
of the foot, cases which were of especial interest in connexion
with the problems of diagnosis.[1] I may add here a mention
of the cases of Ra. (f., 68), in whom severe pain when walking
was likewise connected with spasms of the toes ; of Mrz.
(f., 30), who, after being long confined to bed, was affected
when at length she was able to get up by the remarkable habit
of falling on her knees in the street upon the slightest excuse ;
and that of Db. (f., 37), who walked too quickly, making very
short steps, and with her legs closely pressed against one
another. In all these patients, exercises, continued for rather
a long time, led to the reestablishment of the power of walking
satisfactorily.

In other cases, habit-spasms of the arms were successfully
relieved by similar methods. Ta. (f., 15), who was affected
with rhythmical twitchings of both arms, which supervened
after she had been engaged in tapestry work for a long time,
was completely cured after two months' exercises in which she
practised motionlessness of the arm for considerable and
increasing periods. It is right to mention that in this case the
disorder of movement was akin to the rhythmical chorea of
hysterics, and that suggestion was certainly one of the factors
of cure. But in three other cases of habit-spasms of the hands,
in which a cure resulted after treatment for from four to eight
months, the exercises of reeducation were, I think, alone
operative in the cure. In one instance, where the patient had
the habit of nail-biting, she was cured by the use of what the
Americans call " chewing gum," one habit replacing another.
I have not had any opportunity of applying for the relief of

[1] Nouvelle Iconographie de la Salpêtrière, 1899, p. 353.

nail-biting the ingenious method suggested by Didsbury, which consists in modifying for a time the closure of the jaws, by preventing them from closing completely in order to bite. I have treated five cases of writer's cramp, and found that exercises practised for several months were helpful; the writing became tolerably good, provided that no attempt was made to write fast.

Many spasms of the face and the mouth have given occasion for interesting studies.—Uc. (f., 46), suffering from a spasm of the tongue, was cured by exercises of immobility; but dental treatment, and especially the insertion of an artificial tooth to fill up a gap, played a great part in the cure.—In Abbé Fk. (m., 40), who was suffering from trismus, the moral treatment of his scruples was quite as important as the education of movements [1]; but in three other cases of spasm of the mouth, a cure was achieved solely through prolonged exercises.

Finally I wish to lay especial stress upon the cure of certain cases of spasmodic wry-neck, for I find that the treatment of these cases is very difficult, and requires great patience on the part alike of the doctor and of the sufferer. A young woman aged twenty was cured in five months of a persistent twitching of the head towards the left side, said to have been caused by wearing a heavy hat " which dragged her head to the side." Five other patients, suffering from spasms or twitchings of the muscles of the neck, isolated in some cases and in others associated with spasms of other parts, were cured easily enough by exercises continued for from three to seven months; but a man aged forty, suffering from wry-neck as a manifestation of shyness, was not cured until the treatment had been continued for eighteen months.

5. Instances of the Education of Perceptions.

The disorders of perception which are noticeable in neurotics are more closely akin than is commonly believed to functional paralyses. We are not concerned here with a genuine disappearance of the reception of impressions by the sense organs. What is wrong is that actions and adaptive reactions are no longer correctly and consciously performed. Education can develop the perceptions of a normal person and make them

[1] Névroses et idées fixes, 1898, vol. ii, p; 381.

more precise, so that the individual learns how to react to impressions that hitherto have gone unperceived. Obviously, the perceptive reactions of neuropaths can be modified in like manner. We have just been studying in connexion with paralyses and contractures how the tactile sense and the muscular sense can be educated ; a like development can be observed in the case of other senses. Many authors have recently been studying the education of the sense of hearing in patients suffering from oto-sclerosis, in whom the auditory powers have been reduced. Interesting results have been secured in this field. Still more obvious results can be obtained when we have to do with neuropathic deafness. In my own practice, I have records of an easy cure in six cases of hysterical deafness. In three of these cases I believe that suggestion was the principal factor of the cure ; but in the other three, the education of hearing, in conjunction with regular exercises of the auditory attention (continued for several weeks), were the most active elements in the treatment.

Disorders of sight are, I believe, commoner and more genuine in hysterical patients than most observers are willing to admit to-day. These troubles often disappear spontaneously in the course of the illness, owing to the diminution of the mental depression. Sometimes, however, they come to occupy the most conspicuous place among the symptoms, and they must not be contemptuously disregarded, for in that case they are likely to persist indefinitely. Fixed ideas are almost invariable factors in the production of these symptoms. Suggestion, moral disinfection, must play a great part in their treatment. Still, exercises of vision have, I think, been useful in several of my cases.—Va. (f., 22), suffered for several years from typical unilateral amaurosis. Experiments with Flees' box and with Ducos de Hauron's anaglyphs showed me at the outset that the case was undoubtedly one of hysterical amaurosis, and these experiments were the starting-point in the reeducation. The exercises in binocular vision designed by Javal for the education of sufferers from squint enabled this patient to make a conscious use of her left eye, and cured her long-standing trouble after two months. Jm. (f., 42), who had suffered all her life from a medley of hysterical troubles, had in particular been several times affected with crises of complete blindness, one of which lasted for twelve days. Amaurosis of the left eye was persistent. The cure of this amaurosis was effected in the same way as in the previous case. I shall not dwell here upon the remarkable phenomena which were noted in connexion with this cure, or upon the forms of hemianopic vision which appeared before normal binocular vision was reestablished. I have given an account of these matters elsewhere.[1]

In this connexion, I shall speak of another case of a somewhat different kind, in order to show how the disorder of certain perceptions can have strange repercussions, and how indispensable it is to educate this or that perception. Yb. (f., 61), was sent to consult me because she was suffering from a remarkable phobia. She was unable to go out into the streets without being attacked with vertigo and anxiety. Agoraphobia, as I have often shown, is a very complicated syndrome, and I therefore tried to ascertain the precise cause of the attacks of vertigo. They did not occur when the patient kept her eyes closed, and they were absent or rare when she was standing motionless with her eyes open in front of motionless objects. The vertigo became much more troublesome when she looked at persons who were walking past, and still more so when she looked at carriages in motion ; it was intense when she was herself driving, and she looked out at the objects that flashed by. In a word, the symptom appeared to be caused by the perception of moving objects as the images passed across the visual field. In early childhood, this girl had had a disorder of the eyes, and had been sent to a school for the blind. Her eyes were almost completely cured, and repeated examination showed that, while the vision was considerably reduced in the left eye, it was practically intact in the right eye, the acuity being 8/10. Furthermore, the right eye had an excellent power of distinguishing colours, and a large visual field. Although her vision was thus quite adequate, the girl remained in the school for the blind, where she was given some work to do. Thus living among blind persons, she acquired the habit of making very little use of her powers of vision. Owing to this defective use of her eyes, she came to suffer from a visual disorder which is little known, but which,

---

[1] Un cas d'hémianopsie hystérique transitoire, " Presse Médicale," October 25, 1899, p 241 ; L'état mental des hystériques, second edition, 1911, p. 458.

as we have had occasion to point out, is frequent among persons suffering from depression.[1] I refer to slowness of vision. She perceives objects very slowly by the aid of sight. When there is plenty of time to look at them carefully, she sees them and recognises them very well ; but if the time allowed is scanty, she perceives badly, and is disturbed. This was the explanation of the troubles that occurred in the perception of moving objects, which were apt to seem elongated owing to the persistence of the visual impression, so that they assumed malformed and strange aspects. That, too, was the cause of the imaginary vertigo and of the phobia from which she suffered when in the streets and especially when she was driving in a carriage.

I have noted a similar disturbance in an army officer who had had a gunshot wound in the back of the head. At first he was completely blind, then blindness was replaced by hemianopia. After a while this, too, disappeared, and visual perception seemed normal ; but it was slow, and the patient was greatly disturbed when he looked at moving objects. In both these cases, it seemed to me that the indication was for treatment by reeducation of vision ; and it is noteworthy that, in the girl's case, education of vision was the proper treatment for troubles which at first sight seemed to be nothing more than agoraphobia.

As an instance of the effects of education upon disorders of perception in neuropaths, I may mention the curious case of Madame Z.[2] She was a woman of sixty-five, and had always been extremely neuropathic. Throughout life she had exhibited well-marked hysterical symptoms. For a year she had suffered from paraplegia. She had had hysterical attacks with catalepsy and somnambulism, mutism, contractures of the neck, spasms of the right arm, and various algias. The last symptoms of this kind had been manifested towards the age of fifty. Since then, hysterical symptoms properly so-called had been replaced by arthritic troubles and by symptoms of arterial sclerosis. Three years before I saw her, Z. had had

[1] See my study of the duration of elementary visual sensations, " Bulletin de l'Institut Général Psychologique," 1904, p. 540 ; also an essay on the same topic by Pick, of Prague, " Brain," 1903, p. 470.

[2] The notes of this case were published in the ' Medical Record " on May 11, 1907. See also Etat mental des hystériques, second edition, 1911, p. 470.

severe retinal haemorrhage in the left eye, so that the vision of this eye was gravely affected from the first. After this trouble began, she complained of seeing luminous flashes with the left eye, and of seeing an appearance which resembled iron bars. This was attended with severe pains, and after she had suffered greatly for a year it was decided to sacrifice the left eye, now absolutely useless for purposes of vision, and to divide the optic nerve, while leaving the globe in place, since its aspect was perfectly normal, except that its movements were affected.

It was now, as a sequel to this operation, that there began a strange disturbance of vision, concerning which I made psychological researches. The right eye, which had remained intact, seemed on cursory examination to possess normal powers of vision; there was a sufficient acuity of vision, and the visual field was ample. But the patient complained that she was unable to turn this eye to account, for whenever she tried to look at any object she could only see a strange sort of cloud, composed of vibrating luminous points. Vainly did she endeavour to fix the gaze upon an object, or to follow up a line. Her vision was so much disturbed by the moving cloud that she could see nothing else distinctly. Not only did she find it impossible to read, but even the sight of ordinary objects in the room was so defective that she found it difficult to make her way about. Ere long, this moving cloud began to give rise to vertigo and nausea, so that, if she wished to feel well again she had to close her eyes. These remarkable symptoms continued to increase in intensity for a year, and the despair of the patient, who as I have said was extremely neuropathic, intensified all her other troubles.

A more precise analysis of these disorders enabled us to ascertain the following facts. The vision of the right eye is only maintained at the outset on one proviso, namely that the patient restricts herself to the description of an object placed in front of her, any sort of object, so long as she does not choose it. As soon as she has to fix an object and to accommodate for near vision, and directly there is the slightest effort of attention, the disturbance begins anew. Conversely, she noted certain circumstances in which the trouble was almost entirely suppressed. A particular kind of lighting, from the left side, and a chance position of the patient, brought about a sudden change, and after a few seconds Z. was amazed to find that she could see quite as well as of old. But this restoration of good vision was brief, and she did not know how to regain it. Sometimes she asked to have the left eye, the blind one, firmly bandaged ; or she would press this eye strongly with the fingers. When the useless eye was thus prevented from moving, she would see better with the other for a few moments. She had the habit of using a large reading glass, surrounded by a thick metal mount, and she held this lens obliquely in such a way that the metal rim served, as it were, to prolong the shadow of her nose, and thus isolated the right eye from the left eye more completely.

These observations seemed to show that the right eye was capable of good vision when it was isolated from the left eye ; and that the intervention of the left eye, although it was blind, was the cause of the disorder of vision. To verify these hypotheses, I made a few experiments in which the vision of the right eye was rendered more definitely monocular than ever. I record one of these experiments, a remarkable one. In former days, Z. had practised pistol shooting, and had learned how to aim with the right eye without using the left eye. I begged her, while holding a pistol, or even a simple piece of wood, to repeat the effort at aiming. To her great surprise, she could then see perfectly well the object at which she was aiming, without a cloud, and without the disturbing movements. She even found that it was possible to touch a definite point with the end of the fragment of wood she was holding, whereas she had previously been unable to grasp a large object with her hand. In another experiment I made her look through a telescope, and she could then see objects at a distance perfectly well. Finally, I made her look through a simple paper tube, and in this way she was enabled to read without difficulty. It was necessary that the tube should be very closely applied to the right eye, for if a ray of light entered the eye from the nasal side, the shining cloud would immediately invade the visual field once more. Here was an assemblage of facts which seemed to show that the disorder of vision was mitigated, or disappeared, when the right eye was functioning quite alone, without any participation of the left eye. There is no contradiction between this circumstance and the before-mentioned observation of the fact that the trouble became exaggerated by any efforts in the way of fixation and attention. During visual attention, there is a convergence of the eyes, and the association of the two eyes in binocular vision occurs to a very marked degree. Now we have just seen that, in this patient, it was the association for binocular vision which we had to suppress, if distinct vision was to be reestablished.

How can the above-described phenomena be explained ? Here is a hypothetical explanation. We note that in the normal human being there are two different kinds of vision ; binocular vision, with convergence of the optic axes ; and monocular vision, in which the eyes function independently of one another. Now, when only one eye retains the power of vision, we are not usually inclined to think of these two kinds of vision. At first, we should rather fancy that a one-eyed person could have nothing but monocular vision. Probably that is true enough in the case of those who have lost an eye in early childhood ; but those who became one-eyed in adult life retain the psychological mechanism of binocular vision in all circum-stances wherein binocular vision is ordinarily practised ; and they only employ the mechanism of monocular vision in peculiar circumstances, when they perform one of the actions in which we are accustomed to use one eye in isolation. Any-way, paradoxical as it may seem, the foregoing observations led me to suppose that a one-eyed person may retain the cerebral mechanism of binocular vision when he is reading with attention. These hypotheses may be verified by watching the movements of convergence on the part of the blind eye, or on the part of its stump ; and we may note that a one-eyed person only adopts the mechanism of monocular vision when he aims with a pistol or looks through a microscope. Ordin-arily, this association of the two eyes causes no discomfort, for the reason that the blind eye follows the movements of the sound eye perfectly well, or else because the subject is quite unconcerned about the movements of the blind eye if these should be incorrect. By degrees he will lose the habit of fruitless binocular vision ; but if he be well on in years, and especially if he be a neuropath, he will find much difficulty in relinquishing the customary association.

If we apply our supposition to the case of Z. we shall realise the likelihood that this patient, although her left optic nerve had been divided, was still trying to practise binocular vision whenever she was thoroughly on the alert, when she was paying attention to her vision, when she was endeavouring to follow a line with her sound eye. She was still attempting to bring about convergence of the eyes, to accommodate them each to the other as in old days ; and she was not content to fixate and accommodate with the right eye alone. This obstinate persistence in maintaining a habit can be regarded as having been due to a fixed idea, or rather to one of those psychological states which have become fixed, such as are being continually noted in hysterics. Another reason was that neuropaths are unable to modify their automatic habits. The exhaustion of the visual function brought about by all the troubles, by the suffering and the emotions which followed the retinal haemorrhage, was manifested here by the defective adaptation to a new situation, and the patient had persisted in trying to retain binocular vision. But binocular vision had become impossible to her, not only because the left eye was blind, but also because the left eye had become incapable of movements concordant with the movements of the right eye. It was the inadequacy of the convergence and the accommodation of the left eye which disturbed the fixation and the accommodation of the right eye.

Some attempts at treatment furnished an interesting verification of these hypotheses concerning pathogenesis. I undertook to educate Z.'s vision by developing her powers of monocular vision, and by teaching her how to use in all circumstances the same visual mechanism that we, whose vision is binocular, are accustomed to employ when we aim with a pistol or look through a telescope. I trained her during periods increasing in length to look at various objects and to read through a tube closely applied to the right eye. It was true that reading under such conditions was extremely fatiguing. After a time, the left eye would no longer remain quiet. " My left eye wants to see too," Z. would say. " I feel it at work ; in its efforts to see, efforts which I cannot check, in its efforts to look, it is moving about like a rabbit in its burrow." When this happened the left eye began to exercise its influence over the right eye, and the shining cloud reappeared by fits and starts. This signified that monocular vision, to which the patient was not fully accustomed, was becoming painful ; and that the presence of the tube did not suffice to prevent the reappearance of efforts at binocular vision. After stopping the experiment for a time, during an interval in which the patient kept her eyes closed as much as possible, she could begin to see correctly through the tube once more. Before long I had a queer pair of spectacles made for Z. To the mount in front of the right eye there was attached a small metallic tube, having the size of the orbit, and a length of two inches. Through this tube the patient could see quite distinctly. By degrees we found it possible to reduce the length of the tube, inasmuch as the distal part of it had become needless, so that a length of three-quarters of an inch sufficed. Thus restricted, the tube would not necessarily constrain the patient to monocular vision, but it acted as a stimulus, became a condition favouring the resumption of monocular vision. After a few weeks' practice, this very short tube, or rather this little screen placed in the inner angle of the eye, sufficed to induce the maintenance of monocular vision, and in a manner quite remarkable the patient regained the use of the sound right eye.

6. Attempts at Education in Visceral and Mental Neuroses.

The good effects of education extend, likewise, to other neuropathic affections. There can be no doubt whatever that education can exercise a favourable influence upon disorders which appear to be visceral in character. The reason is that in visceral functions, and especially in the functions of alimentation and respiration, a great many movements under the control of the will play their part; and these voluntary movements can be modified by education. Suffice it to refer to the importance of dietetic regimen, of the regulation both of the quality and the quantity of food and drink. Herein, doubtless, lies a notable part of the subject's education ; but such methods of treatment have more complicated effects, and they will be studied later.[1] What we are concerned with here are the purely educative procedures which can more directly effect a simple modification of movements.

A great many patients, as we have just seen, suffer from spasms or contractures of the lips, the jaws, the tongue, the pharynx ; and it is very important to relieve them of these

[1] See Chapter Fifteen, " Psychophysiological Methods of Treatment."

troubles. I have discussed this matter with a wealth of detail in my record of the case of Marceline.[1] I could quote a great many similar cases, illustrating the same phenomena.

There are many persons who, though they do not suffer from contractures properly so-called, have lost the power of effecting certain elementary coordinations of movement; they are no longer able to chew properly, or they cannot swallow their food properly. These disorders are often combined with a spasmodic affection of the oesophagus, so that sometimes the patient retains his food in the mouth for an indefinite time, or retains it in a sort of oesophageal pouch. Many tics characterised by spitting, regurgitation, and vomiting, are due to the fact that the food has not been properly swallowed and introduced into the stomach. Patients, such as Marceline and Za. (f., 23—a most interesting case), will regurgitate milk a quarter of an hour after it has been apparently swallowed; and it is regurgitated uncurdled, for they have retained it in the upper part of the oesophagus. We must teach such patients how to swallow; must make them repeat the movements of swallowing systematically, until the food has really entered the stomach. In some emaciated patients, when we lay the hand upon the epigastrium we can feel that there is a sort of shock in this region at the moment when the bolus of food passes from the oesophagus into the cardiac end of the stomach, and we must insist upon the patient's making swallowing efforts until we feel this little shock caused by the penetration of the food. In such cases as that of Marceline, we may note the presence of pharyngeal anaesthesia, and the loss of the nauseation (palato-pharyngeal) reflex. I have noticed this especially in patients who have been fed for a long time through an oesophageal tube, and in whom the pharynx has become callous. I think it advisable in such cases to reeducate the pharyngeal sensibility, and even to reestablish the nauseation reflex. When that has been done, the patient will swallow much better.

Much stress has repeatedly been laid upon the danger of aerophagia, which is only a habitual disorder of deglutition, and which plays a great part in hysterical hiccough, eructation, and vomiting. Leven has proposed, as a means of stopping

[1] Une Félida artificielle, " Revue Philosophique," 1909, vol. i, p. 329 ; Etat mental des hystériques, second edition, 1911, p. 561.

aerophagia, that the necktie should be tied tightly below the larynx, in such a way as to make the subject persistently aware of the movements of swallowing. I have on several occasions tried the method in intelligent patients, who were competent without inconvenience to watch thus persistently in such a way. But I think that aerophagia can be checked just as well by exercises tending to reeducate deglutition, such as were successfully practised in Lem. (f., 37). Many patients suffer from habitual regurgitation of food, or from habitual vomiting. I have published notes on a good many cases of the kind and upon their treatment.[1] In many instances, the vomiting is superimposed upon disorders of swallowing and upon aerophagia. Sometimes it is kept up by real dyspeptic troubles, and especially by hyperchlorhydria. Obviously we must begin the treatment by dealing with all these subjacent troubles. Then we must accustom the subject to tolerate the presence of food in the stomach, to resist for a shorter or a longer time the impulse to regurgitate or vomit. Various methods can be employed, and suggestion or moral disinfection will obviously play a part ; but reeducation must certainly not be forgotten. In a dozen cases, several of which have been published, I found that tics of this character can be relieved even in patients who in other respects remain extremely neuropathic.

Constipation is one of the most constant and most troublesome symptoms in these patients, and the muco-membranous enteritis from which they suffer is a strange and obstinate complication—and one whose nature has by no means been fully elucidated. Dietetic precautions, based mainly upon the examination of the stools, in conjunction with various kinds of drug treatment, must play their part in the treatment of these affections. It is none the less true that bad habits have always a great deal to do with their genesis ; and that for this reason in such cases considerable improvement can be brought about by massage, by mobilisation of the stomach, and by gymnastic exercises which move the diaphragm and the muscles of the trunk and the abdomen. Reeducation of defaecation may also be useful here. Paul Dubois is right in insisting upon this point, and I could add a score of cases to those which he records.—Ac. (f., 25) had been suffering since

[1] Les obsessions et la psychasthénie, vol. ii, p. 247.

puberty from a grave form of nervous enteritis. Matters had gone so far that she used to pass mucous and evil-smelling stools every two hours all through the day and the night ; and the amount of urine was reduced to less than ten ounces a day. These physiological troubles were accompanied by various obsessions concerning defaecation, and the patient would no longer leave the house unless she took with her a special utensil which she could use at a moment's notice. The reeducation of defaecation, insistence upon fixed hours for going to stool (under the care of a nurse), and the encouragement of a changed attitude towards her on the part of her family, succeeded within a few months, not merely in transforming the girl's mental condition, but also in restoring the intestinal functions and the nutrition so successfully that within two months her weight increased from ninety-four pounds to one hundred and eight pounds.—In the case of Neb. (m., 32), the treatment also consisted in the education of defaecation. This poor fellow, a typical sufferer from scrupulous psychasthenia, had a dread of being overheard in the water-closet. For this reason he assumed peculiar positions while defaecating, making special kinds of effort while clenching his fists, and so on. As a result of these practices, he completely disordered the act of defaecation, and in the end his whole life was poisoned by the obsession of defaecation. Here a very complicated form of moral treatment was requisite, and in this the regulation and the education of defaecation played an interesting part.

Most neuropaths breathe badly.   I have published a number of observations bearing upon various neuropathic disorders of respiration related to paralyses or contractures of different muscles ; also upon all kinds of respiratory tics, such as polypnoea, coughing, sighing, hiccough, eructation, etc. In other cases, in which such respiratory symptoms are not obvious, if we systematically take graphs of the thoracic and abdominal breathing in neuropathic patients, we shall often find that the breathing is irregular, arhythmical, and superficial, and that the ventilation of the lungs is altogether inadequate. We thus detect disorders in the power of voluntarily modifying respiration, or of quickening or slowing it, and of changing it in accordance with our directions. Such troubles were characteristic in the case of Marceline.[1] I noted them also in the case of Bon., and in several other patients.

Such facts will not surprise us when we recall the intimate relationship between breathing and speech, and between breathing and attention. We note that deaf-mutes breathe badly ; that their respiratory capacity when measured with a spirometer is much less than that of normal children of the same age ; and that their power of blowing is weak. We find the same thing in persons who speak badly, as for instance in stammerers. Nor are we surprised to note similar troubles in cases of hysterical mutism and in all neuropathic disorders of speech. Respiration necessarily undergoes changes when the subject attends to it, and during sleep. Is it not possible that an incapacity for voluntarily bringing about changes in respiration may play a part in producing incapacity for fixing the attention and incapacity for beginning to go to sleep ? I have elsewhere referred to the drowsiness and to the incapacity for fixing attention which occur in connexion with the major respiratory tics ;[2] also to the disorders of respiration and in especial to the diminution of pulmonary ventilation which is associated with conditions of aprosexia, of confusion. Ca. (f., 19), for instance, when she is in one of her states of somnambulistic reverie akin to the crepuscular states of epileptics, has a pulmonary ventilation of only 2.4 litres per minute, whereas in the normal state she has a pulmonary ventilation of 8 litres per minute. All these remarks underline the importance of respiratory disorders in the neuroses.

The treatment of these different respiratory troubles will obviously vary. In certain cases we must deal with the fixed ideas, with certain suggestions, with the contractures which exist more often than we are apt to imagine in the muscles of the neck or the thorax ; but the fundamental part of the treatment will always be respiratory gymnastics. The principles underlying such gymnastics have been frequently explained by specialists. I shall merely add that I think it well, when I have to do with neuropaths, to exercise the patient, not only in normal, full, and correct breathing, but also in modifying the breathing at the word of command, in blowing, laughing, coughing, etc.

[1] Etat mental des hystériques, second edition, 1910, p. 561.
[2] Névroses et idées fixes, vol. i, p. 325.

By such methods we can, first of all, cure symptoms which are respiratory in the strict sense of the term. The polypnoea of several patients, such as Ba. (m., 32), was cured mainly by hypnotism and suggestion; but in many other instances, as in that of Dc. (f., 48), the cure was only brought about by respiratory exercises. In eleven interesting cases of persistent hiccough with hysterical barking, the trouble was cured in this way, although in one of these cases the hiccough had been going on for a whole year. A woman of forty-three was suffering from a persistent spasmodic cough, the main cause of which appeared to have been excessive masturbation; the symptom disappeared after a few weeks' respiratory exercises. Similar results were secured in many cases of the same sort.

In the second place this education of the breathing enables us to relieve various symptoms which are indirectly dependent upon respiratory disorders, such as aerophagia and meteorism, as I have especially had occasion to observe in the case of Nk. (f., 15). Respiratory treatment has also had a successful influence upon troubles of speech, and upon a great many other symptoms. Finally, although I have not yet been able to verify the hypothesis definitely, it seems to me likely that respiratory exercises would have a good influence upon many of the weaknesses of attention and upon certain mental disorders. Unfortunately in most cases of this kind it is extremely difficult to induce the patient to make sufficiently strenuous and prolonged efforts.

Sleep, although it is not ordinarily considered from this point of view, resembles action in many respects. Sleep is itself an action, and as such it can be greatly modified by habit and by education. There is no doubt that in neuropaths we can induce good habits of sleep by training them to go to bed and to rise at fixed hours. A great many observations bearing upon this point will be found in the writings of authors who have made a special study of sleep.[1] A prolonged and rather difficult education was needed to accustom Fb. (m., 16) to sleep without a light in his room; but ultimately the treatment was perfectly successful. It must be admitted, however, that in many cases the cure of insomnia by this method is very difficult.

[1] Cf. Manacéine, Le sommeil tiers de notre vie, 1896, pp. 201 and 210.

Another function which can be benefited by education is the urinary function, which is so often disordered in neuropaths. In many instances, when the urinary disorder occurs in hysterics who are amenable to suggestion, or in psychasthenics who suffer in addition from phobias and obsessions, the treatment is more complicated. But, in many cases, persons who have no serious mental disorder, or who, having formerly suffered in this way, have now ceased to suffer, preserve bad urinary habits which play their part in causing incontinence or retention of urine. One of the commonest of such troubles is undue frequency of urination, which is apt to supervene upon organic diseases of the urinary organs, such as gonorrhoea for instance ; or it may simply arise from the habit of undue precaution in nervous persons, or from a metamorphosis of urinary timidity.[1] The patients try to pass water far too frequently, almost at every moment, although the bladder contains hardly any fluid. The result of this is that they find it very difficult to begin the act of urination, or to perform it correctly ; and in this connexion there arise numerous tics and manias, which culminate in spasm and in retention. Some of these patients form the habit of perpetually passing a catheter, and thereby they are apt to complicate their neuropathic troubles by inducing infection of the bladder. In this case, after we have undertaken the necessary local disinfection, we must teach the patient, by degrees, to dispense with the passage of the catheter, and to urinate correctly, with a sufficient interval between the acts. Quite a number of persons, who used in former days to be described as sufferers from hysterical polyuria, are, above all, as I tried to prove thirty years ago, polydypsics ; and on the other hand Dejerine has recently shown that many of those affected with ischuria are adypsics, that is to say that such persons have an excess or an insufficiency of urine, as the case may be, because they drink too much or too little. In these cases reeducation has a notable influence for good.

Passing over the cases in which suggestion has played a principal part, I think that in a certain number of instances the complete cure of neuropathic disorders of the urinary organs has been effected by education alone. The cure of undue frequency of urination by the regulation of the hours

---

[1] Jules Janet, Les troubles psychopathiques de la miction, Paris, 1890.

of urination is in general quite easy when the diagnosis is accurate. Such a large number of cases of the kind have been recorded, that I need not dwell upon the fact here. In other instances, women who had become entirely dependent upon the use of a catheter, were taught first, and quickly, to pass water naturally after the act had been initiated by the use of the catheter ; then they learned to pass water quite naturally without the use of the instrument. In a dozen cases collected by my brother, Jules Janet, and by myself, men who suffered from neuropathic retention, from urinary stammering, or from urinary timidity, were able after a time to free themselves more or less completely from these tics and spasms. There is no doubt that urinary reeducation was the chief factor in their cure.

Is is possible to make similar observations regarding the genital functions ? According to the theories of some authors it is not possible, for these persons are inclined to consider many of the modifications of sexual behaviour as constitutional, and to believe that treatment is impossible. Such theories have done a great deal of harm in the case of numerous patients who were only too glad of a pretext for persisting in the error of their ways, and for abstaining from all effort. " What do you expect me to do ? " they keep on saying. " I have a woman's soul in a man's body. This is the last great discovery of German science. It will be quite impossible to put a different kind of soul into my body." Such affirmations are childish and ridiculous. Sexual perversions are mental disorders like any others, and their psychological mechanism is extremely variable. They are easily acquired and only in quite exceptional cases are they constitutional or congenital. Fixed ideas, tics, manias, general and local depressions, especially related to certain tendencies, are the principal factors ; and these disorders must be treated like other disorders of the same kind, and can be treated with equal chances of success. All the different kinds of psychological therapeutics will find a place in turn. I have seen a great many cases of sexual disorder cured by suggestion ; and we shall find that other cases can be modified by various forms of excitation ; I cannot overstress the importance of sexual education. Unfortunately, the dangers inherent in the sexual function, and our conventional social customs, render this education very difficult. It is, indeed, a delicate topic, and I shall do no more than give some general indications without going into details.

The first point the doctor must take into consideration is the amount of knowledge of sexual phenomena which the normal individual ought to possess—man or woman, just grown up, at the age. of twenty for instance. It is hardly possible to realise how much ignorance, how much absurd and dangerous error, may exist in the mind of a neuropath. False shame prevents parents from speaking of these questions, and prevents children from asking for information however inquisitive they may be. In intelligent and well-educated families we may find young men like Jean, who at thirty-one years of age asked : " Do women give birth to children through the breasts ? " ; and again : " Is sexual intercourse practised through the navel ? " We shall meet young women of twenty-five who will enquire : " Is there danger of becoming pregnant through sitting in the arm-chair where father has been sitting ? in kissing mother on the cheek where father has just kissed her ? in straining at stool ? and so on." There are still a great many people who find these simplicities exquisitely poetical. What we need to realise is that they are dangerous, and that we do good service to such ignoramuses by giving them the clear notions of elementary physiology which all young people ought to possess. I should like to refer here to an admirable little book which has done me yeoman's service in such cases, written by Madame Leroy-Allais, and entitled : *Comment j'ai instruit mes filles.* I may also recommend Forel's book *The Sexual Question.* But the last-named work is less simple than the other, and is less suitable for the general reader.

Despite the illusions maintained by current moral theories, doctors are compelled to assert that marriage is dangerous for young persons who are too ignorant and too chaste. Without going into details, I may recall the fact that various evils may result from such idealistic practices. Even though these evils are not always serious, there are still plenty of cases of a sufficiently grave kind, such as the onset of vaginismus, hysterical crises, total or partial impotence, phobias and obsessions, which greatly disturb domestic life, and which, in one or other of the partners (and sometimes in both), may induce obstinate neuropathic disorders.

It is doubtless true that the functioning of the sexual organs is not absolutely indispensable, and that a great many persons may remain healthy despite almost complete sexual abstinence. But it is equally true that such abstinence is an abnormal condition, and that after the attainment of a certain age a moderate exercise of the sexual functions is extremely beneficial to the equilibrium of the nervous system Whenever possible, we shall do well to prevent neuropaths from completely renouncing sexual relationship as they so often wish to do, even when they are married. When the conditions are unfavourable to normal sexual relationships, we must not display undue indignation on account of solitary practices, which are far less dangerous and far less important than they are usually considered to be. The terror of masturbation, fostered in the public mind by certain celebrated works, has done more harm by causing phobias and the like, than it has done good by preventing exhaustion. The doctor will certainly do good work by approaching this question calmly, and by giving, without emotion, counsels of moderation.

In households in which one of the two sexual partners is suffering from depression of the genital functions with more or less complete impotence, we can in many instances, when the mental disorder is not too severe, secure definite improvement by a real sexual education. It is very important to isolate the young married couple, so that the abnormal situation may be concealed from the parents and from strangers. I have already referred to those scenes of tragic comedy which occur in our consulting rooms when the indignant father-in-law and mother-in-law bring with them an abashed husband. We must be careful to avoid the presence of indiscreet witnesses, and must deal only with the parties primarily interested in the matter. When one of the married partners is normal and of good will, we must address ourselves to this one of the pair first, and reassure him or her concerning a situation which is often inclined to put people beside themselves. The most usual case is that of neuropathic impotence of the husband. In such instances the young wife is much concerned at having " a husband who is not like other men, who does not know what to do, who can only hurt." We must make her understand that all will come right, and that if she wishes to keep her husband, she must educate him, must simplify the act for him, must prepare him, and must above all save a maladroit person from disillusionments and humiliations.—" Then all the trouble falls upon me ? "—" Yes, certainly, for a time. In the end you will be repaid."—What we have to aim at is something rather strange, and nevertheless realisable and valuable. We have to bring it to pass that the first sexual relationship shall become almost unconscious, and shall be effected almost without the patient's knowing it. An action, in fact, is more complicated, and requires a higher tension, when it is accomplished with consciousness and by attention ; and we must reduce to the utmost this superior part of the sexual act. I have seen a great many cases in which the restoration of peace to the household and the birth of a baby showed the efficiency of the sexual education.

The same sort of treatment is required in other sexual troubles. The only reason why masturbation is really dangerous is because it is so easy, and because unduly frequent repetition is so likely. Anyone who has had experience with neuropathic patients is aware that it is much more often necessary to quiet their fears concerning masturbation than to make them afraid of the practice. Still, there is such a thing as a dangerous excess of masturbation, and the most remarkable instances of the kind are those which occur in certain young women.—Céline, (f., 28), innocently complains, even before the other members of her family, of suffering from a sense of tension, of a deep-seated tremor, with twitchings in the abdomen which make her heart beat, when she sits still for half an hour with her legs crossed, when she is playing the piano, or when she is reading poetry. An extraordinary degree of ignorance, unwholesome agitations, a faulty habit in the placing of the legs, play a chief part in causing such symptoms. It is easy enough to explain them to the subject, and to guide her to better postures. The education in these cases is easy enough.—In other patients masturbation occurs as a sort of derivative as soon as an effort is made or an emotion felt. Lym. (m., 24) masturbates in spite of himself. " I do it as soon as my work becomes difficult."—A woman of thirty does the same as soon as she thinks of going to confession.—These patients are difficult to cure, but for them, likewise, the regulation of sexual functioning is extremely useful. In others, incomplete and persistent genital excitement is the outcome of the longing for marks of tenderness which is characteristic of certain psychopaths.—Consider, for instance, the case of Céline, the before-mentioned young woman of twenty-eight : " I have no confidence in myself ; I am always wanting people to raise my spirits. . . . I wish I had some one who would love me a great deal, who would be always thinking about me. . . . I continually dream of being on his knees as if I were a little child ; . . . this gives me a feeling of great tension, like a violent longing ; I dream of continual caresses, I am fascinated with the idea of kissing, and; then. . . . It is not my fault ; it begins by being moral, and ends in the other thing ; I have too much longing for tenderness ; what am I to do about it ? " I do not believe that in this case the starting-point is really unsatisfied sexual desire. All these patients suffer from depression, and in depressed persons the sexual impulse is by no means exacting. What happens is that the moral depression induces a need for guidance, a need for encouragement, for excitation, for caresses. This culminates in a masturbatory act which is incomplete and barely conscious, and is none the less almost continuous, so that it becomes a further cause of exhaustion. Sexual education will not cure these patients, but it will do them very real service by at least suppressing the final cause superadded to the depression.

Far more often than is usually believed, the various disorders of the sexual life are related to phenomena of depression, either general or local, and, in the latter case, especially connected with the sexual tendencies. I have noted in persons suffering from fits of depression the appearance of masochistic and sadistic reveries.—" I can no longer think of love just like other people and as I used to do myself. I find it necessary to think of a schoolmaster who beats me, who tweaks my nose and pinches my ears, who wipes my nose with his dirty pocket handkerchief ; only this mental picture will give me an erection."—" I can now only love huge and repulsive women who overwhelm me with their weight and their contempt."— " For me love now signifies to examine coffins at the cemetery, to carry them away and force them open, and to look at the face of the corpse."—These fantasies appear in patients whose sexual functions have hitherto been normal, but who are traversing a crisis of psychasthenic depression attended by doubts and phobias of various kinds. They disappear when the patients get better, and when their mental balance is reestablished. The sufferers have an urgent need for being stimulated by the strange or the hateful; they are affected with deviations of tendency analogous to those which exist in the case of obsessions of sacrilege. The fantasies may degenerate into manias and maniacal impulses, but we must not consider them to be manifestations of an abnormal sexual constitution. They must be regarded as symptoms of a curable mental disorder, and normal sexual exercise has its part to play in their treatment.

The group of sexual inverts is a complex one, containing patients who differ greatly one from another, and who have been very inadequately analysed from the psychological point of view. Many of them are merely psychasthenics suffering from scruples, tormented by obsessions and by criminal impulses. They believe themselves possessed by an irresistible impulse towards homosexuality, just as other patients will believe themselves pushed irresistibly towards homicide or theft. I have elsewhere described some remarkable cases of this kind.[1] Others are persons suffering from depression, who are seeking excitation in abnormal action, just as dipsomaniacs and kleptomaniacs seek excitation. Others are persons suffering from timidity, who regard normal love as more immoral and more dangerous than homosexual love. " I have heard so often that intercourse with a woman is a terrible danger for a man." They are timorous, and between them and members of the opposite sex there exists a difference which renders both social and bodily relationships far more difficult than with persons of their own sex. Finally we have to add the factor of a bad education of sexual automatism, whereby the homosexual act is rendered more customary and more simple in abulics, to whom innovation and effort are repugnant. I have collected notes of a great many cases of these various kinds, and I hope some day to publish them all, though the editing of the notes is a difficult matter. The less severe cases of homosexuality, when the patients are

---

[1] Les obsessions et la psychasthénie, first edition, 1903, vol. i, pp. 16, 49, and 590; vol. ii, pp. 30 and 367.

intelligent and when they can be placed in favourable circumstances, are curable more often than is usually supposed.
One such patient wrote to me : " It is really surprising to me
to find myself in love with a young woman, when for twenty
years I have believed anything of the kind to be impossible."
But we have to recognise that among those suffering from
disorders of the sexual impulse, education is an especially
difficult matter when we have to do with homosexuality, and
that we must aim at inducing mental modifications which it
is difficult to class under the head of " education."

These difficulties are yet further increased when we come
to consider the more complicated neuroses in which less
elementary actions are affected. Encouraged by the studies
about which I have just been writing, I tried for some time to
treat neuropaths of all kinds by educational methods, and it
will be interesting to summarise my results. In a certain
number of cases it must be admitted that these results were
encouraging.—Ac., the young woman who was obsessed by
the thought of her stools, disciplined herself by degrees, and
ceased to go to stool so often. When this happened, she
also ceased to think so much about her health. In a good
many patients I have seen hypochondria considerably relieved
in like manner through education. In a great many cases
of phobia, the patients seem to have been improved by educative treatment.—Gc. (f., 19), came to consult me suffering from
a phobia of solitude. She said that she no longer existed,
that she was melting away, that she disappeared into nonentity,
if she were left alone for a moment in a room or in a garden.
Her nurse was told to leave her from time to time, at first for
very brief periods, which were gradually increased, and I
taught her to bear being left alone in this way. After some
months, she was fully restored to health, and the result
certainly seemed to be due to education. Patients suffering
from all kinds of agoraphobia were made to repeat day after
day for months the practice of going out alone, and of passing
through larger and larger spaces, of " traversing very dangerous
streets in which there were no chemists." In many patients
who have a dread of poisons, microbes, crumbs of consecrated
bread, etc., and among those who have the phobia of contact
and a hand-washing mania, a strict education does a great deal

of good. We shall often make a mistake if we yield too much to the patient in order to save him or her from dread and anxiety, and thus permit the performanee of various follies. In many families, I regret to say even in many sanatoria, we find that the phobia of contact has actually been cultivated by such concessions ; and the reader will remember that I have recorded a remarkable instance in the case of Clarisse. It is a good thing to change the patient's environment, for this will assist in bringing about a modification of behaviour. We shall be wise to impose a rigid discipline, involving the almost complete prohibition of washing, or whatever the mania may be, despite the patient's protestations. No doubt the mental state and the obsessions are not instantly modified by this procedure, and the patient will insist that the ideas continue unchanged although the practice is forbidden. It is none the less true that, after an interruption of the kind for a considerable period, the patient will often forget the fears and the manias. In a dozen observations of manias of this kind, I was able to note the suppression of the trouble for at least a year, after some months of strict discipline.

The various authors I have quoted have shown that training in work, even intellectual work, and the acquirement of good habits, are by no means impossible, and that much help will be rendered to the patient by these means. Maurice de Fleury gives excellent advice : " A great thing is not to waste energies. ' Do what you are doing ' the old pedagogues used to say ; do what you are doing, and do not do something else at the same time. If you are playing, give yourself up entirely to play ; but when you are at work, energetically banish everything which is not work, and even banish work of any other kind. . . . Concentrate your mind, put on blinkers, restrict the field of your intelligence to a single object. . . . On no pretext whatever postpone getting to work upon whatever concerns you, for it is the first moments which decide the value of the whole spell. The very greatest geniuses have taken such precautions for fear of wasting their energies." I could quote the cases of a number of patients to whom this advice or similar advice has been of great service. In one of the first cases that came under my observation (it was published in 1896), that of Justine, the woman who for twenty years suffered from a fixed idea of cholera, education to work played a considerable part in relieving her trouble.[1] In the end the patient came to feel the need of work for the relief of her symptoms. " I can no longer remain inactive ; if I do, my thoughts begin to wander in the wrong direction ; but if I set to work, my troubles pass. I can stop the onset of a crisis by spending an hour reading music at the piano."—In other cases, women suffering from the mania of doubt exhibited, as always happens in such instances, grave disorders of conduct. But education to work transformed Ro. (f., 35) and Vkp. (f., 27). They thus came to learn that they really had no notion how to manage their household affairs, that they had wanted to do too much, and to do too many things at the same time ; that they must concentrate their energies, and must do only one thing at a time and finish that before beginning something else. Eb. (m., 31), gradually gave up his perpetual and ludicrous classifications, his manias of abstraction which made his work interminable. The good effects of such educational methods upon physical behaviour and upon mental work are indubitable in many instances. I might reintroduce here numerous case-histories which I have already summarised in connexion with treatment by isolation, and could show that in many of these it was necessary to teach such weaklings the need for a certain independence in the household, the need for resisting claims that would interfere with concentration. It is not always enough to achieve a temporary resignation and liquidation which will rid the patient of traumatic memories, for in many instances the sufferers have to regulate their whole lives by acquiring habits of tranquillity, indifference, and resignation.

But are we, in all these cases, still concerned with education in the strict sense of the term ; or can we say that education, while it certainly plays a part in the cure, really plays the essential part ? I doubt if this question can be answered in the affirmative, and here we touch the limits of the educational method of therapeutics.

7. INDICATIONS FOR EDUCATIONAL TREATMENT.

From the cases that have been recorded, we may perhaps draw certain conclusions regarding the value of educational treatment in the neuroses, and form clear notions as to the

[1] Névroses et idées fixes, vol. i, p. 193.

indications for educational treatment. First of all, the disorders which seem to have been most readily influenced by education are those which concerned very elementary psychological functions. When the trouble is limited to a simple motor function—to the function of walking for example, or to the function of breathing—we have to do with comparatively simple actions, with whose mechanism our anatomical and physiological studies have made us sufficiently familiar. Furthermore, we are concerned with subjects who exhibit little or no psychological depression, who are able to understand what we ask of them, and to make prolonged efforts of attention. This is one of the most favourable conditions, the one in which our success will be greatest. Every one knows that by a carefully designed course of gymnastics a great deal can be done to reeducate a patient one of whose limbs has been mutilated or even amputated. In like manner, we can to a great extent reestablish correct movement in patients suffering from localised lesions of the nervous system.

Just as when a man has lost his right hand, we can teach him to use the pen with his left, so when a tabetic or a hemiplegic has had portions of the nerve centres destroyed, we can teach him a new way of walking. This apprenticeship will obviously be more difficult in proportion as the lesion is more extensive ; but, generally speaking, the functional troubles which manifest themselves in the early days after the occurrence of a nervous lesion are more extensive than really corresponds to the extent of the lesion, and we shall be surprised and gratified to see how many of the patient's movements can be restored.

No doubt things are much less simple when we have to do with hysterical paralyses and contractures, with habit-spasms and other tics, and with the visceral troubles of neuropaths, for in these cases we are far less accurately informed concerning the mechanism of the disordered function. Still, successes are not uncommon, and they show that our hypotheses concerning these symptoms must be fairly sound. When psychological analysis enables us to ascertain precisely what tendency has gone wrong, we shall far more rapidly succeed in prescribing useful education. That is why I laid so much stress upon the remarkable disorder of vision noted in Madame Z., and upon the way in which she was treated by the reeducation of conscious monocular vision. We shall seldom find it possible to be so accurate in our methods ; and in most instances the vagueness of our knowledge of the mechanism of the various forms of functional paralysis, makes treatment by reeducation difficult and tedious.   That is what we find, to an even greater extent, when we try to apply educative methods to the more complicated forms of mental trouble.   The value of educational treatment will be proportional to the knowledge we possess of the mechanism of the disordered function.

A second point is even more important.   Those who have tried to reeducate patients suffering from organic lesions, have noted that the patients' energy and intelligence were more important factors in the result than the actual extent of the lesion.   This is still truer when we are concerned with neuropathic disorders.   Education will be successful in persons in whom the trouble is more or less fully localised to a particular function, and in whom the mental faculties as a whole are but slightly affected.   Those who will benefit by educational treatment will be persons free from marked depression, persons capable of a fair amount of attention, of obedience, of fairly prolonged effort.   On the other hand, when the subject is delirious, or when he is markedly abulic, and incapable of performing the simplest acts when required to do so, we can hardly expect to cure him by simple educational methods. Now, neuropathic troubles are almost always generalised, and are characterised by depression of all the activities.   This fact must obviously restrict enormously the part played by education in the treatment of the neuroses.

The defenders of the method will doubtless answer that persons suffering from depression can be transformed, for we sometimes see them improve under our very eyes, and it is possible to bring about this improvement by education. Cannot we teach people to be more attentive, more " all there," more energetic ?   Can we not teach people how to learn ?

It is indubitable that transformations of this kind do occur in the course of various kinds of treatment, and they sometimes manifest themselves during treatment by educational methods. When they take place, the observer is inclined to attribute them to the education, and to suppose that educational treatment is of great importance in the management of the neuroses. I think there is a confusion of terms here, and that the word " education " is being unwarrantably extended in significance, just as we have seen that the significance of " suggestion " has been unduly extended. If we are to advance along this line of study, we must be more precise in our use of terms. I think we shall do well to use the word " education " in a restricted sense only, when our aim is to upbuild, to render precise and automatic, a particular system of actions. I do not think we ought to use the term education when we are speaking of the development of activity in general, when we are referring to general modifications of psychological tension. Education utilises the energies of the individual, canalises them in a particular direction, so that subsequently it will be easier to economise and augment these energies ; though it does not actually augment them at the time. If a certain treatment enables us to bring about a real increase of energy, a positive rise in psychological tension, we are concerned with a mode of action which is so important and so new, that I think we must distinguish it from methods of treatment hitherto known, and study it under a new name. In the foregoing chapters I have already considered some of the influences which are superadded to education properly so-called, such as suggestion, the discovery and the dissociation of fixed ideas, the economising of energy by repose and isolation. But I think that in these phenomena we can discern, in addition, another very important influence, which can be called *excitation*, the study of which will be undertaken in the next chapter but one. These are the various influences which transform the patient, and which then allow education to take effect.

In fact, even in the cases in which other activities play their part at first, education has its uses. It may only come into play tardily, at a stage when the patient has already made a considerable advance towards cure ; but it will help to render the cure definite, and above all will help to stabilise it. Its essential role is to transform an action into an automatic tendency, to fix it as it were. We do not do enough if we secure, just once, by one method or another, a movement of the paralysed or contractured limb, and then leave the patient to his own devices, for the paralysis or the contracture will soon be just as marked as it was before. We must make the patient repeat the movement, must simplify it, must enable him to perform it with less awareness, under less supervision, and with less effort. When we have obtained the action in an isolated form, we must reestablish the tendency to the action ; and in such a process of reconstruction, education will always play a considerable part.

In a word, we are back once more at the problem of diagnosis, and at the problem of the precise application of curative methods. We must give up indiscriminate talk about education, when we have to do with a neuropathic disorder. Some day we may hope to learn how to distinguish clearly the symptoms for which, and the patients in whom, education is applicable, and to note clearly what place this special form of treatment ought to occupy in the treatment as a whole. It will then be discovered that educational treatment is not all-sufficing, but that it certainly has an important part to play.

CHAPTER THIRTEEN

AESTHESIOGENIC AGENTS

WE always have a hankering after our first loves, and it is very difficult to rid ourselves of the studies which interested us in youth, to recognise them as illusions. In an earlier chapter, I had to make my excuses for continuing to speak to-day of "hypnotism" and "suggestion"; I shall have again to excuse myself in the present chapter for returning to the discussion of complete somnambulism and of aesthesiogenic agents, which are ignored by the present generation of medical men, although for a brief period they excited enthusiasm in those of the earlier generation. I am satisfied that, amid a multitude of errors, the magnetisers and the metallotherapeutists glimpsed some very remarkable phenomena which are hard to explain, and are despised to-day because they are not easy to utilise—but which are real none the less, and are likely at some future date to form the starting-point of important discoveries.

1. THE MAGNETISERS' "CRISES." METALLOTHERAPY.

It is necessary to summarise briefly a history which I have written more than once elsewhere.[1] When we turn over the leaves of the old books written by the French magnetisers, we find here and there descriptions of strange somnambulist states, characterised by a transformation and by a sudden and temporary cure of patients who had been suffering from severe neuropathic symptoms and very grave depression. In the year 1853, writing in his book *Etude du magnétisme animal sous le point de vue d'une exacte pratique*, Baragnon spoke of " the marvellous regeneration which can be accomplished all in a moment; . . . of a resurrection which occurs quite

[1] L'automatisme psychologique, 1889, p. 178; Les accidents mentaux des hystériques, 1893, p. 226; Névroses et idées fixes, 1888, vol. i, pp. 50, 238, and 436; L'état mental des hystériques, second edition, 1911, pp. 368, 549, and 669.

spontaneously, and in which the subject fully recovers consciousness of his ego."[1] We find similar remarks in Pigeaire's book *Electricité animale*, 1839, and in Aubin Gauthier's *Histoire du somnambulisme, etc.*, 1842 (vol. 2, p. 373) ; also in J. P. Durand's *Cours de braidisme*, 1860, p. 97. But the author who has given the most striking description of this phenomenon is, I think, Charles Despine in *De l'emploi du magnetisme animal et des eaux minérales dans le traitement des maladies nerveuses*, 1840. This book was brought to my notice by Gibert of Havre, who was well aware of its importance. The work is entirely devoted to the account of a single case, being the study of the illness and of the treatment of a girl of sixteen suffering from grave hysteria. This girl, Estelle by name, after sustaining a fall which was not in itself serious, but which happened under conditions arousing a good deal of emotion, was attacked by complete paraplegia and anaesthesia of the whole of the lower part of the body, and with dysaesthesic disorders of the trunk. She also suffered from anorexia, and vomited her food unless kept on an extremely restricted and peculiar diet. She complained of a persistent sense of cold, and was always wrapped in rugs, was drowsy and inert, with no signs of voluntary activity, but she was readily suggestible.

After various attempts had been made to induce hypnosis, she passed into a strange condition which Despine called the " crisis." This was characterised by a complete return of the power of movement and of sensibility. " During the crisis, her sensory power is just as good as before she fell ill ; . . . and at the same time Estelle in the crisis is able to run about and even to swim in the bathing-pool."[2] There was an entire change in the condition of the appetite and of the digestion. " One very remarkable thing in Estelle is the nature of the diet during the state of crisis as compared with the diet during the waking state. When she has gone back to the normal state of health, Estelle has a liking to eat almost anything, and she is fond of all the varieties of food she used to eat before she became ill. . . . Furthermore, during the crisis, she eats heartily and with impunity. But since she became ill, she has not been able in the natural waking state to depart from her dietetic regimen of milk and

[1] Op. cit., pp. 154 and 158. [2] Op. cit., pp. 88–267.

eggs without suffering from cramps and vomiting. She really seems to have two stomachs, one for use in the state of crisis, the other for use in the waking state." [1] The feeling of chilliness had also disappeared ; she threw off her rugs and was no longer afraid to plunge into cold water. [2] Her character was completely changed. She had become endowed with a resolute will, and was no longer susceptible to suggestion. [3]

Unfortunately this cure was not persistent, and when she was reawakened—or when the end of the crisis, which never lasted long, came spontaneously—the subject was once more paralysed, anaesthesic, anorexic, uttering continual complaints of the cold, inert and suggestible. She had only a vague memory of the happy period through which she had passed, or she possessed no memory of it at all. At first these favourable crises were of extremely brief duration ; by degrees they came to last longer, and finally a complete cure was effected through a sort of fusion of the waking state with the state of crisis. " This interval of ten months has been for Estelle a period of almost complete fusion of the state of crisis with the waking state. What I mean is that the waking state attended by paralysis of the lower limbs has been gradually confounded with the state of exaltation." [4]

This book is of great interest to students of the history of medicine. We have to note that these studies upon hysterical paralysis and upon hysterical anaesthesia were made in the years 1837 and 1838, and were published in 1840. The important object here is to lay stress upon the remarkable characteristics of the treatment, which consisted in the artificial production of crises attended with complete though temporary restoration of a normal state of health. Other facts of a similar kind have been recorded from time to time in works upon somnambulism. Azam, in his account of Félida X., noted that there were states of " complete somnambulism " in which the pathological disorders and the suggestibility disappeared ; " states in which the idea of the external world and the patient's independence were quite satisfactory ; states of which the subject had no memory when she had returned to her habitual condition of illness." Mary Reynolds, Weir Mitchell's patient, was also subject to " alert

---

[1] Op. cit., p. 47.   [2] Op. cit., pp. 31–39.
[3] Op. cit., p. 37.   [4] Op. cit., pp. 61 and 66.

states," in which there were no morbid symptoms, these states contrasting with the periods of gloom and disorder. In the morbid state she had no memory of the alert state. (Weir Mitchell : *Mary Reynolds, a Case of Double Consciousness*, 1889.) Similar facts have been recorded in most studies of "double personality." They are well described in Laurent's book, *Les états seconds*, 1893. These books describe the same conditions that the old magnetisers used to call "critical exaltations." I think that the magnetisers' researches concerning such conditions formed the inception of what was to develop into the aesthesiogenic treatment.

In order to trace the historical evolution of the ideas we are considering, I think it is proper to associate the foregoing observations with the studies of a school which is to-day almost entirely forgotten, with the researches concerning metallotherapy, and with the studies of Burq. Mesmer's doctrines originated, as we have seen, out of ancient beliefs according to which the stars exercised a great influence upon the human body. The new methods of treatment of which we are now to speak were associated with medieval ideas concerning the influence of metals. These beliefs had already played a considerable part in giving rise to Perkins' treatment by "metallic tractors," which flourished in the United States and in England at the close of the eighteenth and at the beginning of the nineteenth century.[1] They were also influential in giving rise to the experiments of Wittchman, in 1769, and those of Fischer, in 1802. They have a common origin with certain hoary beliefs relating to the action of magnets, beliefs which go back into the days of Ancient Egypt. As early as 1771, Abbé Lenoble made his patients wear magnetised pieces of iron, attached to the wrist and to the chest. In a report to the French Royal Society of Medicine, in 1779, Audry and de Thouret sang the praises of this practice ; and magnets were used in treatment by Laennec, Alibert, Chaumet, Recamier, and Trousseau. Among the magnetisers, some adopted these ideas concerning the importance of metals and of magnets. Charles Despine wrote in 1840 : " I was struck by the remarkable fondness which these patients had

---

[1] A spirited and detailed account of the rise and fall of Perkinism will be found in Oliver Wendell Holmes' Medical Essays, Boston, 1883, pp. 15–38.

for pure gold ; I also noted the obviously different influences exercised upon them by zinc, brass, and magnetised iron. . . . As soon as the gold touched her, her arms recovered life ; but if the glass touched her, it undid the good effects of the gold. . . . For Estelle, pure gold is a veritable lever with which she can move the world." [1]

Between 1851 and 1880, Burq did much to diffuse these doctrines and to give them a more or less scientific aspect. In his thesis for the doctorial degree, written in 1851 ; in various memoirs to academies, penned in 1852, 1867, and 1871 ; and, finally, in his last and very interesting book, *Des origines de la métallothérapie*, published in 1883—Burq studied the modifications resulting from the application of metallic plates to the skin of patients, and also the modifications resulting from the ingestion of the same metals. These experiments were for the most part made upon neuropaths, upon hysterical patients suffering from disorders of cutaneous and muscular sensibility. Gendrin, Beau, and Briquet, between 1846 and 1850, drew attention to the disorders of tactile sensibility in hysterics, which had already been studied prior to 1840 by the magnetisers, as we have learned from Charles Despine's book. But it was Burq who attached great importance to these troubles, and he was instrumental in leading Charcot to teach as he did at the Salpêtrière.

It was not found that all metals had the same power when applied to the skin. Some of them had no effect at all. The patients had " a sort of metallic idiosyncrasy," so that in each patient some particular metal would prove most efficacious. The choice of the most useful metal in each case was determined by various trials, the process being termed " metalloscopy." Burq used a sort of bracelet, composed of several pieces of metal joined by a ribbon. This was applied to the anaesthetic forearm. After a time which varied from two or three minutes to a quarter of an hour, if the metal had been suitably chosen the subject would become aware of various itchings and chilly sensations, or of feelings of heat and weight in the limb. A general sensation of pins and needles would invariably herald the end of the attack and the return of sensibility in all parts of the body ; the phenomena of dysaesthesia always made their appearance during the tran-

[1] Despine, op. cit., pp. 64 and 124.

sition from analgesia to sensibility." [1] As a matter of actual fact, at the same time the subject began to perceive more and more accurately the pinpricks and the various other impressions made upon areas of skin which up till now had been anaesthetic.

Simultaneously with the return of sensibility, a number of other movements could be detected. The circulation was restored, so that the skin lost its pallor. Whereas previously a prick did not bleed, now when the skin was pricked with a pin a droplet of blood would appear, and the skin would redden in the neighbourhood of the prick. The surface temperature of the skin sometimes rose by several degrees ; and whereas the skin had been dry it would now become moist.[2] Finally the muscular power, which had as a rule been greatly reduced in the anaesthetic limb, now became normal. These modifications, though local at the outset, spread continuously, so as to bring about in the end a general transformation of the individual. The paralyses and the contractures, the convulsive paroxysms, and even the visceral disorders, disappeared. If the major hysterical crises were to be checked, it was necessary, said Burq, to bring as much of the patient's skin as possible into contact with the metal. If gold was the most effective metal (and gold was the preference in most cases), the best way to cure all the patient's troubles was to cover the skin with gold pieces.

Burq was convinced that in these cures the restoration of cutaneous, muscular, and visceral sensibility played the chief part. " How can we refuse to recognise that the anaesthesia and amyosthenia which are so common in hysteria are concurrent with all the other manifestations, are the measure of these, and probably their foundation, seeing that the attacks and all the other symptoms disappear with the return of sensibility and of motor power ? " [3] From these theories it was possible to deduce practical conclusions, which the author formulated in very moderate terms. " Assuming that there exists a nervous affection with anaesthesia and amyosthenia, the whole treatment consists in finding a means, of any kind, to restore sensibility and motility to the normal state. Various agents may be employed for the purpose ; for example, we may have recourse to hydrotherapy, gymnastics, electricity,

[1] Burq, Des origines de la métallothérapie, 1883, pp. 36 and 83.
[2] Burq, op. cit., p. 40.   [3] Ibid., p. 38.

stimulants of all kinds, rubefacients, vesicatories, animal magnetism, even novenas—in a word, anything which strikes the imagination ; but, of all possible means, one of the most efficacious is the methodical application of metallic armatures which suit the mysterious individual affinities." [1]

In 1876 Burq reported his experiments to the Société de Biologie, which appointed a commission to examine into their reality. Charcot was the president of this commission, and had the experiments repeated in his clinic at the Salpêtrière. This event had enormous influence upon the teaching of the clinic. At the same time as that in which the ideas of the magnetisers were making their way into the clinic by the paths previously indicated, Burq's theories were contributing to the elaboration of the Salpêtrière doctrines concerning hysteria and hypnotism. Fifteen years later, at a time when Burq's experiments were supposed to have been completely forgotten, and when no one would have ventured to quote the originator of metallotherapy, Charcot was still saying : " The hysteric is not fully cured until every trace of anaesthesia has disappeared"; and Gilles de la Tourette was adding : " The foundation of the therapy of hysterical symptoms is to be found, in my opinion, in the reestablishment of the various perverted or lost sensibilities." In the evolution of ideas, no opinion can be regarded as insignificant.

To begin with, moreover, Burq's teaching was enthusiastically received, and all those who were working in Charcot's clinic were eager to experiment upon the new phenomena. But they took the matter up under unfavourable conditions, just as had previously been the case with the phenomena of magnetism. Not having any idea that they were concerned with psychological phenomena, and failing to understand that their first business should have been to study the mental condition of the subject, and that all kinds of moral precautions were essential to successful researches in this field, they thought only of the physical aspects of their experiments. They believed themselves able to satisfy all the requirements of scientific method by carrying out this physical side of their experiments with the necessary precision. They correctly weighed the metallic plates in chemical balances, and they registered the most trifling muscular tremors with the aid

[1] Burq. op. cit., p. 42.

of Marey's tambour; but they saw nothing wrong in carrying on the experiments in public, amid the chatter of casual spectators, and they would themselves discuss the meaning of the experiments in their patients' presence.

Thus their first studies were directed to the discovery of the physical agents which could be substituted for the metal plates of Burq, and could cause the same effects. Bourneville, Cullerre, Maggiorani, Paul Richer, Dumontpallier (an enthusiast for Burq's metal plates until he became an enthusiast for Bernheim's suggestion), and, above all, Romain Vigouroux, discovered that the metal plates could be replaced by blistering fluids, by magnets, by tuning forks, by electric currents, and in especial by static electricity. Vigouroux summarised these discoveries in his articles in " Progrès médical," 1878, p. 747; and in a more detailed study published in the " Archives de neurologie," 1880–1881, p. 257, entitled *Métalloscopie, métallothérapie, aesthésiogénie*. It was at this date that there began the practice of treating hysterical patients by placing them upon the stool of the static electrical machine. These authors enlarged the scope of metallotherapy, and reached a concept which Burq, as we have seen, was inclined to accept—the idea of treatment by aesthesiogenic agents. " The name of aesthesiogenism," said Vigouroux, " is the general term proposed by Charcot to denote all the natural agents or processes which, like metals, have a special action upon sensation and certain other functions." The various reactions of persons subjected to aesthesiogenic agents were carefully studied. Thus were discovered anew certain phenomena which Burq had already pointed out in a somewhat vague fashion, such as return anaesthesia (variations of sensibility, which appeared and then disappeared once more), the order in which sensation recurred (the reappearance of tactile sensibility before the reappearance of sensibility to pain).[1] Finally, at the close of an interesting account given by Gellé, of the aesthesiogenic treatment of a patient suffering from hysterical deafness, we learn that he discovered, or rather rediscovered, the remarkable phenomenon of transference. At the moment when hearing had become normal once more on the side of the hemi-

[1] Paul Richer, " Progrès médical," 1878, p. 46; Landouzy, " Progrès médical," 1879, p. 60; Walton, Deafness in hysterical Anaesthesia, " Brain," 1883.

anaesthesia, the power of hearing was reduced on the healthy side to the low level which had hitherto characterised the hearing on the diseased side. Soon it was found that such a phenomenon was a usual result of the treatment of hemianaesthesia. Galezowski and Landolt studied the same phenomena in connexion with disorders of vision, and noted the modifications of the visual field for different colours.

This phenomenon of transference had been pointed out long before by the magnetisers, Cabanis having remarked that sensibility " behaves like a fluid, its level lowering on one side when it rises on the other." In my opinion this transference is a real and very interesting phenomenon, when not distorted by ill-directed education. It is in close relationship with the psychological exhaustion and the restriction of the field of consciousness ; and even to-day it deserves careful study. Unfortunately, in the days of which I am now writing it was not carefully studied. The observers were always inclined to ignore the psychological condition of their patients, being concerned only with the objective aspects of the phenomena, and while studying these they complicated them more and more. After making observations upon the effects of the active metals and the neutral metals, they turned to researches upon the effects of the metallic compounds, upon the effects of a neutral metal superposed upon an active metal, upon actions which inhibited one another, and upon those which fixed the transference at this or that stage of development—passing on to researches concerning the most highly involved and incredible forms of transference.

The studies thus elaborately begun, came to a sudden pause. When I turn over the pages of the first volume of the " Archives de Neurologie," 1880–1881, I find that it contains lengthy papers on metallotherapy and transference, among which the most notable are the extensive articles written by Romain Vigouroux. But in no one of the subsequent volumes can I find any reference to the subject. The only exception is that in 1889 I find a brief review by Paul Blocq of Moricourt's book *Manuel de métallothérapie*. All the researches which, in 1878 and 1879, had seemed so full of promise for the future, had passed into oblivion.

There is a very remarkable reason for this sudden collapse. We find it in the first publications of Bernheim, and in the opening of the struggle between the Nancy School and the Salpêtrière School. It is true that for a long time the critics had been contending that the majority of such phenomena were due to the influence of imagination and to that of expectant attention. This outlook was voiced already in the eighteenth century, in the writings of John Hunter; and the idea was again mooted nearly a century later by Daniel Hack Tuke, in his book *The Influence of the Mind on the Body*, 1872. But doctors did not understand the importance of the objection, or the practical difficulties it involved. We are concerned here with a problem analogous to those which Pasteur had to face in connexion with his earlier investigations in the matter of pure cultures and spontaneous generation. The opponents always imagined that it was quite easy to keep their cultures free from the risk of contamination, although in fact these cultures were contaminated by all the germs contained in the air. In the end, a good many investigators abandoned the researches rather than take the trouble to keep their cultures pure

Bernheim's onslaughts were a little rough, but his censures were well deserved. His great merit was that he made doctors realise the risk of suggestion, and the need for a psychological analysis if they wished to interpret neuropathic symptoms. As far as the unfortunate study of metallotherapy was concerned, the effect of his criticisms was that of a thunderbolt. In my opinion, the metallotherapists could and should have defended themselves. They ought to have asked for a more precise definition of the term suggestion; and when an agreement had been reached as to the exact meaning of the word, they should have been ready to abandon the phenomena which obviously belonged to the field of suggestion thus defined, while going on to enquire whether there was a residual group of phenomena which were independent of suggestion, and which were still worthy of examination. But before they could have done this, they would have had to enter the domain of psychological science, which seemed to them difficult and repugnant. They preferred to throw up the sponge, and to go further than their critic Bernheim had done, for he in his first writings had continued to say that the magnet might perhaps have a real effect upon the nervous system. The absolute abandonment of the study of metallotherapy was,

I think, a mistake ; and I consider that Burq's investigations concerning the immediate restoration of health to neuropaths by a reawakening of sensibility and of powers of movement are still worthy of attention.

2. COMPLETE SOMNAMBULISM.

I myself have been much interested in the doctrines of the magnetisers concerning the state of crisis, and in the doctrines of Burq's disciples concerning aesthesiogenism. At the outset of my own studies I was able to observe phenomena analogous to those which formed the starting-point of the before-mentioned theories. The patients who came under my observation at Havre between 1883 and 1889, whose cases were analysed in the records I published during the years 1886–1889, and in my thesis of 1889 entitled *L'automatisme psychologique*, were for the most part hysterical women exhibiting very serious symptoms, such as attacks of delirium lasting for several days, fixed ideas of all kinds, anorexia, vomiting, contracture, and paralysis. One of these patients, Rose, was paraplegic, and was bedridden in hospital for eighteen months. Most of them, too, suffered from disorders of memory and perception, from various kinds of amnesia, and from anaesthesia of the different senses. Wishing to work simultaneously towards the curing of these patients and towards elucidating the pathogenesis of their symptoms, I tried by all possible means to modify these symptoms, to dispel them by hypnotism, by suggestion, and by various educational methods. I endeavoured to make the paralysed limbs resume the power of proper movement ; to induce the patients to feel and to appreciate the impressions made upon their dulled senses.

In some of my patients, and especially in three of them, this practice led to the onset of conditions which seemed to me very strange, for they were in complete contrast with the habitual morbid condition. Sometimes these states appeared gradually, after the subjects had been making efforts to move and to feel, and they were preceded by contortions, and by itching or other forms of dysaesthesia. In most cases they appeared in the course of a hypnotic sitting, and after a period of profound sleep. In especial they were characterised by the complete disappearance of all the pathological phenomena. The disorders of movement, the paralyses, and the contractures, had vanished; the woman who had been bedridden with paraplegia for eighteen months, could walk and run, just like Charles Despine's Estelle; the vomiting had ceased and the patient could take food readily; at the same time, normal sensation was restored all over the body. The memory reached back throughout the whole of the patient's past, extending to periods which hitherto had been completely forgotten. Finally, there were no longer manifest any disorders of will, and suggestibility had apparently disappeared. " This final condition of somnambulism is a state in which the subject, whose personality has hitherto been so greatly restricted, and who in the waking state was so ill, has now become identical with one who is perfectly well and completely normal. . . . This is a condition in which the subject once more exhibits absolute integrity of all the sensations natural to a person in good health, and perfect integrity of memory. In a word, it is a state in which there is no longer any anaesthesia or any amnesia. This state is very important in all respects, especially from the therapeutic point of view.[1] . . . These women, who were so readily hallucinated, who were so passive in the waking state, are, now that they have passed into the so-called sleep, not only in possession of all their senses and of all their memories, but also in possession of all their spontaneity and all their independence. We can no longer impose any suggestion upon them." [2]

In my first studies of these questions I was at great pains to show that this state was not in itself in any way extraordinary; that it was simply the normal condition in which these women ought to have been all the time, but in which they could not continue owing to their morbid depression. I was sorry to find, seeing that I had built such extensive hopes of cure, that the condition of complete restoration was one which could not last long in these patients.[3] If they

---

[1] L'automatisme psychologique, 1889, pp. 114 and 178.
[2] Ibid., pp. 179 and 344; cf. also, Les accidents mentaux des hystériques, 1893, p. 123.
[3] L'automatisme psychologique, pp. 135 and 349; Les accidents mentaux des hystériques, 1893, p. 225; second edition, 1911, p. 382; Névroses et idées fixes, 1898, vol. i, p. 239.

were left to themselves, they relapsed sooner or later, and the anaesthesias and other morbid symptoms reappeared. Another and very important phenomenon now attracted my attention in connexion with these cases. I found that the patients, when they had relapsed into their habitual morbid state, had as a rule completely forgotten the period of artificially induced health. These oblivions made gaps in the continuity of memory, thus giving birth to various modifications of the personality. In a word, the forgetfulness supervening upon the relapse, gave the aspect of somnambulism to the period of quasi-normal health. That is why, in order to denote the periods of temporary restoration, I use the term " complete somnambulism," which had already been employed by Azam to denote kindred phenomena.

These forms of complete somnambulism seem to me to resemble very closely the magnetic crises described by Charles Despine; but I should mention that, at the time I was studying them, I was not yet acquainted with Charles Despine's book, and did not read it till much later. Nevertheless the symptoms of Rose were exactly like those of Despine's Estelle. Although there was no direct influence exercised by Despine's record of Estelle, it is possible that Despine's book had an indirect influence upon my researches, effected in a roundabout way. Despine's book was certainly known to Perrier of Caen, who quotes it in his records. Now, as I have already related, for a good many years Perrier had under his care Léonie, one of the subjects whom I had studied very closely, and one of the first to exhibit to my notice the phenomena of complete somnambulism. It is likely enough that Perrier had induced such states in her, and had made them habitual to her. It is quite possible that the observation of these states of complete somnambulism in Léonie, became a motive leading me to make my researches on the other patients. Ideas are continually passed from one mind to another by indirect and often invisible channels.

I am also inclined to believe that the phenomena have close analogies with those described by Burq and his followers. In these and other authors, we find records of the way in which women suffering from transient attacks of hysteria were restored to a normal condition by the application of gold pieces, and we are reminded of what happened in the cases of Lucie and Rose. The return of sensibility would seem, in both groups of observations, to be the phenomenon which plays the leading part, that which the experimenters particularly wish to produce, and the one which gives rise to all the others. The only differences were in the methods employed to bring about this return of sensation—and the differences were not considerable. That is why, in this historical summary, I bring my own researches upon complete somnambulism into line with the studies of Burq and with those of the magnetisers.

My preliminary observations were confirmed by the researches which I subsequently made in the Paris hospitals from 1889 onwards. In this connexion, I need only recall my studies of a case of allocheiria, in 1890 ; a case of abulia with fixed ideas in 1891 ; a case of continuous amnesia, 1892–1893 ; and the history of a fixed idea, 1894 ; every one of these studies having been reproduced in my book entitled *Névroses et idées fixes*. In all these observations, the patients, who had for a long time been suffering from paralyses, anaesthesias, amnesias, and abulias, of various kinds, were temporarily freed from their morbid symptoms after various kinds of psychological treatment. Marcelle, for instance, who was ordinarily abulic and anaesthetic to an extreme degree, " was at these times transfigured ; her face became bright and intelligent, her eyes mobile and able to look people in the face, her movements rapid ; . . . she herself was well aware of the change, and called the new state a ' bright moment.' There was, in fact, a sort of remission in the illness, a phase in which the brain seemed to resume its normal functioning. . . . This condition corresponds to what I have described elsewhere as complete somnambulism. . . . As I have so often said, it is nothing but a transient reappearance of the subject's normal waking state, which, however, assumes the aspect of a somnambulism because of the subsequent relapse into the state of anaesthesia." [1]

In all these studies, just as in those previously mentioned, I laid stress upon the transitional periods which could be detected between the morbid states and the states of complete restoration of function. The first subjects, whom I studied at

[1] Un cas d'aboulie et d'idées fixes, 1891, Névroses et idées fixes, vol. i, p. 50.

Havre, all showed, in this intermediate stage, signs of profound sleep. Their eyes were closed, and they gave no indications of any kind of reaction. Then, opening the eyes more or less abruptly, they seemed to wake into the alert condition. Some of my patients, like Marcelle, continued to correspond with this type. Others, like Madame D., Justine, etc., on the other hand, exhibited symptoms which were comparatively rare in my earlier observations. They did not seem to go to sleep, but they had various contortions in different parts of the body, and the contortions might even go so far as to culminate in a genuine convulsive paroxysm. This happened in the case of Marcelle, for instance.[1] She continued to complain of sensations of nervous exhaustion, ticklishness, and burning. Several of them, like Madame D. or Justine, complained of severe pains in the head, lancinating pains, tearing sensations, strange feelings like those of broken fibres, like those of bullets bursting in the head.[2]

I also laid stress upon the feelings of the subject at the moment of onset of the alert state ; upon her delight, her gaiety, the pleasure she felt in noting that the light was brighter, that the objects at which she looked had more vivid tints, upon the satisfaction she felt at, as she said, being herself once more, at coming to herself again.[3] Unfortunately, these happy periods were transient. Emotion, fatigue, prolonged intellectual effort, would make the subject relapse into the earlier condition, and then there was, in most cases, amnesia concerning the happy period.[4] The mode of transition from the alert state back into the state of depression was likewise interesting. Sometimes the change took place insensibly. But in most cases it was rather sudden, and the subject presented peculiar symptoms during the transition. Often there was a convulsive crisis, and at the end of this the anaesthesias and other familiar symptoms reappeared.

The part played by aesthesiogenism in the production of complete somnambulism is even plainer in the following observations, which were made at this period by my brother, Jules Janet. After having studied the physical and moral transformations which I showed him at Havre in some of

---

[1] Un cas d'aboulie et d'idées fixes, 1891, Névroses et idées, fixes, vol. i, p. 44.   [2] Ibid., pp. 44, 147, and 165.
[3] Ibid., p. 427.   [4] Ibid., pp. 51, 54, 59, et passim.

my patients, he tried to reproduce them in other patients of the same kind. He noted kindred facts in several hysterics, but he made an especially remarkable study of a young woman of twenty-five, whom he described under the name of Marceline. [1] This was a young woman who had for some years suffered from all possible kinds of hysterical symptoms, and whose chief trouble was anorexia and refusal of food. When, with great repugnance, she had taken a little nourishment, or when she had been fed through an oesophageal tube, she promptly vomited almost everything she had just taken. Thereby she had been reduced to an extreme degree of emaciation and weakness. She also suffered from various contractures, from retention of urine, from different kinds of anaesthesia, and from visual disorders. A few sittings were devoted to hypnotising her ; and to taking advantage of the hypnotic state in order, by means of exercises of attention, to restore tactile and gustatory sensibility. Marceline soon passed into a condition in which she had recovered normal powers of sensation over the whole surface of the body, in which she could move her limbs freely, was able to pass water voluntarily without the use of the catheter, and could eat heartily without subsequent vomiting. " When dealing with a case of this kind," wrote Jules Janet, " we might imagine ourselves to be in the presence of a healthy person in the waking state, for the most practised observer would not have been able to distinguish her from a normal person. She was no longer a neuropath, an incomplete person ; but a young woman enjoying all her nervous functions to the full, showing us all the worth of nerve centres which are perfectly healthy and normal." [2] It was easy to make use of this condition in order to feed up Marceline, so that she rapidly recovered her strength. The condition had been originally induced during hypnosis. Jules Janet regarded it as still being a sleep, and after a certain period he awakened the patient. As soon as she had been reawakened she became inert once more, and exhibited anew all her hysterical disorders. She was incapable of recalling the period passed in the somnam-

[1] Jules Janet, Un cas d'hystérie grave, communications à la Société Clinique de Paris et à la Société de Psychologie Physiologique, " Bulletin Médical," 1888–1889 ; " La France Médicale," April 6, 1889 ; " Revue Scientifique," 1888, vol. i, p. 616.
[2] Jules Janet, " Revue Scientifique," 1888, vol. i, p. 616.

bulist state. Next, of course, Jules Janet aimed at endeavouring to suppress this undesirable awakening, and at leaving the patient in the induced state which, though artificially engendered, was nevertheless to all appearance identical with a normal waking state. " If," I said to myself, " I can leave my patient permanently in this state, I shall have discovered an easy way of curing her hysteria completely."[1] Jules Janet added : " To cure a hysteric of any symptom, we must not only relieve her of that particular symptom, but of all the disorders attending her waking state. We could cure the hysteric, if we could make her live permanently in the new state, in which she became an absolutely complete person, and was not subject to any hysterical symptoms."[2] The attempt was partially successful on several occasions. Marceline remained cured for days and even for weeks in this somnambulist state. But from time to time, either when she was menstruating or as the outcome of fatigue or emotion, she seemed to reawaken ; that is to say, she relapsed into her morbid state, and into a state of forgetfulness of all the antecedent periods when she had been in the alert state. To restore her to health, it was necessary to put her to sleep again and again, and to renew the efforts which had brought about the reestablishment of sensibility. These changes in the visceral functions and in the intellectual functions were very remarkable, and Jules Janet demonstrated them again and again to various persons. Thus a good many students and members of the resident staff of the hospitals, among whom I must mention Paul Sollier, had an opportunity of noting the strange alterations which could be artificially induced in this subject by the modification of sensibility, and also of noting the way in which these transitions were brought about.[3]

To follow the progress of historical developments, we must now turn to the studies of Paul Sollier, published in his work in two volumes entitled *La genèse et la nature de l'hystérie* (1897), and summarised in *L'hystérie et son traitement* (1901).

---

[1] L'automatisme psychologique, p. 135.
[2] Jules Janet, " Revue Scientifique," 1888, vol. i, p. 618.
[3] Concerning the early stages of the treatment of Marceline's case, consult my study entitled Une Félida artificielle, in the " Revue Philosophique," 1910, vol. i, p. 329 ; cf. also, L'état mental des hystériques, second edition, 1911, p. 545.

The attitude taken up by Monsieur Sollier towards Jules Janet made it impossible for me for a long time to quote and discuss the former's works ; but I am glad that Monsieur Sollier, by his letter of protest addressed to Monsieur Ribot,[1] has now enabled me to express my thoughts freely, and to point out the matters in his book which I regard as open to criticism, and the other matters which seem to me worthy of attention.

Whatever the importance of the criticisms, to which we shall have to return, it is necessary to recognise that Sollier certainly endeavoured to record the phenomena which Jules Janet had demonstrated to him, and to verify the value of the theories which had been expounded to him. At a period when nearly all medical practitioners, alarmed at the disasters sustained by Charcot's school, had ceased to take any interest in hysteria and hypnotism, Sollier had the courage to resume the study of aesthesiogenism and of complete somnambulism. The first of the two books just mentioned, *La genèse et la nature de l'hystérie*, was quite isolated when it appeared in 1897, for at that date nobody else was venturing to publish works of this character. The volumes in question, side by side with interpretations which, to say the least of it, are open to criticism, contain a detailed description of twenty hysterical patients considered from the psychological point of view (although the author is under some illusions upon this point) ; and they also contain a study of the effects which aesthesiogenic treatment produced upon these patients. It is true that Sollier, convinced that he is masking the psychological character of his studies by calling them, on page after page, " physiological," believes that he is separating himself completely from those who have previously written on these topics, and that he can save himself the trouble of quoting his predecessors by simply replacing the word "aesthesiogenism" by the word " resensibilisation "—but this little piece of childishness does not modify the nature of his studies, and does not entirely deprive them of interest.

Sollier unhesitatingly adopts the fundamental notion of Charcot's school, a notion formed through the inspiration of Burq, according to which disorders of sensibility are the most essential phenomena of hysteria. He even raises into a dogma

[1] " Revue Philosophique," 1910, vol. i, p. 550.

the principle formulated by Gilles de la Tourette, the fact that localised cutaneous anaesthesia in any region is always linked to a deep anaesthesia of one of the subjacent viscera. Finally, he regards the reestablishment of the lost sensibility as the most vital part of the treatment. The aesthesiogenic methods he employs are identical with those used by earlier authorities. He asks his patients to make efforts of will and of attention, telling them to pull themselves together, to shake off their torpor, to wake up thoroughly. To this end, he orders them to make movements while attending carefully to these movements and appreciating accurately what they are doing ; he orders them to pay attention to all their sensations, to practise feeling delicately in all parts of the body. When this somewhat general instruction proves inadequate, he draws attention successively to each part of the body, saying : " Note the feelings in your foot, your leg ; pay attention to your left hand, become aware of the feeling in your stomach, your abdomen, etc." He goes on repeating these orders for a long time, striving to attract the subject's attention to his own body by all sorts of means. Sometimes he has recourse to static electricity ; often he employs gymnastic exercises to supplement the foregoing commands.

During the period of transformation, Sollier's subjects do not seem to have exhibited the transitional states of sleep which I have so often noticed. They passed through a period of agitation and dysaesthesia. The author lays much stress upon the particular forms of these agitations and contortions, affecting now one organ and now another ; and he is even inclined to assimilate the agitations to the convulsions of a hysterical paroxysm. He also describes minutely the tinglings, the sensations of pins and needles, the twitchings, the burning sensations, announced by the subjects in different parts of the body ; their feelings of torsion or relaxation, of enlargement or diminution of the limbs. He lays stress upon the reactions connected with the awakening sensibility of the stomach—the shocks, gurglings, sensations of pins and needles, lancinating pains, sighings, yawnings, the sensation that the stomach is enlarged, that something soft and warm is running over it, the sensation of thirst (which appears before that of hunger.) He examines the same phenomena, using almost identical words to describe them, in connexion with the abdominal organs, the respiratory organs, and the genital organs.

He lays especial stress upon the sensations which the patients feel in the head. This seems to them large, heavy, and empty ; they feel tearing sensations here, as if bars stretched out from behind or from the front, or wires, were dragging, interlacing, enlarging, forming knots, and then snapping like glass ; as if soap-bubbles were forming, enlarging, and bursting like fireworks. These phenomena, or rather, the talk about them by patients, have already been noted frequently enough, and therefore Sollier prefers to study a somewhat more original point, namely the localisation of such sensations in the head. He is not satified with mentioning the vertex or the occiput, with speaking of pains localised in the fontanelles ; as I have said before, he is concerned with somewhat more precise localisations. In cases of mono-symptomatic hysteria, he always detects a more or less extensive cranial zone which is tender on pressure, and exhibits a more or less marked anaesthesia or analgesia. We have the right, he adds, to suppose that the subjacent region is benumbed. Flaccid paralysis of the right arm is always accompanied by a zone of this character at the level of the middle of the left Rolandic region ; an attack of mutism is accompanied by a zone of cranial dysaesthesia at the level of Broca's convolution ; [1] in a word, the dysaesthesias of the cranial zones are exactly superposed upon the region of the appropriate cortical centres. The observation of these symptoms enables the author to discover laws for other cortical centres, such as the stomach centre. " This is on both sides of the cranium, but always better marked on the left side, five centimetres from the bi-auricular line and from the antero-posterior line, being therefore at the level of the superior parietal lobule in a region which does not contain precisely any known nerve centre." In like manner, according to Sollier, it is possible to discover the cortical centres for the heart, the bladder, the intestine, and the genital organs. Speaking generally, the peripheral anaesthesia and the visceral anaesthesia disappear through the return of sensibility to the posterior part of the brain ; memory

[1] Sollier, La genèse et la nature de l'hystérie, vol. i, p. 385 ; Sollier, De la localisation cérébrale des troubles hystériques, " Revue Neurologique," 1900, p. 102.

is not reestablished until the sensibility becomes normal in the frontal region.[1] These are the observations which have led Sollier to explain all the symptoms of hysteria by a numbing, a sleep, of the cortical centres of the brain, and to formulate what he terms his physiological theory of this disorder.

When the restoration of sensibility is complete, when the patient has been fully reawakened, he usually gives utterance to feeling of astonishment and joy, in such terms as I have frequently recorded : " It is strange how large everything is here ; the furniture and the other objects in the room seem brighter, I can feel my heart beating. . . . It is as if I have come out of a profound sleep, had recovered from a long illness, as if I had been resurrected, as if a new life were opening before me " . . . and so on. These feelings of wellbeing make the patient laugh, and give him a general aspect of gaiety and health which he did not exhibit previously. Side by side with such details, which recall those described in the works of earlier observers, Sollier is more inclined to insist upon less familiar phenomena. All his subjects, on awaking, presented a retrograde amnesia concerning the whole of the period of the previous illness. If the hysterical condition had lasted for two or three years, they awakened two or three years behind the times, for they had forgotten all that had happened while they had been ill. If they had been hysterical since early childhood, they awakened at the age of two or three years, having only the memories, the manners, and the speech, of little children. It was then necessary, by means of a new education, which took the form of perfecting their sensibilities, to aid them to reacquire the lost memories, beginning with the earliest ones and coming down to the contemporary period. The author speaks of this as the regression of the personality, and he refers to the progress that takes place concomitantly with the reestablishment of kinaesthesia.

The patients are then perfectly restored to health. All the hysterical symptoms have disappeared. Normal sleep returns (for the sufferer from hysterical anaesthesia does not sleep, or sleeps only in an abnormal way). This return of normal sleep is a functional restoration of sensibility. Although

[1] Sollier, Coenesthésie cérébrale et mémoire, " Revue Philosophique," July 1899.

the subjects now experience fatigue, they are capable of much more activity than before. Their nutrition is greatly improved, so that they rapidly put on flesh. Unfortunately, like other observers, Sollier has to describe relapses. He calls them "return anaesthesias." These relapses follow various untoward influences, such as menstruation, fatigue, emotion, something that puts the patient out of humour, unduly sustained intellectual work, and so on. Furthermore, there are differences between patients; some of them make efforts to maintain sensibility or to restore it rapidly, whereas others show little goodwill. When a relapse occurs, we must recommence the work of resensibilisation, which is apt to be less difficult than the first restoration was, but may have to be repeated a great many times. Still, though we have these oscillations, striking progress can on the whole be noted. In the twenty cases reported by Sollier (cases of serious and long-standing hysteria), there were about five instances of well-marked improvement; five instances of temporary cure, lasting for a few months; and about a dozen cures which seemed complete, for the cure was sustained for one or for several years. These are interesting results, which must be placed to the credit of aesthesiogenism.

Sollier's book did not do much to restore aesthesiogenism in medical esteem. On the contrary, it seems to have discouraged investigators, perhaps because the work gives so artificial an impression. I have myself been disturbed by seeing how these phenomena can be rendered uniform, and can be arbitrarily systematised by drill. I am afraid I have myself made similar mistakes, and for a long time I have held aloof from such researches. Still, to conclude the history of aesthesiogenism, I can refer to a small number of studies which I published on this subject at a later date, studies undertaken either to round off earlier investigations, or when chance observations attracted my attention once more to phenomena of this character.

From 1887 to 1889, Jules Janet gave a good deal of time to the study of Marceline. After some time had been spent in this way, his attention was monopolised by other work, and he entrusted his interesting patient to my care. Under my care she remained from 1889 to 1901, when she died at the age of thirty-five of pulmonary tuberculosis. Since this lengthy study of a sufferer from hysterical anorexia, who had been under close observation for seventeen years, had considerable interest and was worthy of permanent record, I published full notes of the case under the title *Une Félida artificielle*, in the "Revue Philosophique," 1910, vol. i, pp. 329 and 483. The account was reprinted in the second edition of my work *L'état mental des hysteriques*, 1911, p. 545. Here will be found researches concerning hysterical anorexia and concerning nutrition in these patients whose diet is so greatly restricted—researches made in the physiological laboratory of the medical school. It also contains researches relating to the effects of aesthesiogenic agents upon these patients, investigations in which the influence of suggestion was not suppressed (for that is impossible), but in which suggestion was reduced to a minimum. I shall return to the matter presently, when I come to discuss various hypotheses which have been formulated to explain aesthesiogenism.

I must also make a brief reference to the case of Jm. (f., 42), who was certainly cured of hysterical symptoms by aesthesiogenic agents, her chief symptoms having been those of contracture, which had lasted for several years. The modifications produced in the visual disorders were peculiarly interesting. For a long time she had suffered from amaurosis of the left eye, and, regarding this eye as hopeless, she would do nothing to promote the restoration of vision. Some simple experiments showed me that the trouble was nothing more than hysterical amaurosis, and therefore I tried, during the hypnotic state, to reawaken the vision of the left eye. Vision was restored, although not without a good deal of pain in this eye, which, said the patient, felt "as if it were going to burst." But, to my great surprise, for I was not on the look-out for anything of the kind, the first sequel of the restoration of vision in the left eye was an appearance of disorders in the vision of the right eye, and of remarkable symptoms of hemianopia. Such facts will have to be examined carefully, as soon as any one is inclined to undertake a serious psychological study of transference.[1]

[1] Un cas d'hémianopsie hystérique transitoire, "Presse Médicale," October 25, 1899, p. 241 ; Etat mental des hystériques, second edition, 1911, p. 458.

In a final, and more general, study of the somnambulist influence and the need for guidance,[1] I was able to detect, as a sequel of various methods of treatment, like changes in the behaviour of the patients between two successive sittings. The changes were phenomena analogous to those already recorded. Immediately after the sitting there was often a period of disturbance and fatigue. A good many patients complained of queer feelings in the head, of a sense of torsion, or of explosions ; and they said they felt as if they had been beaten. Some of them, like Irène, had a very peculiar sensation of chilliness. This patient was not really well unless her skin was cold after a sitting, for it was a bad sign if her hands were hot at this moment. We have already had occasion to consider these disorders of circulation in neuropaths. The malaise of which I shall now speak lasted for several hours, and in some patients for several days. After the phase of fatigue, the subject passed into the important phase of *somnambulist influence*, which lasted for very variable times, but was especially characterised by an obvious condition of health and wellbeing. It was in this phase that the subject gave expression to the enthusiastic satisfaction I have already mentioned ; " I weep for joy, and for two years I had not been able to shed tears. I am no longer the same, I am taking up a new life, I seem to have a new head, and I seem to see things for the first time." These feelings corresponded to the temporary disappearance of all the pathological symptoms, the paroxysms, the somnabulism, the delusions, the fixed ideas, the paralyses, the vomitings, and so on; and they corresponded to the development, or rather the reappearance, of the higher mental functions. It was at this stage that the subject, very ill before, came nearest to the normal condition.

Unfortunately, it seldom happened that this condition persisted, especially in the early stages of the treatment. After a time, which varied from subject to subject, and varied in accordance with the degree of illness, there was a complete change. As a sequel to some emotion or fatigue, or simply through lapse of time, the neuropathic symptoms and the signs of psychological depression recurred. In Cora (f., 30), for example, the onset of menstruation was sufficient to bring

[1] " Revue Philosophique," February 1897 ; Névroses et idées fixes, 1898, vol. i, p. 423.

back jealous obsessions : " What will happen if my husband becomes interested in another woman ? " A storm, or a chance meeting in the street, would bring about a relapse in Marceline or in Irène. Sometimes, without any disturbing incident, the patient would relapse, in one case at the end of a week, in another at the end of three weeks, and so on. The relapse was sometimes sudden, with or without a sort of aura, and it then took the form of a hysterical attack. I have described such transitions in Marceline and Irène. In most cases, the transition was a gradual occurrence, occupying a day. Sometimes it happened in the night, and the change was manifest when the patient awoke in the morning. When the change took place during the night, as a sequel to nightmare for instance, an interesting fact could be noticed. The subject would wake up for an instant and would then fall asleep again, but her sleep would now be quite different, would be very light, incomplete and tiring, like that usual in hysterics. In all these varieties, the essential phenomena are the same. All the morbid symptoms reappear pretty much as they were before—the disorders of thought, the inadequacies of action, the agitations, the sentiments of incompleteness—in a word, the whole gamut of psychological depression returns.

I should like to dwell a little upon a recent publication to which I shall have to allude once more when I come to consider the explanation of these phenomena. I refer to the case of a young woman whom I have named Irène.[1] At the time of writing she is thirty-four. Since the age of twenty she has been suffering from serious hysterical troubles and from mental depression. The notes with which I am now concerned relate only to the first two years of her illness, and to these notes I shall have to make certain additions. In an earlier chapter of this work, in connexion with the question of traumatic memories and liquidations, I discussed certain details of this prolonged attack of hysteria. I am now going to return to the matter from another point of view. As we have seen, this girl, who has been markedly neuropathic from early

[1] L'amnésie et la dissociation des souvenirs par l'émotion, " Journal de Psychologie Normale et Pathologique," September 1904, p.417 ; L'état mental des hystériques, second edition, 1911, p. 506.

childhood, found it necessary when she was twenty years old to take sole charge for several months of her mother, suffering from pulmonary tuberculosis. She became completely exhausted, and was finally overwhelmed by her mother's death in peculiarly distressing circumstances. After this incident, she suffered from violent hysterical paroxysms lasting for several days at a time, during which she was delirious, and kept on reliving through the scenes of her mother's last moments, or sometimes describing in words what had taken place. In addition to these crises, she suffered from hallucinations, morbid impulses, contractures (especially affecting the right leg), and various disorders of sensibility (also mainly on the right side), different disturbances of action, to which I have paid particular attention, and, above all, remarkable amnesias.

Although in her delirium she had a precise memory of her mother's last moments, of the death, and of the events which immediately followed—for she kept on repeating her account of them, and dramatically rehearsed the scenes with full details—in her normal life she appeared to have completely forgotten all these occurrences. She seemed to have given up thinking about her mother, whom she had so fondly loved and whom she had nursed with such devotion. Apparently she had lost the power of calling up her mother's personality in imagination. She accepted the idea of her mother's death with indifference, and without conviction, for she had no conscious memory of what had happened. The amnesia extended to the whole three months which preceded the death and to the two months which followed it. In addition the patient had persistently a certain amount of amnesia as regards recent happenings. I have on many occasions drawn attention to this conjuncture of an automatic hyperamnesia during the delirium with an amnesia concerning the same events during the waking state.

Irène spent three months in hospital, subjected to the ordinary kinds of treatment, such as tonics, hydrotherapeutics, gymnastic exercises, static electricity, and isolation from her former environment. None of these measures did her any good, so after a time I tried the effect of treating her by dealing merely with the amnesia, by attempting to educate her in such a way as would recall the apparently lost memories. She was readily hypnotisable, but there was not during the hypnotic state any spontaneous recurrence of the lapsed memories. Under hypnosis, however, I tried to direct her attention towards these memories, to compel her to rediscover them, and to relate them correctly. As in the case of Madame D., the attempt was accompanied by the onset of severe headache. Indeed, in Irène, the pain in the head was excruciating, leading, in some instances during the hypnosis and in some instances after the hypnosis, to fainting fits and vomiting. None the less, memory was reestablished, first of all during the hypnotic sleep, and, at a later stage, after further efforts which were attended with less difficulty, during the waking state. I shall lay no stress here upon the incidents attending this restoration of memory or upon the order in which the memories reappeared. I have discussed these matters elsewhere.

The point with which we are now concerned is that the stimulation of memory had an extensive and very definite influence upon all the symptoms and all the disorders of this neuropath, whose illness was of so complicated a character. Already, during the hypnotic sleep, Irène, after much definite advance in the recovery of memory, entered into a condition which appeared completely new. She opened her eyes, expressed her astonishment to see how much brighter things looked, said she felt happy, and believed herself to be beginning a new life. " It is absurd to say that I am asleep ; I am very much awake indeed. I feel as I did before I fell ill ; it seems to me that I see things more clearly, and that I have grown older. My true personality has returned." She no longer suffered from contractures or anaesthesia, although in the attempts to stimulate her memory I had not made any allusion to cutaneous sensibility. Her activities were transformed. She was no longer timid, and for the first time since she had been ill she began to make fairly resolute plans for the future. If I urged her to undertake further efforts, continually appealing to her memories, she began to writhe, and to laugh uproariously, these being signs of derivation and exhaustion. She would groan and say : " I cannot do any more ; do not go on trying to make me. " If I persisted, there would be an attack of syncope, or a severe hysterical paroxysm, the effects of which were by no means favourable. If I did not press the matter, and awakened her at this stage, the progress that had been manifested was maintained to a considerable extent. From the moment when Irène found herself able to remember her mother voluntarily, she ceased to see images of her mother in delirium ; the crises and hallucinations vanished, together with all the terrors of subconscious origin. Movement and sensibility remained normal. Above all, and this is a point on which I have laid most stress in my study of the case, her actions were transformed and she had become capable of behaving properly. To begin with, doubtless, this transformation was extremely unstable ; and at the least emotional stress there would be a relapse. Still, it became steadily easier to stimulate her memory, the condition of complete somnambulism would last longer and longer, and the reestablishment of health became permanent— for several years at any rate, since of late Irène has had other disturbances which have been cured in pretty much the same way. All that I wished to recount at this stage was the remarkable success of the treatment of a whole group of complex disorders by a simple awakening of memory. Although the procedure varies, the result is the same. The subject enters into a state of complete somnambulism, which lasts for a longer or shorter time, and is followed by amnesia, exactly like the complete somnambulism induced by the awakening of sensibility. That is why I have no hesitation in including the history of this case among the histories of the cases treated by aesthesiogenic methods.

After Irène had been cured of these first troubles, she remained well for several years ; but when she was about twenty-eight some further nervous disorders made their appearance as a sequel to overwork. The new symptoms were much less definitely hysterical in character. As we have often noticed, these patients whose psychological tension is unstable exhibit hysterical symptoms when they are quite young, whereas later in life the symptoms tend rather to take a psychasthenic form. At this later stage Irène very rarely had delirious attacks, but she had again become incapable of work. She suffered from crises of indecision and doubt, which need not be described here in detail. She asked to be treated in the same way as before, and I found that I could induce the same complete somnambulism with the old results. Two facts must be especially insisted upon First of all, even more plainly than before, I noticed that this state could not be induced when the patient was much exhausted. When she was menstruating (and in Irène the flow was often excessive), after several sleepless nights, after a fatiguing journey, when she had remained for two or three days without food, she found it impossible to make the necessary efforts, and the transformation did not occur. Or, if it occurred, it was imperfect. The alert state was not clearly manifested ; it lasted only a few hours ; and the disorders quickly reappeared. Sollier noticed the same thing when he was trying " to reawaken the nerve centres " in his patients, and I am glad to find myself in agreement with him upon a point of clinical observation.

The second point to which I have to refer in my concluding observations upon Irène's states of complete somnambulism, is this. The phenomena which attended the transition at the moment of relapse had assumed a new form. Formerly, as we have seen, the passage from the alert state to the state of depression was effected by way of a major hysterical paroxysm. But now, at such times, there was often a fit of weeping, which would last for several hours, and which appeared to be a sort of attenuated hysterical crisis. In the course of the second period of treatment, the hysterical attacks did not occur in these circumstances, but I was able to note another phenomenon which played an analogous role. When Irène had been temporarily restored, when she had been put back into an active condition, she would remain in this condition for several days, and would have a lively feeling of satisfaction the while ; then she began to complain of malaise and a sense of agitation ; soon she would be attacked by severe and typical migraine, lasting from twenty-four to forty-eight hours. The pain would begin round one of the eyes, usually the right eye, and extend over half of the head. She could not bear that anything should touch her head, could not endure the slightest tap, and could not bear the daylight. These symptoms were accompanied by digestive troubles, vomiting, etc. After an attack of migraine, she felt relieved of her malaise and sense of agitation ; but she had again become impotent to act, hesitant, inert ; in a word, she had passed out of the alert condition which had been induced by aesthesiogenism. The migraine was so closely related to the complete somnambulism which had preceded it, that during certain phases one could induce it experimentally, so to speak. If the aesthesiogenic sitting had taken place on the Sunday, the patient would have an attack of migraine on the following Wednesday or Thursday. Very rarely do we find that migraine can thus be produced at a fixed hour.

I have noticed the same phenomenon in other patients, and particularly in Mab. (f., 35). This case, likewise, was one of depression of all the activities, brought on mainly by war-time emotions and those attending the departure of her husband for the front. Besides localised hysterical troubles, there was inertia, ill-humour, insomnia or somnambulist delirium, anorexia, vomiting, contracture of the right arm, and, above all, hysterical troubles of vision. After aesthesiogenic sittings in which attention was chiefly paid to vision, the patient recovered her normal condition for a day ; but a severe attack of migraine followed, and at the end of this she had relapsed into the previous condition.

All these observations belong to the same category, and seem to me to form a definite natural group. Beginning with the somnambulist crises familiar to the magnetisers, passing through the various aesthesiogenisms of the metallotherapeutists, and coming to the complete somnambulisms which I have studied and to the transformations brought about by the recall of memories, we find an assemblage of phenomena which are throughout of the same kind, and I think we have good reason to seek for an explanation common to them all.

3. The Explanations of Aesthesiogenism.

The historical study we have just been making has furnished us with fairly definite instruction. It has shown us that a great many authors, whose writings differ in time by as much as a century, and who have used very different methods, have nevertheless been able to record essentially similar facts. This leads us to suppose that the facts in question are real, and that they are interconnected by real rather than by fortuitous relationships. Let us try to summarise these facts, dwelling only upon the common elements in the various descriptions. Neuropaths, exhibiting symptoms of the most diversified kinds, can be rapidly transformed so as to lose all their disorders at once, and to return more or less completely to their normal state of health. These transformations are achieved by methods which appear to vary a good deal : by passes ; by the application of various substances to the skin ; by electricity ; by gymnastic exercises ; by commands, and by discourses, relating to sensation and memory. The transformations are accompanied by very characteristic feelings of confidence and delight. But they are transient, and end in a relapse which is more or less speedy and more or less complete, the patient passing back into the antecedent morbid state. Very often the relapse is accompanied by amnesia of the antecedent happy period. Nevertheless these transformations can be renewed again and again, the successive renewals being usually secured with greater ease, so that in the end the patient's health is fully restored. How are we to understand this assemblage of phenomena, or, rather, how can we discover a link between these facts ? This is the problem of the interpretation of aesthesiogenism, the problem we have now to discuss.

The earlier authors believed that the facts could be linked on the supposition that there is an external physical agent influencing the organism ; that the effect of this agent is exhausted after a time, so that the action has to be renewed. At first, the external agent was the " fluid " of the magnetisers ; then it was supposed to consist of slight electric currents produced by the contact of a metal with the skin, this being Burq's hypothesis which was subsequently adopted by Régnard and Pitres. To-day these views have been entirely abandoned, first of all because it was impossible to give a positive demonstration that any such action took place, and secondly because those who inclined rather to think that all the phenomena were due to psychological modifications were fully able to prove that these phenomena could be readily reproduced without the intervention of any of the before-mentioned material agents. Bernheim has summarised this view of the matter very effectively, and with notable moderation.[1] If the criticisms are to be answered, it must be by a reproduction of the phenomena while suppressing, in turn, all the possible psychological influences. Vigouroux seemed for a moment to understand the nature of the problem.

[1] Bernheim, La suggestion, 1886, p. 210.

His plan was to try to bring about transference by the instrumentality of an electromagnet, the current through which was interrupted by an assistant without the subject's knowing anything about the interruption. If this experiment could be relied upon to give successful results, if the transference were produced when the current was passing and were not produced when the current was not passing, although the subject did not know whether the current was passing or not, a definite answer would have been furnished to the psychologists' objections.

Now, the experiment is a difficult one, but when it is performed with proper precautions it invariably gives negative results. I have myself been able to verify this several times. How is it that in the hands of Vigouroux it gave positive results ? " The aesthesiogenic action," he writes, " regularly begins as soon as the circuit is closed in a neighbouring room." [1] When we bear in mind the investigations made by the committee appointed by the Society for Psychical Research (the Reichenbach Committee), and my own investigations, all of which have given results diametrically opposed to those of Vigouroux, we are forced to conclude that the latter did not, in his experiments, take the precautions requisite to ensure that neither the subject nor the operator was made aware of the moment when the current was being closed or opened. Ladame, of Geneva, who made similar experiments in 1881,[2] recognised this difficulty. " It must be admitted," he adds, " that we were not at that time as awake to the importance of suggestive influence as we are to-day, and the results of the before-mentioned experiments must therefore be regarded with a certain amount of scepticism." It is obvious that these authors had not yet come to attach sufficient importance to the psychological problems raised by their experiments.

Another theory is presented with certain physiological pretensions. I refer to Sollier's theory of the sleep and the reawakening of the cortical centres. This theory is of even less value than the foregoing, for it is not an explanation which may be either true or false, but a mere playing with words. No doubt all the writers on psychiatric topics have been willing to admit that certain phenomena were taking

[1] Vigouroux, op. cit., p. 97.
[2] Ladame, " Revue de la Suisse Romande," May 15, 1881

place in the organism at the moment when psychological phenomena were manifested in the behaviour of their patients. " In hysteria," I wrote long ago, " it is not the external organ which is affected, for this is absolutely intact ; the affected parts are the centres which no longer function, or which at any rate are functioning abnormally." [1]   But since the authors who talk about the nerve centres have neither an anatomical nor a histological nor a physiological notion of what is going on in these centres, they are merely appealing to one unknown in order to explain another.   Sollier does not hesitate to do this.   He thinks he is transforming the psychological phenomena by translating them into anatomical terms, or simply by associating them with anatomical terms.   In reality, sleep and waking are psychological terms which only have a meaning when applied to the behaviour of living beings in their totality. An organ, considered in isolation, can be described as motionless, empty, exhausted, or inhibited ; but only by metaphor can we speak of a stomach as being asleep, or of an intestine as waking up.   Nevertheless Sollier is continually talking about cerebral centres which fall asleep and which wake up, and he imagines that when he says this he is really saying something.[2] Unfortunately, it is absolutely undeniable that we are not at present able to formulate any psychological theories of these complicated phenomena.   We can only explain them, or if the word " explanation " be an overstatement we can only clarify and simplify them a little, by linking them up with other psychological phenomena with which we are more familiar.

Formerly people were content with an answer which was vague in substance though exact in form : " We have to do with psychological phenomena." These phenomena were denoted be various names, each author being proud of having some particular term—such names as imagination, expectant attention, suggestion, etc. Perhaps we are entitled to be somewhat more exacting to-day, for we are aiming at greater precision in the use of some of these terms.   The first question which arises is naturally the following.   Is aesthesiogenism merely a phenomenon of suggestion, if the term suggestion

[1] L'automatisme psychologique, 1889, p. 97.
[2] Cf. Pierre Janet, Les névroses, 1909, p. 324.

be used in the sense upon which we have agreed ?   In the minds of the subjects, let us say, certain tendencies have been awakened to reach the stage of an idea, either directly awakened by the words of the suggester, or indirectly by his attitude. The tendencies do not stop at this stage of the idea, to be counterposed to other ideas, to be subjected to the control and the criticism of reflection which takes place in all normal minds ; they immediately undergo development into actions and affirmations, this meaning that they are transformed into acts of will and belief. A suggestion is a tendency which, as soon as it has been aroused to the degree of an idea, automatically passes on to the degree of will or belief, without being subjected to reflection, and is thus transformed into an impulse. Can we detect instances of phenomena of this character in the foregoing descriptions ?

The mere formulation of the definition suffices to show that many of the phenomena we have been discussing do depend upon suggestion. Here is something which must attract our attention at the very outset.   These aesthesiogenic effects occur in hysterics, suggestible hysterics ; and they are rarely met with in patients suffering from other disorders. Nay, more ; they can be induced only by a small number of persons, as a rule by no one else than the doctor who " has influence " upon the subject, that is to say by the person who is ordinarily able to influence these subjects by suggestion. It would be a mistake to believe that any chance comer could hold an aesthesiogenic sitting, even without a patient who is accustomed to such practices.   I have shown elsewhere how difficult it was for me to substitute myself for my brother Jules Janet in the treatment of Marceline.   More than a year elapsed before the subject became accustomed to me, and reacted to my influence much as she had reacted to my brother's.

In the second place, we have to note that some of these types of behaviour are related to certain epochs, certain environments, certain kinds of instruction.   The subjects of Burq and those of Dumontpallier were transformed when they touched gold.   Now I, for my part, have time and again left a gold watch in contact with the diseased arm of a hysterical woman, on the pretext that I wanted to keep my eyes upon the time, but her arm has remained anaesthetic or paralysed

The same thing has happened when I have tried other metals, whereas those very subjects would recover the power of sensation when I stimulated their sensibility or their memory by words. The magnet produced wonderful effects in Charcot's clinic in the early days of his teaching ; and yet, towards the end of Charcot's studies upon this subject, ten years later in the same clinic, the magnet had no effect when I was using it. I have already pointed out that my own subjects in Havre would remain profoundly asleep for a considerable time before recovering the power of sensation, and that when they awakened they came to themselves completely, without passing through any intermediate stages and without contortions. " Probably," I said to myself, " this is an outcome of the influence of Léonie, who had been drilled by the magnetisers." On the other hand, all Sollier's subjects returned to their senses by passing through lengthy gradations, stages accompanied by contortions and manifestations of dysaesthesia. In these instances, an influence had probably been exercised by Marceline, Jules Janet's patient. That was what I was trying to explain in the letter I wrote to Ribot in answer to Sollier's protests. " These things happened during a very remarkable epoch in the history of medical science, when the various observers were influencing one another by suggestion in this matter of hysteria, and when the patients at a particular clinic were drilled, more or less consciously, to imitate some famous subject. In these circumstances, and if we wish to appraise the worth of an author's observations, it is just as well that we should find out whether this author had had the opportunity of becoming acquainted with this or that category of phenomena. . . . In 1897, when Sollier published his book on hysteria, . . . it is likely enough that he had completely forgotten that, seven or eight years before, a colleague had given him a detailed demonstration of absolutely identical phenomena. Indeed, we can be almost certain that Sollier has forgotten, since he makes no allusion whatever to the fact. Besides, if he had been reminded of the matter, he would have declared that it was of no importance, and would not have been able to believe that his earlier studies and explanations could have had any influence at all upon his own observations or upon the symptoms presented by his patients. But those who are to-day studying the affiliation of ideas, those who are able to trace the links that connect the different studies concerning hysteria and the various forms which this disorder has exhibited in this or that clinic, will hardly hold such a view." [1]

The same reflection occurs to us when we detect in all the subjects of some particular author manifestations related to the ideas of this author—manifestations which cannot be noted in the subjects of any other investigator. Sollier, who is interested in translating all the ideas of earlier writers into his own anatomical terminology, is convinced that the cortical centres of the brain play a great part in such transformations, Lo and behold, all his subjects exhibit anaesthesias, pains, peculiar sensations, localised in the neighbourhood of these centres; and he cures his patients when he stimulates these cranial regions. Except in the case of a few investigators who had come directly in contact with Sollier's teaching, no other observer has ever noticed anything of the kind. A few years ago I had occasion to see an unfortunate soldier who, after being subjected to some terrible moral shocks in the war, was suffering from retrograde amnesia, a very complete right hemiplegia, and a large measure of right hemianaesthesia. I asked him if he had any pain in the head: " Yes," he answered, " all over the head, but especially on the right side, the side on which my body is affected." In the course of attempts at aesthesiogenic treatment, which gave only partial results by mitigating the hemiplegia, he said he was suffering from increased pain in the head because he was forced to pay attention to it; and this made him feel very tired, especially in the *right* side of the head. I could quote a hundred examples of the same kind, in which the localisations of cerebral pain were either vague, or had no definite relationship with the cortical centres. To be precise I ought to say that I have sometimes seen pain localised more or less vaguely in the occiput in cases of neuropathic disorders of vision. But, first of all, this localisation is by no means constant; and, when it does exist, I am more inclined to suppose that the painful sensations are connected in some way with the occipital muscles. The muscles of the back of the neck play a great part in vision, and contribute to the direction of sight; in asthenopia they suffer from fatigue and pain just like the

[1] " Revue Philosophique," 1910, vol. i, p. 550.

intrinsic muscles of the eye. I have elsewhere insisted upon the danger of localising these sensations in the head through involuntary suggestions.[1] Braid, long ago, in his experiments on phreno-hypnotism, stimulated the bump of acquisitiveness, and thereupon the patient picked the pocket of one of the audience, stealing a silver snuff-box. Then the stimulation was transferred to the bump of conscientiousness, and nothing could have been more striking than the air of contrition with which the patient restored the stolen article. A good deal of water has run under the bridges since those days, and now stimulation of the same regions makes the subjects speak, or improves their digestion. This unfortunate hypnotism seems predestined to fall into the same traps over and over again !

The same considerations probably account for the retrograde amnesias and the regressions of personality which certain subjects will display again and again in the course of aesthesiogenic treatment. Investigators who do not believe in such phenomena have not had occasion to observe them. In my own practice I have on one occasion detected something of the same kind. Irène, who had just passed back into the alert state, kept on repeating : " I feel strong, I feel younger, as if I were a child once more." She went on to speak of a number of memories of childhood, concerning which she had not hitherto had anything to say. She then relapsed into a long-forgotten patois. Probably this was due to a simple association of ideas, and it was easy to ascertain that the memory of recent events had not been affected in any way. Generally speaking, the subjects in whom sensation improves, experience at the same time an improvement of memory, and do not exhibit a retrograde amnesia.

The experience of this influence of involuntary suggestion can be verified by noting that in a particular subject the phenomena will change when the subject passes from the care of one doctor to the care of another. I related how, when I took charge of Marceline, I tried to diminish the influence of the suggestive factor. I suppressed everything which might seem to give the aspect of a hypnotic sitting to the aesthesiogenic treatment. I ceased to make use of the words " sleep " and " waking " to denote the conditions through which she passed. After a considerable time, amounting to several

[1] Névroses et idées fixes, 1898, vol. i, p. 147.

years, the subject exhibited modifications. The retrograde amnesias which she had used to have when she relapsed into the morbid state, as the result of fatigue or emotion, appeared with less regularity, and they simply extended backwards for a more or less lengthy period without being clearly localised, as of old, to the periods of the alert state.

In a word, it is not enough to say proudly : " I took the utmost care to avoid suggestion, which, already deplorable from the therapeutic point of view, is the most detestable of methods for a psychological investigator to employ." Binet, reviewing Sollier's book, took occasion to criticise his language upon this point.[1] Obviously, it is no such easy matter to do away with the influence of suggestion when we are dealing with suggestible persons. I am certainly inclined to follow Bernheim a good long way, and to recognise that suggestion is a considerable factor in producing the phenomena of aesthesiogenism.

But the explanation becomes far more difficult if we try to go further than this. Are we entitled to say that suggestion accounts for everything in the case of aesthesiogenic phenomena ? Such an affirmation would be perfectly intelligible. We have already seen that suggestion can reestablish sensation and movement, and perhaps suggestion accounts for the reestablishment in these cases. If this be so, all the methods we have just been discussing would belong to the group of therapeutic methods which act by setting psychological automatism to work, and we should have to agree that they are simply advances in the practice of suggestive therapeutics. Yet I am loath to accept this simple solution. As I said in 1889, I have an impression, which may be illusory, that in complete somnambulism there is something more at work than suggestion. This impression of mine must be analysed before we come to a decision upon the problem.

The first point to be considered is that the phenomena of complete somnambulism are very complicated, so that it is rather difficult to accept the view that they are the outcome of a simple suggestion. In the case of suggestion, we said, a tendency is awakened in the form of an idea, and action follows, realising that which was implicit, in the tendency.

[1] Binet, " Année Psychologique," 1898, p. 670

We tell the subject to move, to feel when he is touched, to remember ; and he behaves accordingly. That is what we observe in the case of simple suggestions relating to movement, sensation, and memory ; and the same thing can be observed readily enough in the very subjects of whom we have just been speaking. There are periods in which they are strongly suggestible ; and if at such times I tell them to recover the power of sensation or to recover the power of memory, they do not go further than uttering a cry when pinched or than answering questions correctly. But the interesting and strange fact is that in other cases the same subjects behave differently when we make the same suggestion to them. Now the identical orders are carried out much more slowly, and the action is attended by other and quite unexpected phenomena ; by gesticulations and groans in Marceline ; by periods of sleep in Irène ; then by feelings of euphoria, by fatigue, and even by vomiting in Irène ; after a time, it is followed by changes in nutrition, in urination, in sleep ; it seems to increase activity, to restrict suggestibility ; and, above all, to bring about a total change of behaviour. Have we not here something which altogether transcends the primitive idea of the tendency to feel and to move ?

To all appearance we have ; but the partisans of suggestion can find a good answer. " Your argument," they might say, " is identical with that which the metallotherapeutists and the disciples of Charcot used to employ. Vigouroux said in former days that transference could not be a phenomenon of suggestion, because the subject could not possibly have in his head Landolt's law concerning the order in which colours disappear when the visual field is restricted. Charcot's disciples would not admit that Wittm. could know by heart the postures to be induced by the stimulation of the various nerves of the hand ; all these things seemed to them to be too complex to be the outcome of suggestion. Now, we know to-day that they were wrong. A subject who lives in a hospital where people are always talking about such matters is likely to know better than most medical students the order of the colours prescribed by Landolt's law ; nor need he be a genius to know the position of the hand appropriate to stimulation of the ulnar nerve, the median nerve, or the musculo-spiral nerve, respectively. A suggestion may be extremely complex, so that one single sign, awakening a tendency rich in associations, may bring about multiform reactions. Did we not accept the fact that there are complex suggestions involving changes of personality and the acting of a complicated series of comedies ? It would be enough to contend, in explanation of the before-mentioned observations, that the subjects have understood the suggestion to react to sensory stimuli in the second case in a way different from that in which they reacted in the first. They know that in their doctor's mind the return of sensation implies a certain number of grimaces, followed by the disappearance of all their troubles and the return to good health. They have realised the suggestion as they understood it, nothing more."

We might quibble in this way, in order to show the infinite possibilities of complexity in suggestions. A comedy played by the subject is never so all-embracing as good health itself, and we certainly ask much of automatism if we expect it to realise the idea of health and happiness. If this were all, the practice of suggestion would certainly be much simplified. But I do not dwell upon these considerations, for I prefer to look at the question in a different way. Let us dismiss " the reactions connected with the reawakening of sensibility " ; and let us even dismiss the feelings of euphoria, although these appear to be very important, for they may include complex phenomena of suggestion. But in complete somnambulism, after these initial phenomena, there occurs a notable change in the behaviour as a whole, and this seems to me very characteristic.

What surprises me in this change of behaviour is, not the complicated character of the automatism, but the diminution of automatism and the development of a new adaptation. The patients, as I have said, become less suggestible ; and it is certainly strange that suggestion should render anyone less suggestible, and that simultaneously the practical activity of the subjects should be transformed. Perhaps I may be permitted to return in this connexion to my notes of Irène's case.[1] This young woman, always a neuropath, sorrowful,

---

[1] L'amnésie et la dissociation des souvenirs par l'émotion, " Journal de Psychologie Normale et Pathologique," September 1904 ; Etat mental des hystériques, second edition, 1911, p. 532.

uneasy, and discontented with herself, suffered perpetually from the feeling that her emotions and actions remained incomplete and inadequate. She said that her head seemed always full of affairs which she could not bring to a conclusion. Intelligent and industrious, she was nevertheless incapable of doing anything when there were two or three people in the room. Being extremely shy, she could not eat properly when any one else was there; she wished that she never had need of any one else, and could live quite alone in her own corner. All the disorders of action had been enormously accentuated at the beginning of her illness, and I have taken a good deal of trouble to show that the essential malady underlying the delirious crisis and the amnesias was the complete suppression of action. This patient no longer did any work, and was unable to make up her mind. " You ask me why I have done nothing for so long. I do not know: I am no longer interested in anything. I no longer care for anyone; I am bored to death, that is all." Her social abulia had become so complete that she could not speak to anyone without getting into a rage. I have already referred to the suppression of the activities suited to the occasion, the suppression brought about by her mother's death; and I put forward the opinion that the amnesia concerning her mother's death was a primary factor of this systematised abulia.

Yet now, in the condition which I have termed complete somnambulism (the condition which appeared in this patient directly the suggestion to remember had been made), the most notable manifestation was the change in activity. " The behaviour," I wrote, " has completely changed." [1] Irène has become active and practical once more. She works, has resumed her occupation without boredom and even with interest. She is able to arrange whatever she needs, and to organise her life, whereas in the antecedent condition she was vaguely inert. Another change, very remarkable to all appearance, has been noticed by every one who comes near her. She has become sociable once more. She can now stay in the company of other persons without having those accesses of fear or anger which were continually coming on before, and which prevented her rubbing shoulders with anybody The social abulia so characteristic of this young woman

[1] Op. cit., p. 536.

vanishes in the periods when the mental level has been raised once more.   Finally, what we have called her special behaviour, that which is particularly related to the death of her mother, is also considerably improved ; . . . she now knows how to take practical resolutions, how to choose a lodging unaided, how to regulate her expenses.   In a word, she no longer waits for her mother's guidance as she used to do."   Similar observations, of a yet more detailed character, were made in the case of Marceline.   To make this clear I should have to reproduce all my notes on Marceline's practical and social activities during the period of complete somnambulism induced in her by aesthesiogenic methods.   It must suffice to refer the reader to the lengthy account of this patient which I have published elsewhere.[1]

I think that these phenomena are extremely important. We are no longer concerned with the development of an automatism, however complex in character.   We are concerned with new kinds of activity, not foreseen ; with actions of adaptation and with further syntheses, of which the subject becomes more and more capable in proportion as, on the other hand, she becomes less suggestible.   Are we entitled to say that all this is done by suggestion ?   I think such an assertion is only permissible if we give to the word " suggestion " a very wide significance indeed, so that it comes to include all possible psychological phenomena.   We cannot accept the assertion if the term " suggestion " be understood in the sense to which I have restricted it, that of the development of preexistent automatism.

From another outlook, the interpretation of the phenomena by suggestion encounters other difficulties—if we study the manner in which these transformations take place in the subject. Suggestion, as we understand the term, precisely because it is an automatism, realises itself in a mechanical way, a regular fashion, without the intervention of the rest of the personality ; the realisation is attended by a marked disposition to amnesia and to subconsciousness.   Here, on the other hand, we discern effort on the part of the subject, work which the subject does in order to carry out his task.   No doubt the word " effort " is also a vague term, a word concerning which

---

[1] Une Félida artificielle, L'état mental des hystériques, second edition, 1911, p. 573.

a great many misunderstandings arise. Some efforts are peculiar ways of carrying out movements which can very well be of a systematised character, may give rise to tendencies, and may occur as a sequel of suggestion. But what we are now considering are not efforts at movement, they are efforts to secure adaptation ; they are attempts to perform useful actions, and, above all, to undertake individual researches. I have never seen the phenomena of aesthesiogenism take the subconscious form so common where we have to do with suggestions.

Finally, the circumstances in which these phenomena occur seem to me to present something else of a quite peculiar kind which distinguishes them from suggestion. This is manifest in states of enfeeblement, and even when the subject is more or less stupefied. There result cataleptic paroxysms, automatic movements even during the crises, profound accesses of sleep. The remarkable character of aesthesiogenism is that it cannot take effect when the subject is greatly enfeebled. The magnetisers and the metallotherapeutists had already noticed this. " When the patient is unduly fatigued, when she has recently had a paroxysm, or when one is imminent, these effects fail to occur." [1] Elsewhere I have insisted upon this fact in connexion with my own early observations. Recently I have been able to convince myself once more of the reality of the phenomenon when studying the case of Irène. As I have just said, in her it is impossible to induce complete somnambulism during the menstrual period, and it is also impossible when she has been up all the previous night in order to work, or when she has just come back after an arduous journey. Not long ago she had serious disturbances owing to the emotions and fatigues consequent on the war. She suffered from persistent uterine haemorrhage, and for many weeks was affected with uncontrollable vomiting.

The accesses of delirium returned, and she again became incapable of work or even of any kind of activity. On account of these symptoms she spontaneously returned to consult me, to ask me if I would put her to sleep once more, and if I would give her the same treatment which had always succeeded before. She was, therefore, in the happy condition of confidence which facilitates suggestion, and in actual fact

[1] Vigouroux, op. cit., p. 565.

she could promptly be hypnotised and was very suggestible. But it was impossible to induce complete somnambulism. The attempts in this direction merely led to groaning fits, attacks of migraine, and all sorts of contortions. After the sitting, she did not experience the fatigue of earlier days, nor did she suffer from the vomiting that had formerly characterised this phase, nor did she experience the feelings of euphoria. Above all, it was impossible to detect the characteristic transformation of activity. Not until her health had been to some extent restored by several months' rest and by a few suggestions properly so-called, had the ground been sufficiently prepared, so that a state of typical complete somnambulism could then be induced. But as yet this complete somnambulism did not last long, for it rapidly disappeared after an attack of migraine. Still later, complete somnambulism lasting several days could be produced as of old. We have to do, then, with a phenomenon which requires an expenditure of energy, and which cannot occur in exhausted subjects. This is an important characteristic, to which I shall have to return. We have carefully to note that this characteristic distinguishes aesthesiogenism from suggestion, for the latter does not need this expenditure of force, and it occurs with especial facility in enfeebled subjects.

I must also speak of the way in which the alert state passes off. To begin with, as we have just seen, the alert state lasts only a short time, especially when the subject is very ill ; its duration is proportional to the subject's energy. The effects of a therapeutic suggestion are not restricted in this way. We do not suggest to our patient to relapse regularly after a certain time ; on the contrary we shall suggest that the cure shall be permanent. Next, we have to notice that the relapse occurs by way of a convulsive paroxysm, or by an attack of migraine, etc., which seems to function as a discharge or as a release of tension. At the close of suggestions, nothing of the kind happens. When I have made experiments upon the duration of suggestions, I have always found it difficult to ascertain the precise moment at which the suggestion was no longer acted upon, at which it had been completely forgotten ; and I have never noted the sudden cessation attended by peculiar forms of disturbance which is characteristic of the close of aesthesiogenism.

I think, then, that we are entitled to form definite conclusions as to the relationship between suggestion and aesthesiogenism. Obviously, suggestion plays a very large part here. It determines the form which the transformation takes to begin with ; I even think that it determines the actual start of the transformation, which, in a sense, it originates. It is because we are concerned with suggestible hysterics that we can make them begin this process as the outcome of certain signals or in response to special orders. But here suggestion takes effect upon a peculiar form of action having characteristics proper to itself. Thus it is a suggestion of a peculiar kind, and one which must be distinguished from other kinds.

We are not justified in assimilating aesthesiogenism to the methods of treatment by repose and by the economising of energy, for in the case of aesthesiogenism we are evidently concerned rather with work and with expenditure. I should even say that, in a great many cases, aesthesiogenism involves a considerable amount of work. " It is terrible," said Irène to me, " the amount of work that goes on in me when you have put me to sleep. I am utterly exhausted by it, and the fatigue lasts three days. I have the extraordinary feeling that I have suddenly got thinner, that I am smaller, that I am wasting away." That is why the treatment, as we have seen, is quite unsuitable for exhausted subjects. We can compare aesthesiogenic treatment, not with economies, but with the speculative expenditure which is, to begin with, a loss, but which will in due time bring disproportionately large profits. We should do wrong to advise such speculative expenditure in the case of a person who is absolutely ruined, so that he cannot meet the preliminary demand for funds. In such cases we have to see to it that a little capital shall first be accumulated through economy ; and we must be prudent before we can risk any expenditure.

A more delicate problem faces us when we compare aesthesiogenism with treatment by moral liquidation. Especially does this fact strike us when we look back to the account of Irène given in an earlier chapter. In this patient, the delirious paroxysms in which the scenes of her mother's death were reproduced, disappeared after her memory had been reestablished ; and we considered that the cure of this symptom was due to the liquidation of an event to which the subject had at length definitively adapted herself. But, in that connexion, we alluded to the difficulties of the reestablishment of memory and of the liquidation ; to the difficulties that attended all this modification of behaviour. The liquidation itself, far from explaining the modification of behaviour, seemed to us to be the consequence of that modification. Besides, the other patients in whom we detected the phenomena of aesthesiogenism did not exhibit anything akin to the liquidation of memories. I am inclined to think that the liquidation of a past event is but a particular instance of the labours, of the efforts to attend, which play the leading part in aesthesiogenism ; I think that the moral liquidation, far from explaining aesthesiogenism, is itself akin to this, and presents us with an identical problem.

We have more reason for assimilating aesthesiogenism to education, for it obviously contains an educational factor, just as it contains a suggestive factor. We need not dwell upon these considerations, for they are identical with those we have just met apropos of suggestion itself. Quite obviously, the subjects are drilled in the use of this therapeutic method, so that after a certain time they can apply it much more easily. If such sittings are broken off for a considerable time, the old difficulties arise when we resume them. In certain subjects, aesthesiogenism assumes the form of a genuine education of sensibility. We can see this in the account of the treatment of Marceline.

" The treatment consisted in ascertaining which of the sensations relating to the altered function had undergone diminution or complete suppression. Then it was necessary to try to make these sensations reappear ; that is to say, to make the subject become aware of them once more. For instance, if a leg were paralysed or contractured, we had to examine the cutaneous, muscular, or articular sensations of this lower limb ; we had to ascertain the kind and degree of numbness ; to make all sorts of impressions upon the limb ; pinching, pricking it, electrifying it, and, above all, immobilising it and kneading it. After each stimulation, we had to ask Marceline what she had felt, and compel her to attend closely to her sensations ; encourage her in every possible way to distinguish one sensation from another, scold her when she made a mistake, and begin the whole series over and over again. Above all, we had to order her to move the affected limb, beginning the movement in innumerable different ways. And we had to induce her to perform with the utmost care all sorts of gymnastic exercises of a similar kind to Swedish exercises ; and throughout she had to keep fully aware of the movements which she was making. When she no longer eat properly, we had to go through the same sort of education in the case of the mouth, the lips, and the pharynx ; and we had to spend a great deal of time teaching her to distinguish the taste of sugar from the taste of salt, when one or the other substance was placed on her tongue ; we had to compel her to become aware that the mucous membrane of the pharynx was touched, to make her pay sufficient attention to this disagreeable impression, so that the pharyngeal reflex might be restored to activity. In the same way we had to make her learn how to breathe, how to move the abdominal walls, how to become aware of the movements of the stomach ; we had to make her practise laughing, yawning, etc. ; we had to make her swallow, while herself closely watching and feeling the movements of deglutition, and becoming aware whether the bolus of food had satisfactorily passed into the stomach." [1] The reestablishment of memory was also a long and difficult process in Irène. After we had made her reconstruct the memory of her mother's death, and her own conduct during that night, we had to make her practise the accurate recital of the various circumstances, and to make the recital independent of the attitudes of perception. At first it was quite impossible to make her tell this story correctly without relapsing into crises and hallucinations, that is to say, without associating special attitudes of perception with the relation of the reminiscences. The association of ideas, on which far too much stress has been laid in psychological treatises, is, in my opinion, only a disease of memory. By degrees I was able to make her tell the story with a tranquil distress, that is to say, with an attitude proper to the telling of such a story ; then I was able to bring her to coordinate and classify all these reminiscences. Such exercises can be regarded as genuinely educative in character.

[1] L'état mental des hystériques, second edition, 1911, p. 611.

Nevertheless, if we recall the foregoing descriptions, we shall easily perceive that aesthesiogenism transcends education pure and simple, as we have defined the latter. Obviously Marceline did something more than merely learn to feel when anything touched her skin, seeing that after the sitting she wrote : " I am so happy, without knowing why ; I go out into the streets in order to see happy-looking people, for I fancy that every one in the world must be as happy as I am." I taught Irène to recapitulate certain memories. How are we to explain that this recapitulation led to the suppression of her hysterical attacks, her paroxysms of delirium ; how could it enable her to resume work ? We have come back to the same train of reasoning that we considered in the matter of suggestion, and we are led to the same conclusion, namely that in aesthesiogenism there is an extension of psychological work in excess of the bounds within which education has been effected. Another point, still more important to my mind, is that these patients, as Deschamps has correctly pointed out, are not susceptible to education, and that they repeat the same lesson indefinitely without any improvement. The specific effect of aesthesiogenism appears to be that the patients become susceptible to education, that it enables them to progress. Obviously, then, in this procedure there is something of a peculiar kind, and something which transcends education.

4. Aesthesiogenism and Excitation.

The phenomena induced by aesthesiogenism can, I think, be classed among oscillations of the mental level, among variations of psychological tension.

The fundamental condition of the neuropath is a state of depression, attend by the lowering of the degree to which the tendencies of a higher order can be activated. Neuropaths also suffer from a lowering of psychological tension below the level which was customary to them before they fell ill, and which was essential to enable them to make the adaptations necessary to their particular kind of life. This depression may or may not be complicated by agitation. Whether it is or is not so complicated, depends upon whether the depression leaves the quantity of available energy intact or reduces it.

The condition in which the subject is before aesthesio-genism is undertaken, and the condition into which he relapses as soon as the effect of this practice has passed away, is always more or less characterised by this fundamental depression. " The objective attitude," I have written in this connexion, " was already characteristic. We could divine Marceline's condition when we saw her advancing with small and uncertain steps, her shoulders rounded, her eyes fixed on the ground ; when she spoke slowly and in a toneless voice, without looking her interlocutor in the face, and with a strange air of absorption and reverie." She continued to do her work after a fashion, but quite mechanically, with no heart in it. She did not speak, and did not seem to understand what was said to her. She did not wish to see any one, and had terrible crises of alarm as soon as any one came near her. Her emotivity was incredibly enhanced, and the most trifling incident which necessitated an effort of adaptation gave rise to convulsive attacks, contractures, fixed ideas, and accesses of delirium. I should add that she had a perpetual feeling of intense malaise, of discontent, of self-dissatisfaction, of gloom, and of boredom. No doubt symptoms of a typically hysterical character helped, in this case, to complete the pathological picture, and gave rise to restrictions of the field of consciousness, to suggestibility, to anaesthesias, to amnesias, etc. But the phenomena previously described were fundamental, and these phenomena are found in such subjects.

The condition brought about by aesthesiogenic agents, the condition which has often been described as the " alert state," and which in certain cases constitutes completed somnambulism, is not solely characterised by the cure of the hysterical symptoms, paralyses, amnesias, etc. ; for in it there also occurs a modification of behaviour, which now exhibits characteristics precisely opposite to those of depression. Let us take as typical the summary of what happened in Marce-line's case. In the new condition, her whole attitude was changed ; she stood upright, walked fast, looked in the faces of the people to whom she was speaking, and seemed to have come down out of the clouds. She glanced busily in all directions, for everything within range of vision was extremely interesting to her ; all the objects in the visual field seemed brightly coloured, and had a clearness, a definiteness, she had never noticed before. " I feel as if my eyes and ears had been unstopped." She had become active, and took interest in little works of supererogation. She was gay and frank now, was willing to meet people and to accept invitations, so that every one who knew her was astonished. Although she seemed to have more feeling than before, she was not emotional in season and out of season, but was calmer than of yore. She herself was perfectly aware of the change that had taken place, and realised that her feelings were very different from what they had been. " It seems to me that I am really living now, that I am living a new life, and that I am no longer afraid to look life in the face. I am calmer, I let things happen as they will, and nothing troubles me now. . . . I have risen out of the depths, and shall be able to mend the bad impression I may have made on others ; with a little help I shall certainly be able to go on with my work and to keep my situation." This modification of activity can be summarised in a single word, which has the opposite sense to that of depression, the word " excitation." We must not confuse excitation with agitation, as often happens. That is why, after having tried to define agitation, I must explain the ordinary sense of the word " excitation." Its essential characteristic is a rapid increase in psychological tension above the degree at which the tension has remained for a considerable time. This rise can obviously occur in either of two ways. There may be a real elevation above the level typical of what is regarded as normal. Excitation must, then, correspond to the phenomena which pass by the name of joy—enthusiasm, inspiration, ecstasy. It must play a part in works of genius, in inventions, and in the progress of thought. But this form is rare, and we have little experience of it in our therapeutic observations. The other form of excitation is more familiar ; it is that which we shall find in our patients, the form in which the psychological tension, previously lowered, rises to the level which is regarded as normal.

Excitation, as thus understood, includes phenomena which are the very opposite of those which have been witnessed during depression, namely phenomena of adaptation and calm. The more elevated tendencies, which hitherto the patient has been unable to activate, can now function readily to produce complete action, and they often become more definite and undergo development. The origination of new tendencies may also be witnessed at this time, when new memories and new habits arise. Simultaneously, agitation disappears because the relationship between the tension and the quantity of the mental energies has become comparatively normal, so that canalisation and recuperation of these energies occurs. The emotivity is reduced. Complicated and rapid actions can now be performed with tranquillity ; that is to say, without the accompaniment of inferior, exaggerated, and futile types of behaviour, such as are characteristic of agitation. Convulsive movements, tics, and anxieties have disappeared, and brooding has ceased. A strange thing is that the subject, who is really living more and is attuned to a higher psychological level, seems to be thinking less. Thought and consciousness, far from being essential psychological phenomena, are comparatively extensive in the sick person, and diminish in those who are in good health.

Just as we have observed in the state of depression, these changes are accompanied by secondary phenomena which are internal reactions to the modifications in behaviour. The obsessions, the delusions, the sentiments of incompleteness, undergo transformation into new attitudes of mind, and other sentiments develop in their place—such sentiments as those of joy, interest, confidence, and independence. According to the characteristics of the antecedent troubles, these sentiments present special varieties. It is such modifications of psychological tension which facilitate the activation of superior tendencies and the initiation of the feeling of triumph that gives birth to the sentiments of joy and happiness so characteristic of all the subjects who enter into the alert state. It is obvious that suggestion and drill can modify the expression and the regularity of these sentiments. Nevertheless, I cannot help thinking that they correspond to a real change, to the establishment of a higher level of vitality. It is interesting for the psychologist to note that at this time the subject hardly experiences any sensations of pleasure properly so-called, and is prone rather to feel distressing sensations of fatigue and even actual pains, which are now far commoner than they were in the period of depression. Still the subject is intensely joyful. We must not be too ready to assimilate joy with pleasure and with the absence of pain ; these belong to quite different categories of feeling.

Unfortunately, enfeebled subjects cannot usually, at any rate to begin with, long endure this superior form of existence. More or less speedily they relapse into depression. The moment of relapse is not conspicuous when the process is a slow one. We see a gradual and successive recurrence of the disorders of behaviour and the modifications of the sentiments. Sometimes at the moment of the transition there occur very interesting and peculiar phenomena, indications of the lowering of psychological tension. In the early days of my studies, almost the only one among these phenomena characteristic of psycholepsy which I was able to point out was the hysterical paroxysm. I believe to-day that very various symptoms, such as tremors, motor agitations of different kinds, probably asthmatic paroxysms, fits of weeping, crises of anxiety, and, above all, attacks of migraine, can play the same part.

In an earlier chapter, apropos of liquidation, I referred to the phenomenon of " discharge," which consists in a reduction of the quantity of energy. We are now concerned with the notion of a relaxation of tension. At a later stage we shall have to distinguish clearly between discharge and the relaxation of tension. Here we have to acknowledge that crises of agitation which appear to be perfectly analogous occur in both cases, although weeping fits and attacks of migraine have more often the significance of a relaxation of tension. When we are concerned with relaxation of tension, the level was high before the attack, and permitted of higher forms of activation ; after the attack, the tension is definitely lowered, and exhibits anew the characteristics of depression. We must not be led astray by the aspect of satisfaction which certain subjects manifest after a relaxation of tension has occurred. We have, then, to do with the " beatitudes " related to the suppression of effort, and analogous to the beatitudes so ably described by Mignard in the case of imbeciles and dements.[1] The distinction between " joys " and " beatitudes " was made by me an object of lengthy study in my recent lectures at the College of France upon the degrees of superior activation.

[1] Les états de satisfaction dans la démence et dans l'idiotie, Thèse, 1909.

Nothing can be more instructive than a precise analysis of the mental state of subjects well known to us, studied respectively before and after an attack of migraine. Upon this matter I have collected a great many documents which I hope to be able to use some day. Here I must be content with a few brief indications. In one of my patients, Irène, I was able to note, what I can also note in a great many other patients, that she never suffered from migraine during the periods of definite depression, however long they might last. I have known her pass eighteen months without any attack of migraine, which was a very unusual remission in her case ; but at this time she was in a state of profound depression which made her incapable of action or even of desire. During phases of this kind, the patients continue to bewail their lot, and to regret the cessation of their attacks of migraine, declaring that they were much better when they had an attack of migraine from time to time. The statement is true, for though, in that other phase, they doubtless were liable to distressing falls, they were able between these falls to climb once more, to reestablish their mental condition, and this they are unable to do during periods of prolonged and intense depression. Irène, during the periods when she had no migraine, was no longer susceptible to complete somnambulism, and was no longer sensitive to aesthesiogenic influences. Such patients exhibit no relaxation of tension, simply because they are incapable of tension.

In Irène, on the other hand, the attacks of migraine, became frequent during the close of her period of depression. In this phase, various circumstances could induce " upsets," could cause what we vaguely term emotions (for the word " emotion " is applied haphazard both to ascents and to descents in the psychological level) characterised by efforts to bring about a temporary increase of tension. This young woman, who was extremely shy, and was unable to argue with any one, was compelled one day to reply to an unjust charge, and to defend herself. She did it with a certain amount of courage, and with a fair measure of success, and immediately afterwards she experienced a lively feeling of satisfaction, was full of the joy of life, as always in her period of excitation. But soon afterwards she felt disturbed and agitated ; she was tired, she had become incapable of bearing this tension which was too high for her ; and the very same evening she began to suffer from a severe attack of migraine, after which she was, certainly, tranquil once more, but had again become shy, disquieted, and abulic as of old. During this same period, aesthesiogenic agents could once more act upon her, and could include a more or less lasting phase of complete somnambulism, which contributed greatly to put an end to the depression. But, as a regular rule, two or three days after the séance and the beginning of complete somnambulism, there came an attack of migraine and a relapse.

We may note analogous phenomena at the outset of phases of depression. In Ia. (f., 37), for instance, we could often observe the following phenomena. Some circumstance or other would bring about a great effort, followed by excitation ; then she would have an attack of migraine, and subsequently a more or less lasting phase of depression. One day she was upset because her mother had a sharp attack of haemoptysis. She pulled herself together to deal with the emergency, and cared for her mother so satisfactorily as to be extremely pleased with herself, saying : " I did not know I had it in me." But, two days later, she had a violent attack of migraine, and a new period of depression began. A remarkable detail is that, on one occasion only, in this patient the attack of migraine was replaced by a paroxysm of major hysteria, which, as we have seen, would appear to have similar characteristics to migraine. Migraine, the hysterical paroxysm, and perhaps the epileptic fit also, are phenomena of the relaxation of tension, which occur when the psychological tension has, for one reason or other, been keyed up beyond the point which the subject can actually bear. It is not unlikely that studies of these relationships will one day help us to solve the problem of epilepsy, for there can be no doubt that vertigos and epileptic attacks are phenomena of the relaxation of tension, whose significance is not plain to us because we have not studied with sufficient care the state of mental and psychological tension before and after the symptoms characteristic of the relaxation of tension.

In any case, this depression following a period of mental activity greater than usual, induces a modification which imposes difficulties in the way of the continuity of consciousness and memory. Thus, when we have to do with hysterics who are predisposed to restriction of the field of consciousness, it is often accompanied by disorders of memory, by an amnesia which relates especially to the alert period. The patient who, by the very fact of her depression, finds it difficult to call up memories concerning the extant situation, now ceases to have the power of calling up memories appropriate to the period of excitation. But when she enters into the alert state, she can call up these memories readily enough. We thus witness a series of periodic transformations of activity and memory which enable us, as I have shown elsewhere,[1] to give a simpler explanation of the phenomena of double personality, though this seemed so mysterious in the early days of the study of morbid psychology.

In fact, the alternations of double personality were then associated with a group of phenomena which were commoner and better known. The changes induced by aesthesiogenism in hysterical patients, are only peculiar forms of the oscillations that can be observed in periodic depressions. The excitations we have just been speaking of are no longer so extraordinary if we assimilate them to the excitations which occur spontaneously in these other patients. The earlier French alienists had carefully studied the cases of what they called " folie circulaire," circular or alternating insanity, and they noticed that in the course of the malady these patients often exhibited three successive periods. They had a crisis of depression, characterised by all the phenomena just described ; the state spoken of as normal, which might more appropriately be termed a state of excitation ; and between the two there was a period termed the maniacal phase which had very peculiar characteristics. But it is likely enough that the maniacal phase, which did not always occur, was only a form of depression in which agitation predominated. The essential characteristics of this disease are an oscillation between a state of depression with or without agitation, and a state of normal excitation.

When the passage from one state to the other state occurs rather rapidly, as happened in the case of Lc. (f., 54), for instance, it is possible to note the same astonishment and the same sentiment of euphoria which have often struck us in

[1] Les névroses, 1909, pp. 256–270.

connexion with aesthesiogenism. "At length I find myself in the real world ; at length I am beginning to live again." Finally, when the periods are over, the resemblance to complete somnambulism is often marked. At the present time, in the clinic of my friend Nageotte at the Salpêtrière, I have under observation a remarkable case of this kind, which in many respects resembles the cases of Marceline and Irène. Marianne (f., 34), has for two years been passing at regular intervals through three distinct psychological states, remaining in each of these states a few days only, a fortnight at the most. In the first of these conditions, which always begins rather suddenly at the menstrual period, she is depressed. Taking to her bed, she obstinately refuses to rise, or to do any kind of work ; dreadfully shy, she trembles and hides herself if anyone comes to see her, or if anyone tries to make her talk. She can give an intelligent answer to simple questions, but she does not believe anything that is said to her, and is full of doubts ; she feels unhappy, contemptible, and is sure that she is an object of disgust to every one else as well as to herself. This one of the three phases lasts longest, a fortnight. Suddenly, as a rule at six o'clock in the evening, she passes into a maniacal condition. She will not stay in bed any longer, but gets up, screams, runs all over the place, and tries to break everything. She is now bold and arrogant, and goes on talking by night and by day. After five or six days she grows calm once more and is delighted " to get out of this horrible condition in which one is not a person—to become a person just like other people." She asks to be given some work to do, and expresses the wish to see her parents again. When they come, she receives them most amiably. In a word, she is no longer either abulic or shy, and resumes normal activities. Unhappily, however, this condition does not last long, for in from three to five days the date for the next menstruation has arrived, and she immediately sinks back into the phase of depression. From time to time, especially when a period of depression is nearing its close, there occur sudden oscillations. All at once, in the middle of the day, Marianne will emerge from the state of depression, which has been complete, and will enter into the maniacal state. Or, more rarely, she will pass directly into the normal state. If the last happens, she gets up " delighted to see clearly once more " ; she dresses, says she is cured, wants to resume normal activities, and speaks intelligently. This lasts for two hours ; then she relapses completely, and can no longer believe that even for a moment she has been numbered among the living. Assuredly this is a state of complete somnambulism exactly comparable to those we have already described.

Still, there is a great difference between this condition, and that of our subjects, for all these changes in Marianne occur spontaneously. I could not exercise the slightest influence upon their appearance. On the other hand, in aesthesiogenism the passage to the period of excitation was brought about artificially. Marceline was identical with Azam's Félida, except in one point, which was that she could be made to pass into the alert state at any moment chosen by the experimenter ; that is why I called her " an artificial Félida."

Does this characteristic, however important it may be, suffice to establish an absolute distinction between the neuroses I am comparing ? Is it quite certain that we can never intervene so as to affect the onset of the periodic states ? Since I became interested in these sudden changes, which constitute one of the most remarkable psychological phenomena known to us in the field of psychiatry, I have often tried to effect artificial modifications in this strange rhythm. I must admit that hitherto I have almost invariably failed. Still, I may record here two striking cases.

To be precise, we must recognise that in these two cases we are not concerned with patients quite identical with Marianne. The last-named is a typical sufferer from circular insanity, in the sense attached to this term by the French alienists. A periodicity independent of outward circumstances is an essential element in her illness. Our two other patients would also be classed as sufferers from circular insanity by the enthusiasts of German science who have adopted the conception of manic-depressive insanity, for each of these women has already had several periods of depression. But they are " depressibles," and not typical sufferers from circular insanity, for their crises of depression have supervened at very variable intervals and always as the outcome of exhausting conditions.

However this may be, Jb. (f., 24), who already at the age

of eighteen had a crisis of depression lasting several months, received a profound shock when she married at the age of twenty-one. She was affected by one of those types of genital impotence associated with phobias, which are so characteristic ; and she subsequently entered into a serious state of depression with refusal of food and attempts at suicide. She was sent to the asylum with a diagnosis of manic-depressive insanity, and she remained under restraint for two years. Having noticed that she suffered from paresis and from a certain degree of hypoaesthesia of the left side, and that she was markedly suggestible, I endeavoured, notwithstanding her melancholic condition, to hypnotise her, and to induce her to make certain aesthesiogenic efforts. Under this influence, she would emerge definitely from the melancholic condition for a few hours or a few days, but then relapsed into depression. These initial stages of progress enabled us to send her home to her husband. Stimulation of the genital sense, which acted like a true education, rapidly put an end to the relapses, and ultimately cured the melancholic depression, which had lasted more than two years and which threatened to continue indefinitely.

The case of Kab. (f., 30) is even more definite. This woman has already had two attacks of melancholia, one lasting eighteen months and the other lasting two years. After being exposed to fatigue and emotion (consequent upon the loss of a situation she liked but in which she had been over-worked), she became affected a year ago with a third crisis. I found her in Nageotte's clinic, prostrate in a corner, completely inert. Any attempt to shake her out of herself, only aroused anger ; she would roll upon the ground as if in a fit of hysterics and would relapse into a condition of groaning inertia. I learned that, more than ten years earlier, at the age of seventeen, she had had hysterical attacks, and that she had been treated by hypnotism, and I therefore decided to try whether, in the actual condition of melancholic depres sion, the disposition to hypnotism had been preserved. She was fully hypnotised in three sittings, and there soon developed a secondary condition in which she was much more aware than in what passed for her waking state. This artificial condition underwent development, lasting at first a few hours and then several days. But a relapse, characterised by a violent convulsive seizure and followed by depression, would supervene upon the most trifling incident, as if the development of the melancholic depression were continuing despite these interpositions. After a little while I was able to secure the occurrence of longer periods of normal activity; and after six months' treatment the patient was able to leave the hospital and to resume her work. A previous attack had lasted two years and six months, and it is probable that this one would have lasted at least as long, for in the initial stages the patient's inertia had been greater than ever before. I think that the hypnotism and the aesthesiogenism considerably reduced the duration of the illness. However this may be, I have only quoted these examples for a specific purpose. They show that aesthesiogenism can induce an excitation in the course of depressions properly so-called, when these depressions are not solely hysterical depressions. They confirm our remarks anent the essential character of these procedures. There can be no doubt that facts akin to suggestion play a great part here; but the definitive phenomenon is one of excitation which antagonises the depression.

It does not suffice to recognise that in aesthesiogenism there occurs a certain amount of excitation; for what we have to understand, above all, is the mechanism of this excitation, and how we can reproduce it at will and turn it to account. Upon this matter we know very little. The excitation seems to arise in connexion with modifications of sensation and movement; but it is likely that the connexion may be only casual, for the same excitation can be noticed in connexion with memory, and probably in connexion with a great many other phenomena. Sometimes, trifling modifications of sensibility can induce great excitations; and, conversely, great changes of sensibility may occur automatically without any apparent excitation.

It is probable, therefore, that the important factor is the effort made by the subject to obey the command or to carry out the suggestion aroused by some signal or other. Here, in fact, we have attention and work. We can see this in the signs of effort and in the contortions which some subjects make. We can also see it when we note the time requisite to bring about these metamorphoses. The rapid changes effected by suggestion pure and simple, do not have the same results as those changes which are achieved slowly by a process of genuine labour. " You are trying to make me get on too quickly ; that is what gives me a headache which is enough to drive me crazy." Finally, we can detect this labour in the remarkable fatigue which follows the sitting. Such fatigue is most noteworthy and most regular in those patients in whom there has been real excitation, whereas it is absent when there has been no considerable excitation.

What is this work of which we speak ? We cannot define it precisely. We can only explain it by analogies. Unquestionably it is a characteristic of living beings to have functions of depression and of normal excitation. From the beginning of life, the living being knows how to go to sleep and how to wake up ; and these actions, among other modifications, bring about great changes in the psychological tension. Subsequently, the living being learns how to relax tension during sleep, during play, during confidence, and it knows how to become tense, how to put all its tendencies into a condition of erection when there is difficulty, danger, or expectation. The existence of such functions is also demonstrated by the psychological disorders they present in depressed persons, who become incapable of going to sleep, of waking up, of resting, of adopting the defensive, of assuming an attitude of expectation ; and who, apropos of all these actions, exhibit derivations in the form of emotion. Popular language recognises more clearly than psychological terminology the existence of these phenomena in such phrases as " to be on the watch," " to prick up one's ears," " to be on the alert," etc. At the climax of these phenomena of excitation we have the frenzy of composition and the enthusiasm of the creative artist. An artist said to me not long ago that he had to get into a peculiar condition in order to be able to compose ; that he could do nothing to begin with, but that gradually he got warmed up. " Then," he said, " I live three times as fast as ordinarily ; but when it is over I am exhausted for several days." I cannot help thinking that our subjects do something of the same kind ; and that in them, in certain conditions, an order (or, if you will, a suggestion) to feel or to remember, unleashes special tendencies to effort and even to enthusiasm. The same operations which in the normal human being raise the tension to the point at which creative activity becomes possible, serve in these depressed persons, to raise the tension to a level which is normal in other persons.

This is a strange procedure, which makes an appeal to the most splendid powers of the human genius to enable a hysteric to eat her soup! We are often obliged, in our patients, to have recourse to methods of this kind ; and I have frequently remarked that we may find it necessary to use the most eloquent adjurations and to employ all the devices of oratory to make a sick man change his shirt or drink a glass of water. That is what I pointed out, in especial, in my first studies concerning Marceline and Irène. " My treatment of the patient was something more than a suggestion ; it was an excitation. In psychological methods of treatment, there has not always been enough pains taken to distinguish the factor of suggestion from the factor of excitation, which latter aims at restoring the mental level. I demand from Irène attention and efforts ; I insist that she shall have an increasingly clear consciousness of her feelings. All these things are means for enhancing the nervous and mental tension, for obtaining, if you like to phrase it in that way, the functioning of the higher centres. With her, as with so many other patients, I have often had occasion to note that the really useful sittings were those in which I was able to stir her emotions. I often had to scold her, to discover the directions in which she was still impressionable, to shake her morally in various ways, in order to " buck her up " and to make her rediscover memories and actions. All the methods to reeducate neuropaths about which there is so much talk to-day, are subject to the same law. No matter whether we have to do with gymnastics, with the education of movements, with the excitation of sensibility, with the search for lost memories—the director must always encourage the awakening of attention and effort, the stimulation of emotion, and must then always bring about an increase of tension. When this higher functioning has been achieved, the subject feels a modification of the whole consciousness, which is translated by an increase of perception and activity." [1]

But it is also true that this characteristic of aesthe-

[1] L'amnésie et la dissociation des souvenirs par l'émotion, 1904 ; L'état mental des hystériques, second edition, 1911, p. 542.

siogenism, this appeal to the most lofty sources of excitation, makes its employment a rather delicate matter. The subjects must have certain resources within themselves ; they must be capable of waking up, of pulling themselves together. A good many people are incapable of this, and that is why such methods will not succeed in every case. Even the doctors who in former days were enthusiasts for metallotherapy, were at their wits' end when they had to do with subjects who could make no efforts for the maintenance or recuperation of sensibility. Furthermore, even those who are capable of such excitation, are not always disposed to make the necessary expenditure. They cannot do it when they are greatly exhausted, which means that they cannot do it at the very time when we have most need for the use of this therapeutic method. That is what we were able to observe particularly well in Irène's case. Aesthesiogenism would not work with her when she was " unduly depleted " ; it was essential that she should have recuperated her energies a little before she could make the effort which then restored her definitively.

The reader will realise the complexity of the problems which must be solved if we want to explain aesthesiogenism. In the next chapter we shall have occasion to consider on more general lines the problem of therapeutic excitation. Enough, for the nonce, to have understood that complete somnambulism is not exclusively the result of suggestion or drill, but that there is involved in it, in another and a peculiar form determined by hysteria, a transformation of the mental condition under the influence of an excitation.

5. THERAPEUTIC APPLICATIONS.

The essence of the before-mentioned treatment was to be found in the endeavour to produce complete somnambulism by the excitation of sensibility or memory. If we apply this definition strictly we shall be obliged to admit that only in a very small number of cases is it possible to utilise the treatment successfully.

Apart from the seven cases an account of which I have just been giving, I find among my notes barely six others in which a fairly durable cure of serious hysterical symptoms seems to have been achieved by the systematic and exclusive use of aesthesiogenic treatment bearing upon sensibility and inducing complete somnambulism. I may add three cases in which the patients suffered from amnesia, and in which by excitation of memories there was also induced complete somnambulism. These last cases resemble that of Irène, although the phenomena are less noteworthy. In all, fifteen patients seem to have exhibited the phenomenon which I have called complete somnambulism, and have derived benefit therefrom.

Concerning these patients, I shall give only a few interesting details. Mab. (f., 35) was suffering from a complex of disorders ; nervous paroxysms, accesses of sleep, amnesias, serious alterations of character. These symptoms appeared after an accident to one of the eyes, which brought on hysterical disorders of vision. Simple treatment of the vision, and excitation of the ocular sensibility, were the starting-point of an extensive change in the whole personality. It was remarkable to see this woman—who was not merely suffering from crises of sleep, but who, in the intervals, remained inert, indifferent to everything, ill-tempered with her children— to see how for a few days, after efforts at visual attention, she would resume active habits and return to her normal character. We have already studied phenomena of the same kind in Irène, whose character was transformed after she had laboured to recover the memory of her mother's death. It would seem that general excitation can supervene in various ways, after setting out from very different starting-points.

Nep. (f., 28) had suffered daily for eight months from crises of delirious somnambulism, which came on regularly at five o'clock in the afternoon. The crisis lasted two or three hours, and afterwards the patient had no memory of it. The regularity naturally made us think of fixed ideas and of suggestion. When the patient had been thrown into a condition of complete somnambulism by efforts of attention bearing upon sensibility, she recovered the memory of these crises, and awaited the coming of five o'clock in the afternoon with considerable curiosity, in order to find out whether at this hour she would become ill as usual—but for several days nothing of the kind happened. When she had relapsed into depression, she forgot her crises and no longer consciously expected them. But the accesses of delirium recurred at the

regular hour.   Here we have to do with the reappearance of
suggestibility in the condition of depression.

I must also draw attention to a detail in the case of
Nc. (f., 27). This woman showed very marked reactions at
the moment when cutaneous sensibility returned.   She
groaned, wept, and clasped her hands to her head, while
uttering screams of pain.   She was not an inmate of a hospital,
so she had never seen or heard of such phenomena ; and,
besides, my patients, as I have already said, were not in the
habit of exhibiting such phenomena   If suggestion played
any part in causing her symptoms, it must have been a very
small part.   We have to recognise that among these psychological phenomena we find individual details which cannot be
explained by general rules.

Ob. (f., 24) exhibited a morbid evolution very like that of
Irène. Neuropathic as a child, a sufferer from insomnia,
very liable to headache, she none the less remained fairly
normal until the age of thirteen ; but then, under the influence
of the approach of puberty and owing to emotions caused by
the death of her mother and the remarriage of her father,
she underwent a complete change.   She became very emotional, and upon the most trifling provocation she would
exhibit convulsive agitations.   She was so timid that she
tended to conceal her feelings, and seemed very cold.
Especially she suffered from disorders of memory ; she ceased
to be able to learn, and appeared to have a very poor
remembrance of recent. happenings.   At the present time,
when she is twenty-four, she can give a detailed account of
the incidents of her childhood before she was thirteen, but
seems to know very little of what has happened to her since
that age.   She has psychological scars.   Quarrels with her
stepmother (who did not like her), the departure of her
brother for the army, and the anxieties incident to the war,
greatly aggravated her illness.   At the age of twenty-one she
isolated herself more and more, while complaining that other
people were forsaking her.   She declared that she had
completely lost the power of willing, and wanted to be ordered
about like a child.   She could no longer work, and all her
actions were ill regulated.   She frequently exhibited an
impulse " to change her situation ; to do something else,
no matter what ; to run away, no matter where "—impulses

which are so characteristic of states of depression. At length, one day, eluding observation for a moment, she ran away and threw herself into a river. She was insensible when rescued from the water. When she recovered consciousness she was delirious ; and remained delirious, agitated, and even violent. She could give no explanations, and had no memory of her attempted suicide or of what had happened since. All sorts of absurdities were betrayed by her delirium. She declared that she was Joan of Arc come to save France ; or she would sign fantastic letters with the name of Henriette de France ; and so on. This delirious condition had continued almost uninterruptedly for a year when I first saw the patient. The character of the agitations (which sometimes recalled those of hysterical paroxysms), the alternations between delirium and lucidity, and the localised amnesias, led me to regard the case as hysterical, and to attempt hypnotism. The girl was very suggestible and hypnotisable ; and I tried, exactly as I had done in Irène's case, to revive her memory in the somnambulist state. Quite a dozen sittings were requisite, before, amid efforts and contortions, I could elucidate a detailed account of the period which had preceded the attempted suicide and the story of the attempt itself. It was curious to note how, in this condition, she gave a clear explanation of all the troubles from which she had suffered for so long ; her exhaustion ; her inability to rest ; her dissatisfaction with herself ; her obsessions of shame ; her despair ; her impulse to run away, which had never been understood ; and, finally, her sudden impulse towards suicide. " At any rate, if I were to kill myself I should no longer have to talk to any one, and all my troubles would be over in a moment."

As soon as the return of the memories became definite during the somnambulist state, there was a remarkable change in the mental condition. The patient was obviously improved, became more active, attended better to what was going on, began to feel confidence, and gave expression (as we always notice in such cases) to sentiments of enthusiasm. She was soon restored to a fairly normal condition, such as she had not exhibited since the age of thirteen. I need not dwell upon the periodic relapses, which came at first every two days, then every week, then only after an emotional stress, or during menstruation. For menstruation, which had been in abeyance throughout the period of mental disorder, had now reappeared. This young woman remains a weakly creature, very much inclined to depressive disorders; but for the last year she has been able to lead a normal life and has resumed her work. The case is of great interest because of its close analogy with that of Irène, and because a similar treatment to that used in the case of Irène was more speedily successful here. The treatment of both these cases is akin to the methods of treatment by search for a traumatic memory and to the treatment by liquidation—but the actual liquidation in these instances was secured by means of a state of excitation.

Beside the patients just mentioned I shall place a group of fifteen cases in which the subjects exhibited an imperfect form of complete somnambulism, but in which aesthesiogenism played an important part. It was not employed exclusively, but as a useful accessory to other therapeutic methods. Among these patients were three psychasthenics, who, in addition to obsessions, exhibited hysterical phenomena, and could be hypnotised—though this possibility, in my experience, is rare in psychasthenics. Their mental state was remarkably modified during the period of complete somnambulism, which in them was very short. Qi. (f., 40) in especial, apart from her obsessions and phobias, has always suffered from extreme shyness. Even now, when she is forty years of age, she cannot bear to think that any one is looking at her. " I find it a perfect torment to have to pass in front of a tramcar." If she has to speak to any one, she suffers from all sorts of spasmodic affections and contortions, and can only say a few words after spending some time in efforts, while closing her eyes and turning her head away. This patient, when in a state analogous to complete somnambulism, not only forgets her obsessions, but assumes quite a fresh attitude, looking her interlocutor in the face and speaking without spasms or contortions. She feels stronger and clearer-headed. She says: " The light seems brighter, and the world better." Here we have a remarkable instance of the transformation of shyness, thanks to excitation.

The other patients are hysterics exhibiting various symptoms, which, as a rule, are complex. Not only were they treated by aesthesiogenism. Other methods were also employed, such as suggestion strictly so-called, dissociation of the fixed idea, isolation, and education ; and I cannot therefore venture to say that the cures which resulted were solely due to the method we are now considering. The modification of character brought about by complete somnambulism was very remarkable in the case of Pauline (f., 19). She had always been very timid, and at ordinary times was absurdly secretive, extremely obstinate, susceptible, and jealous. In the artificially induced state, which in her case lasted for several days, she was amazingly transformed, it being especially noticeable that she was frank and confiding. Now, laughingly, she would relate strange incidents that had happened at the outset of her illness ; her proud reveries, the dreadful humiliations she had suffered on account of some inadequate cause, her despair when her mother showed affection for her sisters, her feigning of illness which in the end gave rise to contractures that persisted indefinitely. When we pointed out to her that her character had changed, and that she was behaving quite differently from the way in which she behaved in her ordinary condition, she protested, saying : " I am now my real self, and it was only illness that previously gave me so absurd a character." I am fully willing to believe her, for obstinacy, secretiveness, and jealousy, are phenomena of depression. After a time she was able to remain for months in the better state, and in the end was completely cured.

Notwithstanding these interesting observations, I must repeat that, among my cases, numbering several thousand, those in which complete somnambulism has been obtainable and has had fortunate results are few in number. This can readily be understood if the reader will recall how many conditions must be present to secure such results. We must be dealing with hysterics who are extremely hypnotisable and suggestible, and who have anaesthesias, paralyses, or amnesias of a serious character and of long standing. These patients can be found, although they are perhaps less common than, the metallo-therapists and the observers of Charcot's school used to believe. Still, they are commoner than contemporary doctors are usually willing to admit. But they do not form the majority of the neuropaths we come across in our ordinary practice, and we seldom encounter the conditions suitable for the application of such methods of treatment.

When the appropriate conditions occur, should we make a trial of aesthesiogenic treatment? As a reaction against the teachings of Burq and Charcot, it is the fashion to-day to pay scant attention to hysterical disorders of sensation— probably because too much attention was paid to them in former days. The doctor who twenty years ago was inclined to see hysterical anaesthesia everywhere, is ashamed now to recognise it at all or to take it seriously. I quite agree that it is a mistake to pay too much attention to such disorders of sensation or memory, for this will aggravate the symptoms, and they will often undergo a spontaneous cure when we attend to the general health and to the other more salient manifestations.

It is true enough that in the earlier stages of hysteria, in very youthful patients, and when the disorders are still vague and variable, we must be careful not to direct the subject's attention much to a morbid phenomenon, for we run the risk of making it more definite. But it is not only true of anaesthesia; it is equally true of hysterical cough, nervous vomiting, fits of anger, paresias, algias, etc. In this phase of the disease, the doctor must be discreet and prudent; he must treat the bodily and mental state on general lines, and must lay as little stress as possible on this or that symptom. It is not less true that a hysteric, when she is cured in any way you please, will get rid of her anaesthesias and her paroxysms although we have not paid any attention to them. We have seen many examples of this in the present work. The relief of these troubles is an outcome of the rise in psychological tension, however that may have been brought about.

But it is necessary to point out that the subjects who come to consult us are not always in this condition of primitive ignorance. The young soldier who returns from the front suffering from hemiplegia and anaesthesia, knows perfectly well that he cannot feel anything on the right side of his body, and I do not see how it could benefit him if I should pretend to ignore the fact. I shall not increase his anaesthesia by verifying its existence, for it is already as intense as possible; and I shall not give him a fixed idea of this anaesthesia, for that is what he had before he came to see me. Considerations of this character would prevent our ever undertaking the treatment of a hysterical symptom. Besides, it is not always true that the verification of hysterical phenomena increases them. I referred above to the female patient who came to the clinic suffering from hemianaesthesia. Under careful treatment she rapidly recovered sensibility, notwithstanding the fact that a very large number of persons examined her, who detected this anaesthesia again and again. On the other hand, I agree that if we can readily cure hysteria by any other method, it is needless to have recourse to aesthesiogenism. But there are cases in which hysterical symptoms cannot readily be cured, and in which they continue indefinitely, although the doctors display a magnificent disdain for them. In such cases it is just as well to have in our hands an additional method, which in certain fortunate cases has given remarkable results.

In fact, as we have seen several times in the course of this work, the main difficulty does not lie here. The main difficulty is not to be found in the moral scrupulousness of physicians, but in their ignorance. We do not utilise aesthesiogenic agents more frequently, and we do not turn them to better account, because we do not well know the most essential conditions for this treatment. It is quite certain that the conditions above mentioned, complex though they are, are not all that is requisite. In a great many instances which appear to me perfectly identical with those in which I was successful, I operated, or believed myself to be operating, in the same manner, with no result worth mentioning. The suggestion of sensibility or memory was ineffective, or was restricted in its effects, and did not give rise to that general excitation which is the main constituent of the treatment. Attempts of the kind, which unfortunately always demand a great expenditure of time, were sterile. Excellent manifestations of complete somnambulism have appeared from time to time in my experiments in a manner which seemed too arbitrary. They were analogous to the phenomena of enthusiasm, whose existence we know, but which we cannot induce in a regular manner whenever we need them.

In all the methods that I have just enumerated, which seem to be more or less closely akin to aesthesiogenism, there are probably to be found the germ of a therapeutic method ;

but we do not adequately know the rules that will make of it a method that is readily applicable. We shall, therefore, do well, at this stage, to undertake a more general examination of psychological excitation, of which aesthesiogenism seems to be a particular instance. The study of metallotherapeutics and of complete somnambulism will serve some day, if I am not mistaken, to introduce us to the study of a great problem, which to-day is practically ignored—the problem of excitation.

CHAPTER FOURTEEN

TREATMENT BY EXCITATION

SIDE by side with psychological therapeutic methods which can be accurately defined, such as treatment by suggestion or by rest, we find on all hands forms of medical advice or practice which are difficult to explain in precise terms, and which differ one from another in appearance rather than in reality. I think that these methods of treatment are linked by their tendency to induce personal effort rather than to arouse automatism, to encourage activity rather than rest, to favour social life rather than isolation. I believe that the psychological phenomenon which plays the leading part here is the phenomenon of excitation, whose importance has been indicated to us by our study of aesthesiogenic treatment

1. HISTORY OF TREATMENT BY EXCITATION.

Philosophers and moralists have often advocated optimistic doctrines appealing to the courage and energy of mankind. The Stoic morality was based upon this confidence in human powers, of which we are apt to despair too readily. " You are saved this very moment," said Luther, " if only you are willing to believe it." The earlier alienists used to insist upon the importance of work in the treatment of mental disorders. " It is often far less by drugs than by moral means," wrote Pinel, " that we can effect a happy diversion in the gloomy thoughts of melancholics." [1] Among the moral methods most important in the treatment of insanity, Leuret gave a leading place to work.

Passing to consider contemporary philosophers, we find that William James was more eloquent than any one else in insisting upon the profound resources of the human mind, which, he declared, were not utilised sufficiently. He was fond of protesting against the depressing habit of fear. As Bourdeau

[1] Pinel, Traité médico-philosophique sur l'aliénation mentale, 1809, p. 348.

has well shown, James, before he became the apostle of pragmatism, was the psychologist of effort and the educator of the will. He had a disdain for undue contemplation, and he thought that we should seize every possible opportunity to develop action. Bourdeau writes : " He did not wish us to allow the motor energy of motion to evaporate. He said that when we come away from a concert, we should see to it that the charm of the music continued to act in us, so that it might find expression in some deed of courtesy and goodwill. To perform every day some action containing even an infinitesimal ingredient of asceticism and heroism, some action which goes rather against the grain, is to insure ourselves against the hours of anguish and defeat." [1]

William James, although he recognised that Mrs. Eddy's Christian Science was packed with absurdities, considered that it embodied a useful application of the foregoing principles. " We are just now witnessing . . . a very copious unlocking of energy by ideas, in the person of those converts to ' New Thought,' ' Christian Science,' ' Metaphysical Healing,' or other forms of spiritual philosophy, who are so numerous among us to-day. . . . The common feature of these optimistic faiths is that they all tend to the suppression of what Mr. Horace Fletcher calls ' fear thought.' " [2] James thinks that the same principle is at work in the writers who have analysed the mystical " revivals " which are so common in the United States. They have noticed in the course of these great religious ceremonies, that rapid conversions take place, and that the converts manifest signs of euphoria, and a metamorphosis of the whole personality ; the subjects pass rapidly, if not from vice to virtue, at least from a torpid and gloomy existence to a healthier and more courageous one. The curious thing is that these writers have imagined that they can discern a proof of the truth of religion in the psychological phenomenon of excitation—though this phenomenon is really trivial enough in the instances they describe. We have studied more remarkable forms of it after aesthesiogenic sittings, and we know that it can manifest itself in a no less lively fashion

[1] Bourdeau, La philosophie affective, 1912, p. 31 ; cf. James' famous essay on Habit, reprinted as the fourth chapter of vol. i of The Principles of Psychology, London and New York, 1890, p. 126, etc.

[2] James, The Energies of Men, " The Philosophical Review," January 1907, p. 17.

after so petty a thing as a glass of champagne. But it is not our business here to study the dogmatic conclusions which the theologians have essayed to draw from this phenomenon.[1] Enough to say that James, when giving a description of these sudden conversions, says that the authors in question have helped to make the phenomenon of excitation more widely known, and to throw light on the advantages which can accrue from it for the reestablishment of moral health.

It is doubtless true that doctors used hardly to think of founding a definite method of treatment upon this phenomenon of moral excitation; but they were not ignorant of its power, and they often declared that it must play a certain part among other methods of treatment. We find allusion to treatment by work and by effort in all the writings of the French alienists of the nineteenth century. Brémond's remarks have become famous: " If you cannot have an ideal, you should at least have a stimulating passion. Sterne was quite right in saying that it is better to do the most useless thing in the world, than to remain for a quarter of an hour without doing anything at all. Cultivate rare tulips, become an autograph collector, breed rabbits, be a fisherman, turn eggcups, cut out silhouettes for your children, hunt butterflies, or collect postage stamps. The one thing that matters is that you should have a passion for something." [2]

Forel, in many of his books, insists upon the importance of lively interest, and upon the value of stimulating work. He advises that we should have various occupations which shake up the mind and raise it above the level of its ordinary work.[3] Those who have the largest number of interests in life are not plunged into despair by the loss of one of the objects of their affections; they do not relapse into " the narrowness of an exclusive egoism." [4] Forel's study of the moral treatment " of bachelors, of old maids, of celibates, of widowers, and of childless widows " is worthy of particular attention. He shows us how necessary it is to have our lives well-filled, and to provide nutriment for our sentiments and our passions.

We find the same ideas in the writings of many others who

[1] Cf. Leuba, A Psychological Study of Religion, 1912.
[2] Brémond, Les passions et la santé, 1893, p. 121.
[3] Forel, L'âme et le système nerveux, 1906, p. 313.   [4] Ibid., p. 312.

think that they are merely advocating suggestion. Bernheim does not hesitate, in this connexion, to speak of the excitation of the attention, and of " psychological dynamogenism." [1] A fortiori, these ideas play a notable part in the moralisation method of Paul Dubois, for the great merit of such works as his is that they contain more ideas than might appear from the ill-defined terminology, and they set forth the still undifferentiated germs of all the psychological methods of treatment. " The return to optimism is often difficult in patients whose life is seriously troubled, but such a return is essential. . . . I have myself found in mental weaklings a power of resistance which I should never have expected, and which only needed to be awakened." [2] He records cures achieved through a return of religious faith ; and he lays stress upon the education of the character, which must be rendered more energetic and more tense, for that is far more important than the cure of this or that nervous symptom.[3]

Finally, in the various books on gymnastics and physical culture, it is not difficult to discover numerous allusions to the good effects of excitation. Movement, as Lagrange has pointed out, does not merely strengthen our muscles; it also activates respiration, digestion, and nutrition.[4] The good effects of gymnastic exercises upon the mental condition of patients are also perfectly clear. " The will plays its part in every movement, and the will, like every other faculty, is perfected by the habit of exercise. In these exercises, the patient finds the revelation of a faculty of which he had ceased to be conscious, the faculty of making efforts. He proves to himself that his organs have not completely lost physical energy." [5] Long ago, Briquet pointed out that gymnastic exercises restored the moral energy of hysterics. [6]

Pitres expresses similar ideas.[7] Tissié speaks of the treatment of phobias by Swedish exercises.[8] All these authors recommend that the majority of such patients should practise exercises suited to their age and taste, such as bicycling, horse-

[1] Cf. H. Aimé's thesis, Etude clinique sur le dynamisme psychique, Nancy, 1897 ; " Presse Médicale," 1897, p. 180.
[2] Dubois, Les psychonévroses, 1904, p. 517.
[3] Dubois in Parker's Psychotherapy, III, ii, 31.
[4] Lagrange, Les mouvements méthodiques, etc., 1899, p. 100.
[5] Ibid., p. 442.   [6] Briquet, L'hystérie, 1859, p. 113.
[7] Pitres, Leçons cliniques sur l'hystérie, 1891, vol. ii, p. 58.
[8] Congrès des aliénistes et neurologistes, Bordeaux, 1885.

back riding, rowing, and various other forms of open-air exercises. They point out that these exercises contribute to moral redintegration just as much as to the increase of bodily strength.

I should like, at this stage, to refer to my own researches concerning the reeducation of the will and of attention. In the study of one of my earlier cases, that of Marcelle, I pointed out the importance of these methods of treatment.[1] I think, however, that I applied them more adequately in a subsequent case, that of Justine. Notwithstanding the fact that her leading fixed idea (that she was becoming infected with cholera) had been overcome, the patient, owing to her suggestibility and to the weakness of her mental synthesis, was continually relapsing into all sorts of fixed ideas. In order to raise the level of her mental activity, I tried to make her undergo a sort of gymnastics of attention. Mental work could not be performed without arousing resistance, and sometimes serious symptoms; but before long it produced noteworthy results.[2] At the same period I was describing this effort of education and attention as an essential method in the treatment of hysteria,[3] in order to counteract suggestibility and mental debility. Notwithstanding the great difficulties of this method of treatment, I have been able in favourable circumstances to make the patients' parents help me. I was thus enabled, by degrees, to make these patients study history, translate foreign languages, work at painting, music, etc.; in this way I have achieved many remarkable and encouraging results, so that it seemed to me regrettable at this time that the institutions to which the patients were sent could not in certain cases become real educational centres.

In my work *Les obsessions et la psychasthénie*, 1903, when dealing with the prophylaxis of these disorders by the education of children, I referred to the importance of muscular exercises, and even of exercises presenting a certain amount of danger. "Infants and young people should learn, and should learn at

---

[1] Un cas d'aboulie et d'idées fixes, " Revue Philosophique," 1891; Névroses et idées fixes, 1898, vol. i, p. 1.

[2] Histoire d'une idée fixe, " Revue Philosophique," February 1894; Névroses et idées fixes. 1898, vol. i, pp. 156 and 195.

[3] Traitement psychologique de l'hystérie, in Robin's Traité de thérapeutique, 1898; L'état mental des hystériques, second edition, 1911, p. 676.

their own cost, to pay attention to reality, to watch the instruments they are using and the movements they are making. Danger plays an essential part here. When it has been overcome, the young folk acquire self-confidence ; their mental level is raised by satisfaction because difficulties have been conquered. As Marro has well said, the fact of having been in danger is to the mental organism what the fact of having resisted an infection is to the physical organism ; it creates a power of resisting further and more serious dangers. Quite early in their lives, we must, in all sorts of circumstances, leave these young people to themselves, let them go about alone. Necessity will compel them to adapt themselves to circumstances, to become practical ; and this will provide an antidote to scruples and phobias."

With regard to the moral treatment of confirmed illness, I insisted upon the simplification of life, this being in conformity with the observations made in the present work concerning rest ; then I devoted myself to the study of the uplifting of psychological tension by the reeducation of emotion. We are not concerned here with the vague and elementary emotion which in the last resort constitutes the anxiety of phobia, but with the more definite emotion which is related to circumstances and is well appreciated by the subject. Next, I insisted upon the guidance of efforts, and above all upon the work of attention. In these maladies, lack of attention plays an essential part ; it is against this that all the patient's efforts must be directed. We must choose various kinds of mental work suited to the age and social position of the patient, but must always endeavour to make the patient do work which is more or less interesting and which presents a certain amount of difficulty, so that it shall not be done too automatically.[2] It is not difficult to realise that all the methods of treatment which give rise to sthenic emotion, which cultivate work, effort, and attention, have as a common characteristic that they raise the psychological tension, and contribute to what we have defined as excitation.

At about this period there developed a remarkable therapeutic method which is, I think, little known, for I rarely see it analysed or discussed. I refer to the method of Roger

[1] Janet, Les obsessions et la psychasthénie, 1903, p. 686.
[2] Les obsessions et la psychasthénie, 1903, p. 718.

Vittoz, of Lausanne, which simultaneously derives from the before-mentioned studies upon the need for reeducating the attention, and from the methods of the disciples of the New Thought in the United States. An account of the method will be found in a book by Vittoz which summarises his earlier studies,[1] and in an essay by M. W. W. entitled *A Patient's Outlook on Psychotherapy*.[2] The patient is trained to concentrate his thoughts persistently upon successive objects. To this end he sits down with his eyes closed, the left hand on his knee, and must think only of this left hand. He tries to imagine it precisely, to feel its presence although it does not move, and by attention to arouse in it some slight sensation. He continues this exercise for twenty or thirty seconds to begin with, then for a whole minute. Then in like manner he fixes his thoughts on one foot, then on the other foot. In other exercises he fixes his thoughts upon a number, 8 for example, upon its shape, and its factors, without allowing any other thought to distract his mind. Then he passes on to the number 2, 3, or 4. " You obliterate 2 from your thoughts, replace it by 8, and so on." Throughout this period the doctor incites the patient to attend carefully. " You are letting your thoughts wander ; I am made aware of it when I merely touch your forehead."—" It is not my fault ; my thoughts wander of themselves "—" You must pull your thoughts together energetically. . . . Call up in your mind the word ' timidity,' and rapidly replace it by the word ' courage.' "

The patient who has thus been taught to concentrate his thoughts upon simple objects, knows how to guide his thoughts, how to rid his mind of obsessions ; he knows how to forget the pain he has been feeling in his knee by thinking of the knee itself. He knows how to perform a mental action attentively and precisely. " Try to take firm decisions which you will not have to recall, and to do so even as regards the little things of life ; avoid indecision, and avoid arguing with yourself." The patient will cease to suffer from distraction ; he will cease to forget where he has put the objects of which he is in charge. The reeducation of practical behaviour will rid him of the phobias and the obsessions which were the conse-

---

[1] Traitement des psychonévroses par la rééducation du contrôle cérébral, 1911.   [2] Parker's Psychotherapy, III, iv, 79.

quence of this disorder. I think that the methods recommended by Vittoz are sometimes rather strange, but the underlying principle is sound.

Quite a number of other French writers repeat the same sort of ideas, though perhaps with less precision, and without trying to explain the technique of reeducation. Still, reeducation is the central idea of Payot's book [1]; and it is the central idea of the excellent and sometimes more practical advice of de Fleury. The latter writes: " We can derive real advantages from our most undesirable defects, such as vanity and jealousy; we can transform the direction of the energy that animates a fixed idea, so that it becomes a factor of creative energy. . . . We must be careful to avoid giving our patients too distant an objective, for neuropaths are lethargic, and suffer from a sort of myopia of the mind which renders them incapable of seeing anything which is not close at hand. . . . There seems to be a series of hand-to-hand combats between the invertebrate will of the idler and the moral energy of the physician who cares for him." [2] Camus and Pagniez believed that we could learn to will " by the repetition of more and more difficult voluntary actions." [3] Paul Emile Lévy, who is likewise an optimist, is convinced that he will be able to make all the lunatic asylums close their doors, to put an end to isolation, suggestion, and various other disagreeable methods of treatment, by the education of the will and of effort. He considers that all patients, when properly guided, will be able to carry on this education and to make the necessary efforts in their own homes.[4] Grasset draws a distinction between a lower and a higher form of psychotherapeutics, though his reason for doing this is not very clear. Moreover, he likes to speak of treatment by suggestion as an inferior form of treatment—which is a rather childish thing to do. Still, he describes very well under the name of " superior psychotherapy," a form of education which aims " at the culture, the increase, the perfectionment of the will; at self-mastery; at the moral unity of the ego, of the normal and complete personality." [5] Dejerine and Gauckler, in the book they have

[1] L'éducation de la volonté, 1894.
[2] Introduction à la médecine de l'esprit, 1897, p. 262.
[3] Isolement et psychothérapie, 1904, p. 144.
[4] L'éducation rationelle de la volonté, son emploi thérapeutique, 1898.
[5] " Revue des Deux Mondes," September 1905, p. 373.

devoted to the discussion of the ideas of Paul Dubois concerning moral education, of course reecho their master in showing that "the personality must aspire towards the thing to be fulfilled, the ideal to be satisfied. . . . The patient who has rediscovered an aim is no longer a neurasthenic." [1] They teach that the emotional reaction of the personality can become sthenic when it is well accordant with the personality.[2] It is useless, they say, to flee the emotions. The one requisite is to learn how to appraise them. Appraisement will only be possible in so far as the whole personality of the patient has been renewed in a monoideist direction, has been guided towards a practical, philosophical, or religious goal." [3] In all these books we find the same philosophy, but its expression is unfortunately vague, and the reader cannot but feel that he is being presented with rhetorical formulas, which may be instinct with a general truth, but which are difficult to apply.

These works by French authors being fairly well known in my own land, I shall give more space to an account of some little books most of which were published in the United States. They have found readers here, and I think they are worthy of attention. They belong to the trend of thought which is generally known by the name New Thought Movement. The attempts at the moral treatment of disease which pass by this name are really the progeny of the doctrine of the celebrated P. P. Quimby, Mrs. Eddy's teacher. This school had been almost forgotten, but its ideas were revived owing to the success of Christian Science, and in competition with Christian Science.

During the last few years, the New Thought Publishing Company has issued a great many booklets which, from the theoretical point of view, do not appear strictly scientific, but which have a very practical aim, and a lofty moral inspiration. A good many of them have been translated into French, and they have more readers among patients than among medical practitioners. The titles of some of them are suggestive, and give a good notion of the character of the contents. Here are some: Happiness and Marriage; Hygiene of the Brain and the Cure of Nervousness; Experiences in Self-

---

[1] Les manifestations fonctionnelles des psychonévroses, 1911, pp. 424 and 546.   [2] Ibid., p. 319.   [3] Ibid., p. 544.

healing ; Training of Children in the New Philosophy ; The Will to be Well ; The Power of Silence ; Your Forces and how to Use Them. I have space only to mention a few of the names, and to deal with a few of the ideas in this vast collection.

The writings of Horatio W. Dresser and Henry Wood were quoted by William James, who had a great esteem for them. In the books of Hiram Jackson and Richard J. Ebbard we still find reference to the use of hypnotism and suggestion (though of a rather peculiar kind) superadded to moral advice. P. M. Heubner, in his *Perpetual Health, How to Secure a New Lease of Life by the Exercise of Will Power*, insists rather upon efforts of will. The Rev. Samuel Fellows' articles in Parker's *Psychotherapy* (III, ii, 79 ; III, iii, 78) betray the same inspiration. This author mentions various remedies which will ensure sound sleep ; and he reveals to us " how to live a hundred years and be happy." The writers believe in the power of religion for the lengthening of our days ; they advise us to keep before our eyes examples of happy longevity, and to say to ourselves that we feel younger and younger every day. Excellent advice, but perhaps it is not always easy to carry out.

Thomas F. Adkin has published a work upon *Vitaeopathy*. He says : " As I practise it, it is a combination of personal magnetism, magnetic therapeutics, and suggestive therapeutics. . . . I begin treatment directly I look at the patient. The way I fix him in the eyes, and the way in which I grasp his hand, mean : ' I can cure you ; I want to make a good impression on you.' I keep on repeating this phrase to myself. . . . By thus fixing your gaze on the root of the nose, just below the base of the brain, you become fascinating and pleasant, and you convey the mental suggestion : ' You are better ; you will go on getting better from hour to hour.' Add the use of passes, watch the tone of your voice, space out the syllables you utter, . . . be persistently courteous and encouraging. In that way you will cure a great many patients by encouraging them to live, and you will earn a lot of money." The writer is amusingly simple and frank ! What he has to say is typical of this system of treatment which aims at encouragement and is inspired by the cult of success.

William Walker Atkinson, joint editor of the " New

Thought Magazine," has written a book entitled : *Thought-Force in Business and Everyday Life, being a Series of Lessons in Personal Magnetism,, Psychic Influence, Thought-Force, Concentration, Will Power, and Practical Mental Science* (Chicago, 1901). Its aim, the author tells us, is to make widely known the secret forces of the mind. " Do you want to be energetic ; do you want your thoughts to be energetic ; do you want to be brave ; do you want your thoughts to be courageous ? Then say to yourself vigorously : ' I can do so-and-so.' Never say to yourself : ' I cannot do so-and-so.' You can do whatever you will to do—if only your will be sufficiently active. Success and wealth are not reached by pure intelligence, but by the practical exercise of the will. The objection may be made that will power varies much from person to person. No matter ! Your business is to develop your own will power. You must learn to believe in yourself, to become aware of your own potentialities. To this end you must perform definite exercises necessitating the concentration of thought upon some specific object. For instance, one such exercise is to concentrate your thoughts upon some one who is walking in front of you. Fix your eyes upon the back of his neck, and try to make him turn round by the effort of your thought. Think as vigorously as you can that you want him to turn round and look at you. Picture to yourself that he is at the other end of a tube starting from your eyes ; form a concrete image of this tube. In another exercise, one which aims at the development of your personality, you must imagine this personality to have a concrete form ; must imagine that there is a wrapping which ensheathes, protects, and isolates it ; must imagine that no external force can affect it in any way whatever. . . . To develop your will power, you must place yourself in conditions of absolute tranquillity, must become perfectly relaxed and motionless. Then, for five or ten minutes, you must breathe slowly and deeply, must concentrate your attention on yourself, and must keep on repeating to yourself : ' I have no fear ; I wish to remain perfectly free from fear ; I want to rid myself of fear ; I order fear to vanish.' Fix in your mind the written aspect of these two words ' without fear ' ; analyse the state of mind of a fearless man ; repeat these words again and again."

We find similar ideas and similar practical recommendations in a little book by X. Lamotte Sage, entitled *Personal Magnetism, an advanced Course of Suggestive Therapeutics* (New York, 1902). Notwithstanding the title, there is nothing in the book about magnetism or suggestion. For some reason best known to himself, the author chooses to term " personal magnetism " the guiding influence which one mind can exercise upon another. That which most people call a " sympathetic, seductive, dominant " personality, he calls a " magnetic " personality. He writes :

" A subtle and invisible influence emanates from one whose will is firm and strong. This influence controls others far more powerfully than any spoken words could control them. Resolve every day to have a vigorous will, and make up your mind to control others by your will. Determine to succeed. . . . We can develop our personal magnetism to such an extent as to be able to influence 95 per cent. of those with whom we come in contact. The acquirement of this personal magnetism is of supreme importance, for it will give you health, influence, happiness, and wealth. To attain such a power, you must practise certain preliminary exercises, some taking the form of breathing exercises, and others the form of solitary meditation. Above all, you must write out in large letters, learn by heart, and continually repeat, certain important phrases. You must fix your mind on these phrases as you are going to sleep at night, and the instant you wake in the morning. Here are some of them : ' I have succeeded, I shall succeed, I must succeed, nothing can hinder my success, I shall make a success of my life, I cannot fail.'—' My will is strong, no one can resist my influence, I can control others ; they will all love me, and will do whatever I want them to do ; I shall compel them to love me.'—' I shall control myself, I shall never be cast down, morose, or shy.' If you practise such exercises regularly, they will develop your will in a surprising way ; they may seem trifling, but their cumulative effect will be marvellous. . . . Before a business interview, fix your mind on the person whom you wish to influence, make up your mind that he will not be able to go against your wishes, that he will do whatever you want, that he will sell you this, or will buy from you that. If, when you go to see him, you have these suggestions firmly implanted in your mind, your power will be practically irresistible. You must

never be without this energy, this self-confidence ; you must
be animated with it when you shake hands, so that your grasp
shall manifest the strength of your splendid will."

All this is extremely American ; it is a treatment of depression by the persistent affirmation of energy. I have been
surprised to learn of late that these little books have been
read in Paris by patients on the alert to discover anything that
may promise them the energy they lack. Working-class
women attending the Salpêtrière clinic have, I find, made a
practice of carrying about little pieces of paper on which, in
a large hand, were inscribed formulas they would continually
repeat to themselves. " I am strong, very strong, my will
shall be very strong before men, and shall yield only before
God ; no one will be able to resist my influence, I am determined to succeed, I am sure of succeeding." Unfortunately
I have to add that these were poor depressed subjects, painfully
timid women, who had never succeeded in anything at all.

The last book in this category I wish to mention is
W. Turnbull's *Course of Personal Magnetism*. It contains a
remarkably interesting psychological notion of desire, and of
the resources in the way of energy which wishes can procure
if we only know how to use them. Desire in all its forms is,
says the author, a mental current highly charged with energy.
When you yield to desire, you scatter energy, and you
consequently reduce your power of attraction, you discharge
magnetism which you ought to have kept in store. The
force of desire is manifested in a great many mental trends,
such as impatience, anger, prodigality, slackness, and, above
all, vanity. The last trend is the one which is the most
enfeebling, and the one which is almost universally present.

When you feel the current of desire, refuse to yield to it.
By a conscious effort of will you must arrest the enfeebling
discharge, and at the same time you will create a condition,
of attraction which will exist for just as long as the desire
remains unsatisfied. For instance, you feel a desire to do
something which will spread an idea of your importance, of
your talents, of your superiority—this is the desire for approbation. The desire impels you to go against your will, your
judgment, your good taste. It is a mental current which
you can turn to your advantage, instead of allowing it to
discharge itself with a deceptive crackle like the spark of the

static electrical machine. You must repress your desire for approbation, and then you will experience an increasing sentiment of dignity and power. . . . From this point of view nothing is so important as the capacity for keeping a secret. When you know a piece of news, hold your tongue. " A secret is a unit of mental magnetism stored up in the battery of your brain. The keeping of this secret produces a force which will breed force, just as money put away in the bank breeds money ; the more secrets you keep, the greater will be your reserves of energy. . . . Temptations of all kinds are benefits in disguise. If we store up our forces, we strengthen our battery of mental reserve power and increase our personal magnetism. You should not talk of your troubles ; you should not ask for sympathy or flattery ; you should discover the energy that animates your wishes, and be careful not to squander it."

I think that these are very remarkable reflections concerning the balancing of the mental budget. We shall have to return to them, and to show their importance. All the writers of this group have, if I may say so, the same defects and the same merits. They obviously tend to exaggerate a good deal, and they are remarkably simple-minded. They lack both psychological and clinical accuracy, and they do not record any cases which might enable us to check their affirmations. But it is quite true that they have a clear notion of the latent forces of which William James used to speak, and that they make an interesting appeal to psychological excitation as the essential treatment of depression.

Certain other schools were likewise encouraged by the success of Christian Science. The theosophists, whose doctrines I am unfortunately not in a position to study here in detail, have often expressed similar ideas concerning the cure of our weaknesses, as we may see in Annie Besant's book, *Thought Power, its Control and Culture*, 1901.

In the United States, we find a group of doctors and psychologists, quite independent of these various sects, who have studied the same problems in a more scientific and more experimental manner. The various methods of treatment recommended by the members of this school may be spoken of generally under the name of " work cure," proposed by R. C.

Cabot in contrast to the " rest cure " at one time so much in favour in Philadelphia.

Philip Coombs Knapp, of Boston, pointed out as early as 1897 that the best way to cure workers suffering from traumatic neuroses, was to keep them as long as possible at their work, or to send them back to work as soon as possible, instead of making them rest indefinitely, as doctors were inclined to do at this time. Schwab, of St. Louis, declared that among his neuropathic patients there was a need for social life, a need for serious occupation, a need for an ideal outside the domain of their sufferings. He tried to form a circle of some of these patients, to occupy them, to arouse their interest in writing little literary works, to induce them to organise their lives ; and, in many instances, depression and the feeling of incessant fatigue disappeared. Lewellys F. Barker, of Baltimore, when treating neuropaths, is especially inclined to appeal to their interest, attention, and capacity for effort ; and he lays stress upon the valuable effect of stimulating emotions. He says that we should be less concerned with driving away worry and despair, than with the positive step of cultivating hope and love. Joyous emotions, according to him, are the most potent stimulant of body and mind. There is an important future awaiting the therapeutics that appeal to the emotions.[1]

Morton Prince, of Boston, was the editor of and one of the contributors to a very interesting little volume from which we have already made a number of quotations. The other contributors, like Prince himself, are doctors with a special knowledge of psychology who have interested themselves in psychotherapeutics.[2] As introduction to this work he penned a remarkable study entitled *The Psychological Principles and Field of Psychotherapy*, in which he showed that psychological healing must transcend the routine prescriptions of suggestion and rest. " The point of view, the attitude of mind, the beliefs, the habit of thought, must be modified by the introduction of new points of view, of data previously unknown to the patient and drawn from the wider experience of the physician ; by instruction in the meaning of symptoms and in their organisation and causes ; by the suggestion of expectations that justly may be fulfilled ; of ambitions that ought

[1] Barker, On the psychic Treatment of some of the functional Neuroses, 1906.   [2] Psychotherapeutics, a Symposium, 1910.

rightfully to be entertained ; of duties to be assumed but too long neglected ; of confidence and hope ; and, above all, by the suggestion of the emotion and joy that go with success and a roseate vista of a new life." [1]   The same volume contains an essay by Boris Sidis, who adopts a philosophical standpoint, and restates some principles of William James.   This author, Sidis, had already shown an interest in conditions which he termed " hypnoidal," and in which suggestion was at work. In the essay we are now considering he shows that in these hypnoidal states, hidden forces can be awakened.   We tap untouched reserves of energy.   " Far less energy is used by the individual than there is actually at his disposal."   The more complex the organism, the greater is its need for such reserves of energy.   " We must loosen the grip of some of the inhibitions and lower the thresholds, thus utilising a fresh supply of reserve energy. . . . The patient feels the flood of fresh energies as a ' marvellous transformation,' as a ' new light,' as a ' new life,' as ' something worth far more than Life itself. " [2]

I must not forget to mention the authoritative part played in this field of therapeutics by Professor J. J. Putnam, of Boston.   He expounded his views in lectures delivered at the Lowell Institute in March 1906 ; in his *Considerations concerning Mental Therapeutics* [3] ;   and in his contributions to Parker's *Psychotherapy* entitled *The Psychology of Health* (I, ii, 24), the *Philosophy of Psychotherapy* (III, i, 17), and *The Nervous Breakdown* (III, ii, 5).   He also insists upon the importance of effort and work, saying that the best prophylactic against the neuroses is a systematic education which will teach the patient to distinguish true fatigue from false, and will enable him to form a just estimate of his powers.   Sacrifices, responsibilities, effort in self-discipline, efforts to achieve mental progress, give a more comprehensive outlook on life.   Above all, it is important that people should feel themselves to be in relationship with other minds, that they should feel that they are working with others and that they are working for the benefit of society.   Putnam describes a remarkable attempt made by the Massachusetts General Hospital to establish social

---

[1] Psychotherapeutics, a Symposium, 1910, p. 35.   [2] Ibid., pp. 126–132.
[3] Studies of the Neurological Department of Harvard Medical School, 1906, vol. i.

relationships among neuropathic invalids, to encourage them
to make joint efforts, and to communicate enthusiasm to one
another. He says that the success of Christian Science in
this line shows the value of the method.

Finally, Putnam tries to communicate his own enthusiasm
for philosophical studies. He does his utmost to counteract
materialistic and pessimistic doctrines ; he tries to show that
scientific and philosophic concepts of evolution are able to
give us splendid hopes. The nervous troubles which are so
common to-day, will not, he says, continue to develop ; and
in the next century people will have a more stable mental life
than ours. As F. W. Myers already pointed out, nervous
troubles are not always a sign of degeneration, for sometimes
they may be an indication of efforts to effect a new adaptation.

It is interesting to note how widely these ideas have been
diffused. We find an almost identical statement of them in
Alfred T. Schofield's little book.[1] According to this author,
the principal requisites for cure are an increase of hope, faith,
cheerfulness, activity, mental work. At all times, he declares,
the best remedies have been religious sympathy, altruism,
philanthropy, and ambition. We learn from Coleridge that
the best doctor of nervous disorders is the one who can best
inspire the patient with hope.

R. C. Cabot may be regarded as one of the leading advocates
of the work cure. Upon this topic he contributes a remarkable
series of essays to Parker's *Psychotherapy*, essays entitled
The Use and Abuse of Rest (II, ii, 23) ; *Work Cure* (III, i, 24) ;
The Analysis and Modification of Environment (III, iii, 5).
We have already seen that this author is opposed to treatment
by unduly prolonged rest, which, he says, leads to impoverishment. In connexion with our studies upon isolation, we have
noted his observations concerning the influence of environment
and the maladjustments of family life. He says that rest and
peace of mind can be more often secured by a remodelling of
the patient's life than by sending him to a sanatorium.

The most essential part of his outlook is his conception
of idleness and work. Cabot states that the morbid fears of
the neuropath, the patient's mistrust of his stomach, his talka-
tiveness, and his sexual disorders, are the outcome of not

---

[1] Nervousness, a brief and popular Review of the moral Treatment of
disordered Nerves, 1910.

having enough to do. There is a period of growth when young fellows must have something dangerous to do, and their life explodes if we try to confine it in a bottle. How often do we see that people who have led an active life decay rapidly when they retire. Their health breaks down as soon as they abandon the work which has been a natural prop to them. Nervous troubles make their appearance in a woman of forty because her children have grown up, so that they no longer give her any occupation, and she does not know what else to do with her time. To cure nervous patients, we must get them back into the common stream of life, set them to work which will enable them to forget their own sensations. Work will even distract us from misfortune. A woman, immediately after her husband's death, had to take charge of important business affairs. Not only did this enable her to bear her misfortunes, but she was fain to admit that her new life was much happier than the old one had been. Work brings success; the experience of success is one of the happiest in life, and is able to bring health to the neuropath. The doctor must try to find for his patient some pecuniarily profitable occupation, for it is paid work that is the most helpful. Finally, work has social consequences. It brings the worker into contact with fellow-workers, promotes comradeship and cheerfulness, encourages a sense of freedom and responsibility, so that work can even transform the insane, as has been noticed in the Gheel colony.[1] We have to study the patient's earlier career in order to deduce the best methods of guidance and reorganisation. The physician's task would be incomplete, were he to fix his attention upon the immediate symptoms, and were he not to try to regulate the future of those for whose care he is responsible.

Although the various studies I have just been summarising are many of them interesting, their perusal leaves a somewhat confused impression, so that the reader cannot help asking himself if they are not philosophical studies rather than medical investigations. We are reminded of Paul Dubois' method of moralisation, and indeed several of the before-mentioned authors acknowledge their obligations to Dubois. But there is a certain advance upon Dubois, there is the recognition of a notion to whose establishment I have myself

---

[1] Cf. F. Meen, Comptes rendus du Congrès d'Amsterdam, 1907, p. 795.

contributed, namely that neuropathic disorders, and even the majority of mental disorders, depend upon a fundamental alteration of activity. The fault is not so much a disturbance of sensibility, memory, or the reasoning powers, as it is a disturbance of the functions of synthesis, apprehension of the real, and psychological tension. The remedy is not to be found in reasoning, or in moralisation properly so-called, but in the exercise of the most exalted functions, by sthenic emotions, in a word, by excitations. That which aesthesiogenism attempted to do in a manner which, though more precise, was much more restricted, these authors are trying to do in a more general and more practical way. They are trying to enter the field of excitation in which aesthesiogenism was the pioneer.

But it remains true that these studies, in their initial stages, are inadequate. From the psychological point of view they provide hardly any precise indications concerning this phenomenon of excitation, which they aim at utilising. They speak of reserve energies without explaining their nature, their importance, or the way of mobilising them ; they speak of sthenic emotions without explaining what distinguishes them from ordinary depressive emotions. It is difficult to discover in these studies a psychological description of excitation. From the clinical standpoint, the physician remains unsatisfied. The clinician's criticism will be, that his real patients, those suffering from periodic depression or from psychasthenia, those affected with a crisis of doubt, are absolutely incapable of effort, hope, the faith that moves mountains. This incapacity is the very essence of their disorder. It is futile to go on dinning into their ears that they would be saved if they would only believe and hope. Such a truth, such a glimpse into the obvious, is of no use to them whatever. You cannot endow them with these fine virtues by exercises, for they are incapable of being trained. The subjects in whom such methods are successful, are merely idlers suffering from boredom, and not really sick people. If some of them have been ill, the methods in question only cure because the trouble was already on the highroad to cure. —I am afraid that such criticisms have a large measure of truth in them.

That is why I cannot close my account of this particular development without an explanation of treatment by excitation, any more than I could do this in the case of the previous methods of treatment. We shall have first to consider certain clinical studies which will serve, to some extent, to supplement the foregoing.

2. ACCIDENTAL STIMULATION IN THE COURSE OF DEPRESSIVE CONDITIONS.

The problem which faces us in connexion with all these attempts at therapeutics is the problem of excitation, the problem of an excitation that is artificially induced by the doctor. Before considering it, we shall do well to arrive at clear notions concerning the natural excitation which occurs spontaneously in the course of the evolution of nervous disorders. This leads us to consider once more the oscillations of the mental level to whose importance I already drew attention a dozen years ago.

The natural evolution of mental disorders introduces to us a remarkable phenomenon, and one about which we cannot reflect too earnestly. I mean, spontaneous cure. No doubt there are certain individuals who, having once fallen by the way, can never get on to their feet again. In these, the psychological tension gets continually lower and lower, and we have to watch the sad spectacle of a slow but progressive decadence. This is what has given rise to the notion of hebephrenia or dementia praecox. We are usually concerned with fairly young patients, in whom a depression of the psychological tension has occurred during the flowing tide of adolescence. Their depression speedily becomes extreme, and impairs the functioning, not only of the more exalted and more recent tendencies, but also of the more elementary and more ancient tendencies. They pass rapidly from psychasthenic depression with doubts and obsessions, to obstinate asthenic delusions and negativisms; then on to asthenic dementia and complete mental impotence, which soon becomes incurable. Apart from these special cases, we find others in which the subjects, after passing rapidly into a condition of psychasthenic depression, seem to remain indefinitely at the same level. A good while ago I described the case of Boa. (f., 20) as a typical instance of psycholepsy, for, after reading

---

[1] Les obsessions et la psychasthénie, 1903, vol. i, pp. 525-543.

an article in a periodical, this young woman passed rapidly into a condition of depersonalisation and persistent doubt. Twelve years later, she seemed to me to be almost exactly in the same condition as when I first saw her. I could quote quite a dozen similar instances. They are exceptional, however, for in most patients depression manifests itself as a crisis with a definite beginning and a definite end.

We are told that such patients invariably relapse. It is not true. Quite a number of persons have a serious crisis of depression in youth, recover from it, and never relapse. With regard to those who do relapse, is the relapse inevitable ? Perhaps it is in certain instances, when, owing to the evolution of the disease, after a good many relapses, and thanks to the development of an ill-understood kind of automatism, period-icity has become an essential part of the disease. But the remarks which apply to certain forms, as to circular insanity, for instance, must not be extended haphazard to all forms of depression. Most of the patients are persons with inadequate powers of resistance ; they are depressibles and not cyclo-thymics. They relapse when they again come under the influence of causes similar to those which led to their first illness. All that we can say is, that a great many things may, in them, occasion relapse. Still, they have been cured in the interim, and the more or less frequent relapses do not invalidate the essential fact that it has been possible to reestablish their mental level.

When we study these restorations of mental level we usually give the name of " cure " to those which last for a considerable time, such as a year ; and we do not pay much attention to those which are brief, lasting only a month or a few days. But this distinction is not a very accurate one, for the relapse often depends upon special circumstances, and it may be a mere matter of chance which has determined the duration of the good periods. It is quite likely that the temporary eleva-tions in the course of the disease, and the durable elevations at the end of the crisis, are of the same nature, and we must pay the same attention to those of both kinds. I have pointed out before that such " lucid intervals " can be detected in all periods of the disease, but that they are more frequent at the beginning and towards the close of great crises of depression. " Again and again," said Claire, " the light ceased to pass away from me ; it drew nearer to me, I don't know why. When this happened, I knew that I had been making a fool of myself, that I had not really done wrong ; and I no longer suffered from self-torment.   I seemed to have become reestablished ; I had a feeling of faith in God, and returning hope. . . . But only twice did I find my way back completely to the light ; the memory of this kept me going for a long time, for it had shown me the road." [1]

When these ascents are rapid, they resemble a sort of transient intoxication, and they give rise to peculiar feelings of exaltation and ineffable happiness, analogous, though inverse, to the sentiments of incompleteness from which overscrupulous persons suffer.   I have described many phenomena of this kind.[2]   Here are some examples.—Rb. (f., 28), who for six months has been complaining of a persistent feeling of depersonalisation, who is continually tormenting herself with the question whether she has not been transformed into some other and unwholesome being, and who is constantly meditating upon death, is herself greatly astonished by these sudden transformations which appear in the course of treatment by rest and isolation.   " It is extraordinary !   All at once I become myself, I recognise the sound of my own voice ;   my disquietudes have vanished ;   I have confidence, peace of mind, feel quite cheeky."—Noémi, tortured for a year by obsessions of death, suddenly recovers calmness and happiness. " I was cured all in a moment ;   death no longer existed.   I felt a great exaltation, and a superabundance of life.   Last Tuesday morning, I don't know why, perhaps because the sun was shining or because my thoughts were so cheerful, I went on singing for a whole hour, and felt as if I should like to embrace every one, to love every one, and to cry my affection from the housetops."—When these exaltations are excessive, they seem, as we have already pointed out, to exhaust the subject's energy, and to become themselves one of the causes of the subsequent depression.   Dh. (f., 22), has intoxicating feelings of happiness and joy, which make her quite ill.   " In these sensations of joy there is an intensity of feeling which gives me a positive heartache.   The visit of one of my girl friends has caused me so much delight that I have been quite

[1] Les obsessions et la psychasthénie, vol. i, p. 528.
[2] Ibid., vol. i, p. 380.

overwhelmed. Even the next day I could hardly control myself or speak, and all my gloomy thoughts had returned."

I may remark in passing that certain strange theories concerning religious conversion, the theories to which William James attached so much importance, are based upon the study of phenomena of this kind. It is likely that the alleged converts of whom he speaks, and whose ecstatic feelings he describes, were merely patients suffering from depression (though the nature of their malady had not been recognised), who, in the course of religious observances, or under some other strong influence, manifested more or less durable phenomena of excitation, and became inspired with feelings of ineffable delight. Perhaps these phenomena are not of much importance to the theologian, but they are certainly important to the psychiatrists.

Some of these elevations of the mental level must be related to the phenomena we have studied. They must be the outcome of rest, liquidation, economy, usually achieved without the physicians having been aware of the fact. But in other cases we have to recognise that such transformations are brought about by circumstances which compel the subject to act, and to expend energy. The strange thing is, that these circumstances and actions seem, at first sight, to be exactly the same as those which we have previously regarded as obvious causes of fatigue and depression. Here we encounter a paradox of which an ample demonstration must be given, and we shall do well to set forth our observations concerning excitation in the same order as that in which we set forth our observations concerning depression.

Religious Ceremonies. In reviewing the dangerous circumstances of life, we noted to begin with that the first communion in a great many children, and religious practices in many adults, were apt to give rise to doubts, over-scrupulousness, and melancholia. Now, it is easy enough to point to cases in which the effects have been the very opposite. That is what we find in the studies of William James to which I have just been alluding. This author speaks of numerous cures of nervous disorders through religious conversion or religious practices. I shall not dwell here upon cases that have come under my own notice in which a cure was induced by entering a convent, for here the influences at work are more complex. Suffice it to recall that I have seen a good many children and adults regain courage and recover rapidly after hearing a sermon, going to confession, or resuming religious practices which had been discontinued for a considerable time. This is equally true of all religions, and we may say that it is no less true of all superstitions. In four cases I have noted the beneficial influence of spiritualistic beliefs and practices. A hypochondriacal woman, of an authoritarian disposition, with delusions of persecution, was most satisfactorily transformed (to the advantage of her relatives as well as of herself) when she had been accepted as a member of a small circle of theosophists. Those patients who are cured by religion do not often come under medical observation, and we should doubtless hear of them far more often if we were priests or pastors.

Social Functions. Society life is the cause of a good many illnesses taking the form of excessive shyness ; but it can do much good in many other nervous cases.—I have already related how Jean was transformed during a fortnight by a formal dinner to which I compelled him to go.—Sb. (f., 27), abulic and phobic, affected with an insane longing to choke herself by swallowing handkerchiefs or pillows, had no trouble of this kind when she was in very agreeable and amusing society. " I am only well when I go out in good company, and all my troubles return as soon as I am alone at home." —Lydia was cured of a severe crisis of depression the evening before " a great ball where I had to make a fine appearance." Recently the same patient recovered from another and serious crisis in order that she might attend a party given in honour of a friend of hers who had become engaged to be married. —Bs. cannot sleep well unless he has been dining out.— Héloise is transformed by having to make the preparations for a big dinner party.—These phenomena enable us to understand why so many psychasthenics are fond of town life and dread country life.

College Life and Examinations. Intellectual work is by no means invariably harmful.—A talented painter, Rv. (m., 40), can check a crisis of depression by working hard in spite of fatigue, and in spite of severe headache which gets worse when he begins to work.—Tb. (f., 20) knows how to cure her crises of doubt and over-scrupulousness when the first symptoms appear. She simply has to study hard.—Kx. (f., 26), though exhausted and affected with phobias, goes to concerts or lectures, and this often enables her to rid herself of her troubles, "which would have been much worse and would have lasted much longer if I had stayed at home and rested." [1]

Even examinations, which people look forward to with terror, and which seem to be responsible for so much mental depression, will not always be found to deserve their bad reputation. " I never feel so well as at examination times ; an examination day has always been for me one of the jolliest days in my life, for then I am quite free from my over-scrupulousness," says Ud. (m., 25). " After an examination I am generally quite cured for several weeks."—Bkn. (f., 26) is extremely sorry that the examination period of life is over for her. " I was much happier when I had to pass examinations ; it prevented me from being ill, and it did me a great deal of good."

Holidays, Travelling, and Sport. In contrast with what I have said before about the bad effects of travelling and holidays, I must now mention cases in which these have had a favourable influence upon patients. A good many crises of depression in university students will pass off in the month of August during the holidays.—Wkx. (m., 29) is generally much better during this month, which he spends among friends in an inland watering place. " The voyage distracts my mind, and frees me from my customary anxieties. I can only keep myself going by excitation."

Various kinds of sport induce fatigue, and must therefore be considered very dangerous by all of those observers who attach so much importance to fatigue as a determinant of depression. But among my own notes, I find an account of more than twenty cases in which moving about, and even violent exercise, have had a most salutary influence. Patients like Lise, affected with grave obsessions, are well aware of this. " Moving about relieves me of fixed ideas, and motionlessness and rest are dangerous." [2] Horseback riding, boating,

[1] Les obsessions et la psychasthénie, vol. i, p. 532.
[2] Ibid., vol. i, p. 530.

and bicycle riding, will check brooding and morbid anxiety.
—Emma, when in despair after the breaking off of a love
relationship, will climb crags or have " a craze for long
bicycles rides," and she finds that these do her a great deal
of good.—Ms. (f., 35) can only be set right by long walks.
—Tt. (m., 30) cures his crises of depression by long motor
journeys, driving the car himself. " The work of driving a
a car, which seems so fatiguing, is what rests me better than
anything else."

Professional Occupation. Professional work has been
continued by a great many patients throughout a crisis of
depression. Certainly this does not do harm in all cases.
On the contrary, I have noted a good many instances in which
it has done good and has contributed to a cure.—Wkx. complains that his work as a journalist has sometimes made him
ill. It may be so ; but he omits to note the numerous instances,
which have been obvious enough to me, in which his professional
work has supported him and encouraged him, or in which it
has brought him little successes which have transformed
him for months.—Byc. (m., 50) is well aware that he has never
been so perfectly restored as when he has had to put his
shoulder to the wheel and do the work of ten persons at once.
—Though Daniel was so much upset by his work as a soldier,
I could counterbalance his case by twenty others in which
a soldier's life did the patient unmistakable good. But this
is a special matter to which I shall return when I come to
consider the question of moral guidance.

Changes in Mode of Life and in Occupation. One of the
most remarkable modifications occurs in connexion with
change of domicile and with changes in the mode of life and
occupation. Though I have reported six cases in which a
change of domicile was the starting point of serious depression,
I have in my case-book the notes of six other cases, no less
striking, in which a change of domicile effected a cure.
Patients will often say to us : " As soon as I change my
environment and my habits, I become completely free from
my obsessions, and my digestion works much better." The
last remark recalls to my mind numerous cases in which
muco-membranous enteritis, which is so common in patients

suffering from depression, ceased to give any trouble during a voyage, or after a change of environment. We can note the same thing in the case of migraine.

The excitation caused by such changes of environment is very plain in those who suffer from accesses of doubt, for these patients will then recover the sentiment of reality.— When Zb. (f., 23) returns home after being away for a time, she recognises her parents as real, although before the change nobody had seemed real to her. Her brother, who was very ill, made a strong impression upon her. "I found him especially real, and I recognised him better than the others." —Anna (f., 24), who suffered from an extreme and persistent sense of unreality, was delighted when she went to a strange town to find that the houses and the trees were more real than in her former environment. In her case it was possible to turn this momentary elevation of tension to good account therapeutically.

Struggles, Quarrels, Dangers, and Sufferings. Incidents in life which render a struggle necessary, and those which arouse the violent efforts of anger, have worked many cures.—Xb. (m., 26) no longer suffers from tics and no longer stammers when he is angry.—Rk. (m., 20) is freed from his characteristic doubts when he is out of temper.—Lydia, like Dm., tells me that a domestic quarrel does her more good than a strychnine tonic.—I have known quite a number of women patients in whom obsessions have disappeared for several days because they had a quarrel in a tram-car or a scene with their husband.

Actions which render considerable effort necessary may also have a good influence. Patients discharged from hospital and suddenly obliged to look for some remunerative occupation, will occasionally recover at this time in a quite unexpected way.—Ar. (f., 50), always hypochondriacal and querulous, found it necessary to render aid to a young soldier who fell down in front of her door. She cared for him with great attention for several weeks, and to the amazement of her family "she did splendidly."—I have never forgotten a very remarkable incident which surprised me much at the time. Bn. (f., 40), who had become affected for the third time by severe depression, had been ailing for several months, and still seemed to be a long way from the end of the crisis. She was dining with her niece, a young woman nearing the end of pregnancy, when the niece's labour-pains began unexpectedly. There was no one else in the house who could give any help, and all the work of caring for the young woman during child-birth was thrust upon Bn. She felt intensely excited, and thereby was completely restored, so that there was no longer any trace of the previously severe melancholia.—In a great many psychasthenics, acts of attention have a peculiarly stimulating effect. Plo. (f., 30) says : " I have never been able to make up my mind to do anything on my own behalf. I cannot make a beneficial effort unless it is under the delusion that I shall please some one else by what I am doing."

It must be plain from the foregoing observations that the more or less serious dangers to which patients are often exposed will not always have disastrous consequences. The picturesque writer Töppfer, when describing his travels in Switzerland, writes : " It is a great pity that danger can be so dangerous. If this were not so, we should be inclined to seek danger simply for the delight it brings, for the sake of the joyous feelings which accompany deliverance from danger." [1] Marro, in his work on puberty,[2] says : " One who has overcome a difficulty is like one who has passed through an infectious disease ; he has been immunised. "

Elsewhere I have referred to the astonishment with which I noted that one of my patients had come extraordinarily well through a truly alarming catastrophe. The case was that of a young woman who was easily overwhelmed by even trifling emotion, and who became affected by a severe crisis when surprised in any way, even when the surprise was agreeable. On one occasion she was shipwrecked, the vessel running on the rocks in the middle of the night. She remained calm, and showed remarkable courage, rendering valuable service to the women and children among her fellow-travellers. For several months after this incident she remained in excellent health. I have seen a number of similar cases.—Zc. (f. 30), a melan-cholic suffering from depression and with ideas of suicide, tumbled into a well accidentally (so she said), and was almost asphyxiated before being rescued from it. She was trans-formed by the accident. " The cloud has been lifted ; at

---

[1] Töppfer, Voyages en Zig-zag, 1885, p. 215.
[2] La pubertà, etc., see Bibliography.

length I can see clearly again ; I feel that I shall be able to begin a new life." It is true that the depression returned, but not until two months had elapsed.—Wkx. was restored to health for a week thanks to a duel.—Gx. (f., 28), who was continually suffering from hysterical paroxysms, was cured of these after having seen some one fall down in an epileptic fit. Of course this was the inverse of what we usually see.—Justine was transformed because she saw her husband in danger when he was stopping a runaway horse.—We may class among these dangers, the case of one who is trying to carry out a theft. The incident of V. (f., 50), which I have published elsewhere, is typical. We shall have to study this patient's case in connexion with morbid impulses. Enough here to say that for a month V. had been suffering from intense and obstinate melancholic depression. Then, in a large shop, she picked up something and went away without paying for it. The emotions accompanying this theft were so delightful that she felt perfectly well on going out.[1]

During the war I have had an opportunity of making a number of similar observations. By quite a dozen persons, whom I had only known as sufferers from weakness, pusillanimity, and crises of depression, unexpected bravery was shown in wartime. Ba., Francis, and Wkx. became admirable private soldiers or officers, and were themselves amazed at the way in which their phobias and obsessions vanished. Cea. (m., 40), who in civil life has been excessively depressed and gloomy, recovered a healthy poise amid the terrible dangers of the war. " When there was a frightful bombardment going on, the only result was to make me feel the need to write, and it was during these periods that I wrote the best pages of my book."

Finally, and this is a strange thing, physical and moral suffering will often have a stimulating effect in such patients. Georges Dumas describes the transformations which mental suffering will induce in melancholics : " It is mental suffering, not simple sadness, which causes delusions ; mental pain is tonic, stimulating, and evocative. . . . The melancholic who passes from sadness to pain is aroused and stimulated." [2] I may add references to some of my own cases.—" This acci-

[1] La kleptomanie et la dépression mentale, "Journal de Psychologie Normale et Pathologique," 1911, p. 97.
[2] Dumas, La tristesse et la joie, 1900, p. 94.

dental burn has done me a lot of good," said a woman patient who was suffering from depression, doubts, and depersonalisation. "For several days I have felt inclined to burn myself again, in order that I might once more feel a real sensation."—Claire used to say : "I long for emotions, and even for sufferings. I want a distressing emotion which will shake me out of myself, for that picks me up more than any reasoning can do." [1]—Agathe, having been to the dentist, who hurt her a great deal, felt much better, was freed from headache, and no longer saw "rain falling" in front of her eyes (muscae volitantes).—Anna, previously mentioned as affected with morbid doubts, cut her hand while peeling an apple : " I was so much amazed to feel that this hurt me, that I recognised myself as a normal person, and I recovered my personality for two days."—Francis was morally restored by getting his foot crushed : " A real pain does me such a lot of good ; joy does not affect me nearly as much as pain."

The Illness or Death of Near Ones and Dear Ones. We can assimilate to the foregoing facts the moral suffering caused by the serious illness of near ones and dear ones. Under this head I can class the notes of sixteen cases which show us how patients in a serious condition of depression were suddenly improved when they had to watch night and day at the bedside of some one whom they loved.[2] I must also refer to a remarkable improvement in health after the death of the parent, although this misfortune, as we have seen, has in other cases caused serious illness.—" After my father's death," said Claire, " I was greatly distressed, but my real distress caused me far less suffering than the imaginary reproaches of my conscience. I was more energetic and had more will power. The remarkable thing is that I never slept better, for my sleep was calm and free from dreams and nightmares." The same things happened in the case of Justine, that of Sb. and that of Noémi. The last named was freed from her anxieties and obsessions concerning death immediately after the death of her mother. " It was a sort of dismissal, a delightful discharge, an oasis in the desert. The obsession had vanished, and I had a renewed pleasure in the trifles of existence.

[1] Les obsessions et la psychasthénie, vol. i, p. 538.
[2] Ibid., vol. i, p. 537.

Betrothal and Sexual Relationships. I have referred to illness caused by betrothal, but I can adduce just as many cases of cure of illness by betrothal.—Lo. became ill when she married, but her betrothal had done her a great deal of good.[1] —The same thing happened in the case of De. (f., 19), who for years had been obsessed by a dread of the growth of superfluous hair, but who was cured when she became engaged, and could laugh at her former fancies.—Mu., a woman of thirty, abulic and suffering from morbid doubts, was transformed when she became engaged, and did not relapse until the engagement was broken off. I could give many similar instances.

I have also referred to all the trouble that might arise in connexion with marriage and sexual relationships. But I have to show now " that one emotion in particular can act as a remarkable stimulant, the sexual emotion. When these patients experience complete sexual excitation, they recover their energy and their mental unity."[2] I have at least twenty cases in my books to justify this statement.—In relationship with a woman whom he admires and loves, Cea. (m., 40) recovers, at any rate for the first few months of the intimacy, all the enthusiasm and all the facility in literary composition which he used to have during the greatest dangers of the war. " I had all the animation I had felt under heavy gunfire, I was full of love, ease, and delight ; I felt myself a demigod with a heroic temperament."

Simple sexual excitation at sight of a beloved individual will sometimes raise the psychological tension. My notes concerning the remarkable woman patient who always believed herself to be " in a black sepulchre " are very amusing in this connexion.[3] This good woman, though already fifty-six years of age, had a tender passion for a young man who was a student in the hospital. " It is only when I think of him that I am really on earth. When he passes before me, my heart leaps, and I no longer recognise myself ; everything is rose-coloured instead of draped in black ; everything really exists, the sun has come back, I am a woman like others, I really exist instead of being dead. Two hours later everything is black again, and I am dead once more at the bottom of a tomb where there is nothing alive. How stupid it all is ! "

---

[1] Les obsessions et la psychasthénie, vol. i, p. 536.
[2] Ibid., vol. i, p. 537.   [3] Ibid., vol. ii, p. 352.

If we consider love adventures solely from the point of view of mental hygiene we certainly cannot always condemn them.—Fjj. (f., 40), like many others, is well aware that she can only be reestablished in health by fresh love adventures. "This is the only thing which has never failed. Sometimes I try religion, or works of charity, but they are a poor substitute, I always have to come back to the one treatment which really does me good."—Ec. (f., 42) has passed through a number of severe crises of depression. For months she had been inert and plaintive, suffering from digestive disorders, anxiety, insomnia, etc. Then she suddenly got better and her husband was delighted. But this was at the very moment when she had begun a liaison with the husband of one of her women friends. "These mysterious assignations occupy my mind and distract it from its troubles; prevent my thinking of my unfortunate marriage with a good fellow who is so unromantic. . . . When I had seen my beloved that day, I could digest my food well and I slept all night." The intimacy lasted for three years, during which time the patient had no relapse. Unfortunately her lover died, and the depression promptly recurred. After a few months of suffering, Ec. thought she would give religion a turn, and formed the habit of going to see a priest every day. This was the beginning of a fresh intrigue, with renewed "mysterious assignations." The melancholic crises vanished once more. After a year of perfect health, the patient had a fresh stroke of ill luck, for the priest, who was uneasy in the situation, decided to break off relationships and to leave the country; thereupon Ec. fell seriously ill once more. I know perfectly well that erudite psychiatrists will say that in this case the whole story was one of a series of relapses in a case of manic-depressive insanity, and will think that this magical term can save us from having to make such indiscreet reflections. I wish that the word would explain everything, but I cannot help recording, for the interest of psychiatrists of a future day, how singular was the coincidence of the cures with success in love adventures, and the coincidence of the relapses with the close of these!

Héloise (f., 42), a good observer, when she was in the midst of a severe crisis of melancholic depression with persistent insomnia, digestive and circulatory troubles, etc., wrote to me the following letter : " Yesterday, Sunday, I went out driving with some friends, and I dined with a particular friend of mine. He saw me home, treating me with respectful affection. When I went to bed, none of my arteries were beating too strongly or too quickly, and I fell asleep promptly, without taking any sleeping draught. The night's rest was calm and restorative. Although my dinner had been anything but a wholesome one, when I awoke this morning I felt perfectly well. Why have I been thus transformed ? I do not know, but such is the fact." The case is that of a woman whose need for tenderness and intimacy I have already described. She has a constant longing for love, to win affection and admiration, but she rarely succeeds in fulfilling this desire ; or at any rate she does not feel that she succeeds, for her depression prevents her having self-confidence, and compels her to worry herself perpetually. Under the influence of sexual excitation, she becomes more capable of intimacy and self-confidence, and is able to realise her dream, or to believe it realised. Thereupon, all her troubles simultaneously disappear.

Pepita (f., 47) suffers from impulses which may be described as real erotomania. We shall have to study this again presently. The impulses in question have involved her in catastrophes. She has compromised herself with persons of bad character ; she has lost her jewels and large sums of money, and has imperilled the honour of her family. But here we are considering the matter from a strictly medical and therapeutic point of view. The actual fact is that this terrible adventure cured her for two years of a very serious condition of hypochondriacal depression, attended by circulatory disorders—a condition from which she had suffered for several years. " I saw the danger," she said to me, " but I love danger and emotion. With him, there was something new every day ; every day there was some fresh entanglement to get out of, there were new combinations to invent . . . everything attracted me towards him He was a queer fellow and in poor health ; I was his mistress and his mother ; I was responsible for him. He understood me, he was as gentle as a dove, he would feed me with his own hands—or else he would beat me ! There were frightful scenes, horrible scenes of violence ; every day I was afraid he would kill me if he fancied I looked at any one else. But that was life ! No doubt things turned out badly in the end, but I had passed hours in my life never to be forgotten. All my life I have loved adventure, mystery, the unknown ; I need these things ; I need lies, need a life in the midst of intrigues . . . I cannot live a stuffy and monotonous domestic life ; when I do, I feel as if I should go off my head." Unfortunately, she seemed to be right, for she relapsed into illness as soon as her adventure was liquidated, whereas she had been perfectly well during the period of danger. Psychiatry must on no account ignore these important facts.

Children. I need not adduce fresh examples to show that maternity, which is so dangerous so some women, is a safeguard to many others. In a dozen of my cases, young women were cured because they had to devote themselves to taking care of little children.—Qi. was well aware that she had been saved by her son.—Aj., who became very ill at the age of thirty-seven, realised that the reason was that her children had become too old. " When they were quite little, I had to undertake on their behalf maternal duties which were a support to me."—Whilst some women relapse because of their children's first communion, others get better at this period, and acquire a better understanding of religion. Whilst many women are depressed at their daughter's marriage, Héloise improved enormously when she received the visit of a young man who was in love with her daughter.

In a word, all sorts of occasions can be the starting-point of favourable excitation. I may summarise the foregoing remarks in a rather trivial fashion. We know that most of these neuropathic patients pass through a bad time early in the morning when they first awaken, that they usually get better as the day goes on, and that they are at their best in the evening. It is possible that complex influences bring about this gradual daily change. Food and light may play their part. But we must also take into account the accumulation of actions, many of them of infinitesimal importance, which the patient is compelled to do, and which gradually produce a condition of excitation as the day nears its close. Whereas we have previously seen that actions, and especially actions that are difficult, exhaust and depress, we now see that in other cases the same actions may have the very opposite kind of influence. We here encounter a contradiction which raises an important psychological problem.

3. IMPULSES THAT TAKE THE FORM OF A SEARCH FOR EXCITATION.

After having studied the cures which occur accidentally in the course of states of depression, I think we shall do well to pay special attention to certain kinds of behaviour which the patients themselves regard as a salutary treatment, and to which they attach enormous importance, so that at all hazards they are continually trying to repeat such behaviour. The impulses with which certain patients are affected seem to be related to the search for stimulant forms of activity which can restore the psychological tension. I have elsewhere insisted upon this conception of the impulses : first of all, from the general point of view, in my study of the pathogenesis of some impulses ;[1] and, subsequently, in a more specific fashion, in my study of kleptomaniac impulses in persons visiting large shops.[2] The question must be reconsidered here, in order that we may ascertain whether these impulses can give us valuable therapeutic hints.

Patients who suffer from depression of the psychological tension have, as every physician knows, obsessions which express and symbolise their sentiments of incompleteness and their disorders of the will, linked, so to say, to some particular difficulty. But a great number of them are likewise affected with obsessions and impulses of another kind. They are constantly telling us that they think of a desire to perform certain actions, that they long for certain situations ; and they declare that the performance of these actions would do them all the good in the world, and would restore the integrity of their moral energy. " I am in an unfinished state ; I need something which will give me the finishing touch, the sacred fire." The more intensely they suffer from depression, the more strongly do they feel the urge to perform this liberating action. Whereas the impulses related to the ordinary obsessions, such as the imaginary impulses to crime that occur in patients suffer-

[1] On the Pathogenesis of some Impulsions, " Journal of Abnormal Psychology," April 1906, p. 1.
[2] La kleptomanie et la dépression mentale, " Journal de Psychologie Normal et Pathologique," 1911, p. 97.

ing from obsession with over-scrupulousness, are hardly ever carried out, or are realised only in the form of quite insignificant actions—these impulses to perform actions that are stimulant, and are regarded by the patient as salutary, are very often realised, and may give rise to dangerous types of behaviour.[1]

Impulses of this kind are very various, and they cannot all be enumerated here, but I shall group some of them under three heads ; impulses to perform elementary actions related to the inferior tendencies ; impulses to perform social actions of a somewhat higher type ; and impulses to perform moral actions depending upon tendencies of a rational order.

The Search for Elementary Excitation. Among the most typical impulses of the first kind is *dipsomania,* the impulse to consume alcoholic drinks. Equally typical is *morphinomania,* together with other forms of *toxicomania*—the impulse to take morphine or other toxic drugs. But I shall not dwell here upon these particular impulses, for the absorption of the poison complicates the psychological effects of the action. The various toxicomanias will have to be considered later in connexion with the topic of drug treatment. Enough here to recall that what the drug addict is especially in search of is something that will raise psychological tension.—Dr. (f., 33) gives this explanation of her dipsomaniac crises : " I feel very weak and sad ; I lose all hope, I think of suicide. If I drink, it is to set myself up once more ; I am driven to drink by terrible anguish of mind. I drink to lift the shadow which has fallen upon me, and this feeling of deep shadow is so terrible that it overcomes all other considerations. When I drink, it makes things worth while once more, and I find that I cannot live without such a feeling." [2]

I must also mention here *impulses to eat to excess,* although similar difficulties arise in this connexion—the effects of the food that is taken complicate the result. A great many subjects in the early stage of depression have too hearty an appetite.—Ed. (f., 60) recognises by this fact that she is about to relapse into gloom. Very often a slight depression induced by fatigue or emotion will bring on such an exaggeration of

[1] Les obsessions et la psychasthénie, second edition, 1908, vol. i, pp. 56 and 59.
[2] Cf. L'alcoolisme et la dépression mentale, " Séances et Travaux de l'Académie des Sciences Morales," September and October, 1915.

appetite, and I have seen it in neuropathic children at the time of the first communion.—In some cases, this exaggeration of appetite reaches the pitch which is termed bulimia, then taking the form of an impulse to eat continually, and incredibly large amounts.—Fc. (f., 26) never leaves the house without taking with her a large bag stuffed with food, in order to provide for her most pressing needs. "I have to eat continually; bread, ham, chocolate, sugar. Whenever I have a chance as I go about I steal onions, green stuff. Nothing else keeps me alive; if I did not take this precaution, I should fall down after ten steps." It is interesting to note that the bulimic impulse replaced the impulse to drink wines and spirits which the patient had had when she was eighteen during a first crisis.

These impulses to the activation of an elementary tendency can arise without the absorption of any stimulant substances. In my first study of the topic, published in 1906 in the " Journal of Abnormal Psychology," I referred to the remarkable case of an *impulse to seek for and induce pain.* I have described also the strange feeling of happiness, akin to religious ecstasy, which a young woman of twenty, Nea, procured for herself by pouring boiling water over her hands and feet.[1] She knew perfectly well how absurd this behaviour was, and in a remarkable letter she apologised for what she had done, but she added : "What was I to do ? I knew that this would make me feel alive once more, that this would restore me to myself, and I could not resist the impulse." Such an impulse is rare in so complete a form, but it exists in a mitigated form in a great many psychasthenics, who feel an urge to pinch themselves, or to bite their hands till the blood comes, simply in order that they may feel something.

In the same article, I refer to the case of Ms. (f., 35), who, after having suffered from crises of bulimia, suddenly ceased to demand vast quantities of food, and became subject to another impulse, that of *dromomania.* She went on walking for an indefinite time. "I know perfectly well that I must walk at least thirty miles on the high road in order to feel transformed. Then I am more at my ease, and I begin to become a living person."[2] This impulse to walk sometimes

---

[1] Les obsessions et la psychasthénie, second edition, 1908, vol. i, p. 58.
[2] Ibid., vol. i, p. 56.

gives rise to vagrancy of a peculiar kind—which I call "fugues."
Hc. (m., 51) has made several of these extensive fugues.   In
one of them he walked all the way from Paris to Lille.   " This
impulse to vagrancy," said he, " always develops in the same
way.   I become intolerably bored.   Everything seems heavy
and tiresome ; everything is dead ; the world is worthless,
and I myself am worth less than nothing."   (Here we have
sentiments of incompleteness, feelings of depression.)   " I
then feel the need of moving actively about, I have an irresistible and almost insane desire to do something which will
cure me quickly and infallibly of this intolerable torpor.   I
try to take precautions against myself, to prevent myself from
starting off.   I lock myself into my room and throw the key
out of the window.   But this is of no use.   I take off the lock,
I don't know how, for I can never recall the early days of my
crisis."   (In this patient, the beginning of the attack takes a
hysterical form, so that he has no more memory of what has
happened than if he had been in the hypnotic state.)   " All
I know is, that I come to myself several days later on the
high road.   I am bubbling over with enthusiasm ; it is a lovely
night ; the country is beautiful ; everything is for the best
in the best of all possible worlds ; all I want is that some one
should give me work to do, and I am convinced that I should
do it splendidly.   I have not the grit to stop all at once so
pleasant a walk, and I continue my peregrinations for several
days, always rejoicing that my cure becomes more and more
assured."—Akin to this impulse towards vagrancy, this impulse
to move the limbs, are the different forms of mania for sport
described by Tissié of Bordeaux.   I have myself recorded
several examples of the kind.

One of the most important manifestations of the impulse
to secure elementary excitation is the *search for sexual excitation*,
which gives birth to the various forms of erotomania.   In this
connexion, we must be careful to avoid confounding with the
genital impulse, properly so called, all the impulses to search
for love, to search for adventure, or to search for devotion—
for in these latter the genital functions often play a very minor
part.   In true erotomania, the patient seeks excitation mainly
in the actual practice of coitus, independently of all the social
actions which pave the way for the act of intercourse.   These
impulses may take the form of solitary masturbation, homo-

sexual coitus, or heterosexual coitus, with very little regard to the personality of the sexual partner or the circumstances attending the sexual act.

I shall not repeat the descriptions I have already given of these impulses. It will be enough to lay stress upon two characteristics. First of all, the impulses only arise in periods of depression, and after a certain number of symptoms of depression have already made their appearance. In the second place, it is obvious that the patients seek solace in these activities, and believe that they will find a cure therein. In actual fact, such genital activities often provide an excitation which frees them from some of their troubles, temporarily at least. Women will behave quite properly at times, when they still retain a fair amount of interest in their daily life and in their households. " They go on the loose because they no longer take interest in anything."—Ib. (f., 23), after a series of fatigues and emotions, became slow and inert ; she felt herself to have been abandoned without any guidance ; she no longer knew how to live. " I cannot go on living like this, without interest in anything or anybody." She gave herself up to complicated love affairs, and would have as many as five lovers at once. " For a long time this has sufficed to make me happy and able to work hard."—Jca. (f., 25) says : " The doctors make me tired with their remedies and their regimens. When I am really in love, I no longer suffer from enteritis. The doctors know nothing about that ; they do not know anything about real life."—Pepita, at the age of fifty, still cures herself in the same way of her crises of visceral congestion and enteritis. She says : " I am only really well when I am man-hunting.'

The search for genital excitation, like the impulse to drink, may be combined with the need for walking and for physical agitation of which we have already spoken, and may give rise to fugues. Yd. (m., 32) is greatly upset when reprimanded at the office. In his case the latent period of emotion, the period of incubation, lasts from twenty-four to forty-eight hours. At the end of this period, he can no longer keep quiet where he is ; he feels an urge to go out, to breathe freely ; he can no longer work, he is stifled if he sits in the office or in his own house. Soon, then, we shall find him in the streets of Paris, wandering about by day and by night at the doors of the studios and at the gates of the barracks, " searching for an ideal friend." He finds his way into the slums ; exposes himself to terrible dangers ; plunges into debauchery. After two or three days of this kind of life, he emerges, worn out but serene. " I am cured of all my black thoughts, and am able to work hard once more, for my physical and moral distresses have disappeared. "

The Search for Social Excitation. The more exalted tendencies, the social tendencies, can also, in depressed persons, become the starting-point of various impulses. In the previous chapter, apropos of isolation, I described the impulse to dominate, the impulse to search for love, as well as the impulse to tease and torment others, the impulse to disparage others; and so on. I need not return to these matters. In that chapter, after describing some of the impulses, I studied the effect they had upon the patients' associates, and showed how depressing an action they exercised upon the other members of the family. Now we have to consider these same impulses, and certain kindred impulses, from another point of view. We have to enquire to what extent the patient regards them as advantageous to himself ; to what extent he finds in them, or believes himself to find in them, a source of excitation.

Such satisfaction is obvious in persons of a domineering temperament. They are absolutely delighted when they can secure servile obedience from others, and when they can humiliate others. " You are quite right when you say that this is very distressing to my daughter, and that I make her cry ; but it does not matter much to her, and it does me a great deal of good."

I need say little more about the frequent morbid impulses which take the form of *detraction, ill-nature,* and *cruelty.* I have already pointed out that, underlying this urge to degrade others and to make others suffer, there is, above all, concealed the urge to uplift oneself.—When Lox. (f., 40) finds it impossible to speak of another woman without saying that the latter cannot keep her house properly and fails to look after her children, this is because Lox. is thinking of herself in contrast, and wants us to realise that she is an admirable housekeeper and that her attention to her own children is unparalleled. When such detractors say that the merits of other persons are really merits of no importance, it is because they are afraid that they themselves lack these particular qualities.—When Gh. (m., 30) tells us how self-seeking retail traders are, and how they will move heaven and earth to gain a halfpenny, that is because he is himself incapable of gaining a halfpenny, and because he is forestalling possible criticism. Such detraction is invariably a form of boasting.

The mania for *teasing* and *tormenting*, and the mania for *making scenes*, are sources of enjoyment and excitation to many patients. " Scenes " says Ud. (m., 25), " change the current of my thoughts and do me an infinite amount of good. The floods of tears I shed, and the floods of tears I make others shed—without them I could not work, I could not live. They do me all the good in the world."

Love, as we have seen, consists for the majority of such persons of an assemblage of acts of complaisance, of efforts to interest, of compliments and of flatteries, which, substantially, are nothing more than excitation. That is why depressed persons are always wanting to be loved. That is why they are perpetually tormenting those with whom they associate to embrace them and to caress them. " She is always playing the martyr, and she continually raises beseeching eyes to me asking ' you do love me, don't you ? ' "—Gh. (m. 30) spends all his days following young working women about the streets, hoping to make a conquest. He wants a woman to love him, to cajole him, to console him. He has no friends, and he needs some one who will understand him. He will be satisfied with a kindly look and a promise of love. " This would buck me up, and give me new courage. I remain for hours in a sort of vague stupor, awaiting the sweet sensation of warmth which preludes recovery. If I spend my time going up and down the streets, it is in order to draw from certain persons' looks a little of this warmth. Then I feel well ; I am no longer shy ; I no longer stammer. Then, wherever I go, I am well received."—Another patient says : " Why does not my husband look at me when I sit opposite him at a dinner party ? Why does he not become uneasy when I talk to another man ? Why does he not pay me compliments upon my new dress ? If he cannot do this, I must really find some one else who will do it, and do it well ; for that is the only thing that will restore my peace of mind."—Héloise, a woman of forty-five, says : " I am lively, cheerful, can laugh like a child. I am still as bright as a little girl, and can play with every one like a kitten. Why does no one notice it ? Why does no one pay me compliments ? I have such a craving to be adored, that I feel as if I must die for want of it. I need to be complimented ; I cannot live without this. If people pay me compliments I become natural, amiable, reasonable, just like any one else. When I am with my husband and my daughters, who make light of me, I nearly go off my head."— Another patient says : " My need is that some one would need me."—Another : " I want to be some one's god."—Another : " I do wish that some one would come and look me up ; I'm sick to death of having to run after other people."—Another : " What I want is that I should have an effect upon some one ; that my arrival should produce a vivifying effect, and bring joy and sweetness. This has been my dream since early childhood."

Another point has to be considered. One who succeeds in inspiring love, has made a conquest, has triumphed over some one. " Love," says Emma, " is the only thing which sustains a woman's life, for it is the only thing in which she can really succeed by her own unaided energies. I need to flatter some one, to cajole some one, in order to make a conquest. This is an important operation in the case of my friend, Mr. X., a rather ferocious person of a superior type, cold and correct, with the reputation of being a misogynist. When I am able to say to him, ' You are my ivory Christ ' without his being outraged, I have achieved a signal success. It does me so much good to work towards this end. It relieves me of doubt more than all your remedies."

Why do these patients continually demand that their lovers should have exceptionally fine qualities ? Simply in order to increase their own sense of security, and their own feeling of triumph, for it is more advantageous and more flattering to one's self-esteem to be loved by a person of superior type.—" It is not enough to be able to flirt," said Emma, " One must be able to flirt with persons of superior type ; that is what bucks one up ; one cannot live without that."—Héloise : " The more lofty the object, the more does pride aspire to the conquest of it. I should be crazy with joy in my humility, to be the chattel, the mere chattel, of a man of note ; to see him shine ; to spare him all trouble ; to spoil him ; even to endure that he should deceive me, provided only that he was happy. He must have need of me, and must at the same time be superior to me. There is no contradiction here. God is superior and independent, and yet he needs the love of his creatures. If any one were of no account, he would be nothing more to me than a leech, and I could not love him ; I should feel him to be inferior, to be a weakling like myself, to be seeking his own ends. My ideal is to find a strong being, one who is self-poised, one who himself needs to give, to lean down, to accept these tendernesses which are not incompatible with strength. This being must have a need to share ; he must need that I should need him ; he must need to give me joy, and must not claim anything else." What a strange and involved kind of self-deception is this ! How she deceives herself concerning what she really desires, which may be defined as " to be loved for one's own sake." This poor woman, very intelligent, but extremely depressed, does not dare to say simply that what she wants is to meet a being who is very rich, who possesses everything, and who is capable of giving her her heart's desire without asking anything in return.

This need for approbation and for social success which underlies the majority of amorous impulses, can also be manifested in isolation in numerous other ways. These patients, without concerning themselves with love properly so called, make a claim for perpetual congratulations and everlasting praise from the society in which they find themselves. To secure this, they are obliged to make a show of themselves, to attract attention, even by eccentricities ; to extol themselves at every moment.—Zoé (f., 26), when she had been depressed by the death of her mother, endeavoured to attract attention, a thing she had not done before. She uttered lamentations that her mourning prevented her from showing herself off to advantage ; she was constantly fishing for compliments, even regarding the shape of her legs.—Bfa. (m., 27) recognised that his character had completely changed, that he was making himself ridiculous among his comrades by his absurd desire to show off and to ask for incessant compliments.—Héloise, in her most serious period of depression, exhibited a remarkable aspect. She had a perfectly childish vanity which conflicted strongly with her vigorous intelligence. She passed her time in explaining at great length that she occupied a splendid position, was very rich, had all sorts of fine acquaintances, was possessed of many merits and perfections, was full of devotion to others. " Morally I have a beautiful nature and am perfectly loyal, which is rare among women ; I am capable of everything that is grand and fine when I know that this will be appreciated." She would retail the names of all the great persons who had overwhelmed her with letters and attentions, would speak of all the declarations of love she had received or was about to receive, would enumerate all the little compliments which had been paid her. She felt moved to come and tell me that her masseuse had complimented her upon her shoulders. " If I have so much need of compliments," she said, in excuse, " it is because nothing but compliments can make me feel like other people, whereas everything which humiliates me is bad for me and throws me back into my morbid self-depreciation."

All this display of extraordinarily simple vanity is a product of disease. It is necessary to recognise the fact, and to realise that the vanity will disappear as soon as the depression passes off. Then we are astonished to see these women in quite another character ; they become so discreet that we can hardly recognise them. The disposition to demand a great deal of attention, and to display ridiculous vanity, used to be attributed to hysteria ; and Charcot would speak of these patients as " the patients with the red ribbons." There is a misunderstanding here. The trait in question is characteristic of depressions of the mental level below a certain point, although the intellectual integrity is unimpaired. If hysterical people often present this trait, it is because they are depressed and not because they are hysterics.

The same persons will constantly try in every possible way to secure social success. In this connexion I may mention a form of illness which is not very well known, the impulse which leads certain patients to undergo overwhelming fatigue in order to succeed as conversationalists, or to shine at social functions. Sometimes this impulse will manifest itself in any environment, and will be exhibited towards any chance comer.—Pepita wants to please every one, even in the street, " even to please a good old woman whom I meet by chance." She tries to make a conquest of any stray person she may encounter.—We find the same impulse in a yet stranger form in Kb. (m., 29). He says: " I have always had a horror of making enemies, and I need to win sympathy at all costs." For some time he has been tormented by a strange impulse to talk to all and sundry and to produce a good effect on them by his conversation. Since his occupation makes it necessary for him to take a great many journeys by rail, he resolves before he starts that he will not say a word during the journey. But directly he gets into a railway carriage, he loses his balance and feels irresistibly impelled to begin talking that he may astonish his fellow-travellers, and may make a conquest of the compartment. He forgets that he is only a petty commercial traveller. He assumes the role of a great politician whom he admires, adopting this man's tone and phraseology. Thus he exposes himself to a thousand disagreeable adventures, and when he returns home he is in despair because he has made himself ridiculous once more.—Similar phenomena occur even more frequently in society life. A great many women know that they need rest; but they cannot rest, for they prepare for their parties as if these were battles, and every visit exhausts them for several days. " At any cost, I must do everything that will make me perfect in the salon, and will enable me to resemble Madame Récamier or Ninon de Lenclos." The same impulse recurs in the perpetual and vain search for reputation and glory.—Some, like Gp. (m., 30), who is gloomy, discontented, and ashamed of his body, will engage in dangerous sports which give them no pleasure, in which even the bodily movement gives them no excitation, simply in order to make themselves remarkable for their courage and to win fame. Others are obsessed with the idea of immense wealth, and are animated by an impulse to pile up money " in order to make a splash which will astonish the world." Others combine these various impulses, exhibiting a strange mixture of grandiose and childish ambitions.—Ye. (m., 28), who had been intelligent and brilliant up to the age of twenty-one, became exhausted by sexual excesses and a prolonged attack of gonorrhoea. First of all he suffered from brief crises of psycholepsy, from the age of twenty-one to the age of twenty-six; then he passed into a condition of depression which was more or less masked by agitation and by ambitious impulses. This young man, though he had been a reasonable fellow, now launched out into a number of risky financial enterprises in which he wasted his means. He tried to justify himself by expounding his schemes in interminable discourses. He said : " I want to undertake all kinds of things at once, and to make an astonishing success everywhere. I want to resume my studies and to write important works on history, literature, philosophy, political economy. . . . I want to make a voyage round the world, for I have some negotiations I must undertake in order to find capitalists who will help me to carry on a number of great mining enterprises and to arrange for the drainage of various marsh-lands. . . . I shall become a great advocate and I shall make myself a reputation in parliament. . . . I shall undertake important patriotic tasks, which will need the possession of a considerable fortune, will need relationships with various persons of note and the finest attainable moral and intellectual qualities. . . . I shall have a son who will succeed even better than I shall do." We must not, by such a farrago, be led astray ; we must not be content with a diagnosis of agitations and delusions. He is fully aware that he is exaggerating, that he is absurd. He knows that he is really ill, and that his main desire is to find some one who will go on listening indefinitely while he talks. " When I say that I want to become a great man of business, an amazingly successful man of the world, substantially what I want is merely to become a man once more." His main trouble is a state of depression, and an impulse to restore his mental level by boasting.

The Search for Adventure and Danger. In most cases, neuropaths are very timid, and we are rather astonished to find that some of them have a strange taste for danger. Aj., like Irène, is fond of being in a noisy crowd, takes pleasure in passing along streets where the traffic is congested. " I want to see accidents, I want to see dogs being run over ; this does me good even though it makes my head ache." In amorous impulses, which are of so complicated a character, we can detect a psychological factor which, when isolated, may undergo a marked development. I refer to this same impulse to seek adventures and dangers. Emma is well aware that such a factor is at work in the excitation which love assignations give her. " Oh, yes ! the flesh is weak, but that is not the main point. The alarm and the shame which the most trifling peccadillos entail are so delightful that I never get tired of yielding to this temptation. It is agreeable because I feel that it is wrong. This fills me with fear, with remorse, makes my heart beat fiercely, and in the end brings me a peace of mind and a confidence in life which last a long time." These are phrases which the moralist will find it difficult to understand; but the psychologist knows well enough that painful depression, with its doubts, its disquietudes, and its anxieties, does not vary directly with remorse, and that it existed before the wrongdoing. On the other hand, wrongdoing and remorse may stimulate the mind, may dispel depression and restore tranquillity.

The lure of adventure and danger often decides the behaviour of depressed individuals. I have already described patients who fling themselves into adventures which conflict with common decency, who tell us that they need the experience of impropriety, that they need to get out of the ordinary rut, if they are to be able to breathe freely.[1] Since I first drew attention to this I have had occasion to watch more serious instances of the same phenomenon. These impulses to seek adventures are a sub-variety of the impulses to seek excitation, and therefore they are more easily realised than the imaginary criminal impulses of over-scrupulous persons. For this very reason they are more dangerous. Cdo., a woman of thirty-one, who for a long time had suffered from neuropathic disorders, but whose behaviour had been perfectly correct in a very conventional environment, suddenly ran away from home, and after five days she was discovered by the police in a brothel of the lowest kind. She had no amnesia ; she related her misadventures and her miseries during these five days ; she fully realised the madness of what she had done, regretted it, and begged us to charge it to the account of mental disorder. But she felt obliged to admit to her doctor that she had been in search of happiness and had found it. " At any rate I was alive for a few hours. I found my own personality, and I did not pay too dearly for my discovery."

Pepita's case, to which I have already referred more than once, was even stranger. She was a woman over forty. Her husband was in a good position. She had two charming chil-

---

[1] Les obsessions et la psychasthénie, vol. i, pp. 541 and 552.

dren. Her social circle was wealthy and strait-laced. But for two years she carried on a double life which would hardly have been thought possible outside a novel. At home she was the respected mother of a family, but was gloomy and plaintive because she continually felt ill and unhappy. Simultaneously, outside the home, she was engaged in the most complicated intrigues. She had secret correspondence addressed to her at all sorts of accommodation addresses. Almost every day, and very often at night, she spent her time with and shared the life of a ne'er-do-well, who was a thief and was addicted to absinthe and ether. She cared for him tenderly when he was worn out by debauches and when he was dead drunk. She made unheard of exertions to get money for him in the most complicated ways, pawning or selling her jewelry and trinkets. She borrowed large sums of money wherever she could, and engaged in commercial enterprises which bordered upon frauds. When, after two years, her double life came to light, her family were positively amazed.

Cases as remarkable as this are not to be met with every day, but the same temperament explains the behaviour of a good many patients. I think, for instance, of those who take to smoking opium. " It is not that I find it particularly pleasant," said Emma, " but I like to do extraordinary things ; it is so jolly to let one's whims run away with one."—Similarly with those who have a passion for litigation. " Look here," said Héloise, " these law-suits, and the emotions they arouse, have thrilled me through and through, so that I find it impossible, now, to spend my time doing needlework while sitting under a tree with father and mother."—The same taste is exhibited by persons who have a passion for gambling. Marro has pointed out how this passion plays a great part in depressed persons.[1] Lydia and Léa have a passion for losing money in all the lotteries. " I know it costs more than other remedies, but it is much the best cure."—Finally, we can see like tendencies in all those who detest a bourgeois existence ; who have a love for playing a part in a tragedy ; who believe themselves to be budding Pascals.

Akin to the impulses we have just been considering are others which are perhaps less familiar, but which are very interesting in connexion with the study of stimulant impulses.

[1] La puberté, 1902, p. 282.

I refer to the impulse to steal things in large shops, what is known as *kleptomania*. In an earlier work, I have recorded a good many cases of the kind.[1] One such case was the remarkable one of a woman who had been depressed and saddened by a very strict regimen, and who had a mania for drinking coffee to the accompaniment of eating stolen rolls.[2] Since then I have had clearer proofs of the stimulating influence of theft, and have penned a special essay on the subject.[3]

The important detail in Madame V.'s case is that I had known her for several years before she gave any sign of this particular perversion. When she was fifty years of age she was subject from time to time, after emotion and fatigue, to crises of depression taking a melancholic form and attended by insomnia, constipation, complete abulia, inertia, and obsessive over-scrupulousness. It was a typical instance of recurrent melancholia. I had watched her in two such crises—one of which lasted six months and the other eight months.

Eighteen months after the end of the latter crisis, the old symptoms recurred. There was the same insomnia, the same constipation, the same over-scrupulousness, the same feeling that all her perceptions were, so to say, veiled. I expected a crisis of depression fully identical with the previous ones, and having a duration of about six months. But, to my great surprise, within a few days she said that she was perfectly well again, and she no longer came to consult me. Seven months later, her son arrived, utterly aghast, to tell me that his mother had been arrested, red-handed, while stealing in a department store. A search made at her house had disclosed a vast quantity of stolen articles which she had never used, and from which even the price-tickets had never been removed.

The poor woman explained that during the early stage of the crisis of depression, the beginning of which had come under my notice, a lady friend had taken her on a shopping expedition. She was quite uninterested ; and, simply in order to buy something while she was there, she picked up from one of the counters a little brooch which her friend wanted her to buy. She looked round for a salesman in order to settle the purchase, but did not see one disengaged at the moment. Her friend failed to notice that the patient had not paid for the brooch. Holding

---

[1] Névroses et idées fixes, 1898, vol. ii, pp. 197 and 202.
[2] Ibid., vol. ii, p. 194.
[3] " Journal de Psychologie Normale et Pathologique," 1911, p. 97.

the article in her hand, she followed her friend to another part of the shop. After taking a few steps, she became uneasy, for she fancied that she might be regarded as a thief and was greatly moved by this idea. The emotion thus aroused was the first strong feeling she had had for a long time. She could think of nothing else than this remarkable fact, and went on walking about the shop, overwhelmed but deliciously thrilled. In fact, she was infinitely better, and when she returned home (taking the stolen brooch with her) she was able to work once more, and to look after her household affairs. She had recovered energy and good-humour, and was filled with the hope of cure.

This unlooked for excitation only lasted for one or two days. Depression returned, and Madame V. could not help recalling the emotion she had experienced in the shop. Though in general during her illness she was unable to make up her mind to anything, she found it quite easy to go back to the same shop. " I went there to see if I should feel just what I had felt before." Having arrived there, despite a vigorous moral resistance she gave way to the longing to attempt a new theft. She succeeded perfectly, and cured herself thereby for several days. Since then, she had been continually inveigled into repeating the cure. " I could not get on without doing this thing which would bring me relief."

To summarise what happened, I may repeat that she had had two attacks of mental depression, the second exactly like the first, one lasting six months and the other eight months. A third attack, beginning in the old way, was checked for eight months, during which time the patient was dominated by the impulse to theft, and the depression came on once more as soon as the impulse was checked. This case affords a clear demonstration of the intimate relationships between the impulse and the depression. It is obvious that the impulse derived its force from the need for excitation, a need which developed in the course of depression ensuing upon sentiments of incompleteness.[1]

Instructed by this case, I looked for the same characteristics in other cases of kleptomania and found them in seven instances. The most typical of these was that of Mc. (f., 25). She had had a first crisis of depression at the age of nineteen. After this,

[1] " Journal de Psychologie Normale et Pathologique," 1911, p. 103.

she remained inert and querulous for six weeks, began to drink to excess, and to give herself to casual lovers. " I went on the loose to distract my mind, and found the remedy very successful." In a second crisis, which supervened when she was twenty-five, she tried another remedy, for instead of giving herself up to sexual irregularities, she took to stealing in large shops, the excitement of this playing the same part.

In two other instances, theft was complicated by the addition of another form of social acitivity which was found equally stimulating.—Nd. (f., 17) stole all sorts of little objects, penholders, scissors, thimbles; but she promptly gave them away to schoolchildren, in order to pose as a lady bountiful. After these little successes she was relieved of the intolerable sadness from which she used to suffer when menstruating.— Oc. (m., 38) practised thefts of a much graver character, stealing hundreds of francs from his employer's till. He did not save up this stolen money, but used it in treating all his comrades and even casual acquaintances. " I paid for their fun." The strange thing was that he drank very little himself. He had no need of alcohol to raise his spirits, for the success of his trivial generosity and the emotion attached to spending the stolen money, caused him "a delightful excitation, which relieves me of my timidity, my stammering, my cowardice, and gives me the pleasure of feeling myself for the moment a real man." [1]

Another case of kleptomania, that of Len. (f., 38), shows us how the impulse to theft which had played an important part in several crises of depression, was replaced in subsequent crises by more or less serious *attempts at suicide*. Having noted the fact in this instance, I was led to enquire whether, in other cases, attempts at suicide might not have been undertaken for their stimulant influence. The circumstance is difficult to verify, but I have no doubt that it occurred in a remarkable case which I reported to the Société de Psychologie. —Pd. (m., 17) was suffering from intense gloom, with inertia and indifference. He himself spoke of the condition as " a crisis of boredom." In order to relieve himself of this condition, he tried, so he said, drink and going on the loose, for six months, without success. Then he made up his mind to kill himself. Directly he had definitely determined upon suicide, he felt much

---

[1] Cf. " Journal de Psychologie Normale et Pathologique," 1907, p. 348.

happier. The thought of death, thanks to the emotion by which it was attended, proved far more stimulating than all his previous excesses. When writing pathetic farewell letters to his friends, he felt enormously better. He found it delightful to fire a shot from his revolver at his image in a mirror. When, at length, he shot at his material body, inflicting a very trifling wound, he had at that moment a genuine delight such as he had not experienced for a long time.[1]—It is clear that in ordinary cases the impulse to suicide has no such character, but it is quite possible that this happens occasionally.

We may assimilate to the cases just described, those of the patients who feel a *need to frighten themselves*, to cause themselves moral suffering, by perpetually keeping before their mind some painful thought or some gloomy spectacle. I have often had occasion to point out phenomena of this kind in connexion with the mania for going into lofty and dangerous places which is so characteristic of many patients suffering from obsession. Georges Dumas, in his book, *Troubles mentaux et troubles nerveux de guerre*, records a number of interesting cases of this kind. He writes : " The impulsive ideas of crime which he hardly ever puts into effect are useful to him through the emotion he experiences when he dreads performing the crimes, although he knows perfectly well at the bottom of his soul that he will never yield to these impulses. . . . In the doubt and vagueness of his thoughts, he felt the need for a strong emotion which would readapt his mind to reality. . . . He thought of the horror of the pinewood, feeling simultaneously fascinated by it and terrified by it ; he struggled against returning to this wood, but he was well aware that he would be vanquished in the struggle, and the presentiment of his defeat toned him up even while it made him suffer. . . . There, filled with voluptuousness and horror, he refreshed his depressed nervous system and his enfeebled will by looking on the dead." [2]

The Search for Intellectual Excitation. I must point out that in these patients we sometimes find a group of impulses of a loftier kind, impulses to the exaggerated exercise, and sometimes to the quite unregulated exercise, of the loftiest

[1] Cf. " Journal de Psychologie Normale et Pathologique, 1907, p. 347.
[2] Op. cit., pp. 28 and 31.

tendencies of the human mind; religious, moral, or scientific tendencies. We shall find the same characteristics in these impulses, as in those we have just been studying. In certain scenes of religious enthusiasm, as in the revivals described by William James, it would seem that sexual excitation is adjoined to religious excitation. I do not think that this occurs as a general rule; in many instances we can note that a cure of depression has ensued upon practices or feelings that are purely religious in character. It is obvious that many patients regard religion as a means of refuge from their depression.—Madeleine, the ecstatic of whose case I hope to publish a detailed study, suffers from constitutional depression, and is persistently liable to crises of doubt and abulia. In order to find comfort, she pursues God in order to implore him to succour her. " I feel that it is in a successful prayer, in a successful communion, that I shall find my lost joy." She does, in fact, rediscover this lost joy, for her crises of doubt are interrupted by periods of religious ecstasy and of intimate delight experienced in the contemplation of the divinity.

The search for moral perfection can play the same part as religious practices, and it is easy to show that it may become impulsive in depressed patients. Moral declamations are common.—" I have reached a point at which I have need to perform some great action. That will cure me."—" I am never so well as when I have done a good action. The 'ideas' of Plato, the chastity of the early Christians, that is what pleases me just now, it is to these that I would gladly turn."—Yd. (m., 33), who is now a sexual invert, and who tries to cure himself by lifting young scamps " up to the rank of gentlemen," began by suffering from crises of moral exaltation in the course of his first attacks of depression. He wanted to reform his life, wanted to become better than any one else. " This hope which fills my heart enables me to live."—It would be interesting to ascertain whether a similar mechanism may not play a part in obsessive over-scrupulousness.

The same characteristic is more conspicuously displayed in impulses to devotion. In most cases these impulses to devotion are really nothing more than a form of impulses to dominate or of impulses to love.—Héloise is constantly talking about her devotion, which is " trustworthy, discreet, and tender; a little flower which never fades and which always smells sweet."

But when we press our enquiries, she is willing to admit that she is animated with a false need for devotion just like a false hunger. She says: "I make a great fuss about my need to devote myself; and yet I know perfectly well that if I want to devote myself to any one, I need merely stay with my mother, who is now very old. Here is an object for devotion ready to my hand, but this would be too simple."

Yet there are cases in which the impulse is more genuine, in which the subjects really long to devote themselves to some one—to unsuitable objects, indeed, but until they are completely exhausted, and without securing any advantage to themselves, simply that they may obtain moral gratification and achieve the excitation which is brought to them by a disinterested action that is useful to others.—Lydia and Léa, who are greatly depressed and are tormented by the phobia of fatigue, recover their energy directly they are called upon to take care of a sick relative.—"The only thing that does me any good," says Ep. (m., 38), "is to make others happier than I can make myself. When I feel that some one has need of me, I regain self-confidence."—Noémi only recovers energy when she has charitable deeds to perform. She has successfully founded charitable societies, and in work of this kind she can expend a lot of energy. "The only refuge I can find is in philanthropy; it is the refuge of imbeciles, and it is among philanthropists that one finds most imbeciles. I devote myself to this because I am incompetent to do anything better; but it must be admitted that this is sometimes an excellent remedy for me."

Id. (f., 45) is impelled to devote herself to little children now that she has lost her own. She has a persistent desire to care for poor children and would like to adopt one, although her husband is opposed to the idea. "The sight of a child for which I can do something has a tranquillising effect on me; I become quite a different person as soon as my interest is aroused in a child. When children come to my house and I take care of them, it is as if a veil had been torn away; it has the effect on me which David's harping had upon King Saul. Although in general I can do nothing, can finish nothing, cannot write a letter, cannot play through a piece on the piano, cannot go for a walk, I can do any amount of work for children, for I feel then that I have something to do, and that

I do it well."—This devotion to little children, which is quite a common characteristic, may depend, as in the case we have just been considering, upon the excitation of maternal tendencies in a woman who has lost her own children. But it may also be connected with a phenomenon of which we have already seen a manifestation in connexion with the search for love, with the search for an easier form of devotion. It is this degrading of devotion in depressed patients which explains the common impulses to devotion towards animals and the strange impulses of zoophilia. I have elsewhere published an account of two typical cases of " mania for cats," and need not return to the matter here.[1]

Reverie is a symptom of depression, for it is a form of activity characterised by diminished tension, and one which replaces a real and more difficult activity. But at the same time it is a means of excitation, for it renders possible the development of certain successful activities. The " serial story," which I cannot study here fully, is not simply a story which the patient relates to himself ; it is a form of behaviour ; it is a manner of imaginative living ; with sketches of attitudes, gestures, and internal conversations ; it is another life than real life, and one lived in more favourable circumstances. Kindred attitudes to those which we should assume in reality before this or that person, or before this or that object, give us the feeling that the person or the object is actually present. Conversations in which we ask ourselves questions and give ourselves answers, while changing a little from time to time the mode of speech and the accent, give a semblance of reality to this artificial life. In such a " serial story " we find the same degree of faith that we have in play or in many religious sentiments. We have a faith in the agreeable and comforting character of the operation as a whole, without stressing the reality of this or that detail.

This " serial story," which is carried on to a more or less developed degree in the majority of normal individuals, undergoes a very extensive development in enfeebled individuals whose psychological tension is inadequate for satisfactory accommodation to reality, and who find it preferable to live after their own fashion in an artificial medium which is more

---

[1] Cf. Névroses et idées fixes, 1898, vol. ii, p. 145 ; Les obsessions et la psychasthénie, 1903, vol. ii, p. 446.

to their taste.   In almost all such cases I find that the serial story has played a very great part in the life, especially during the first years of the illness when the depression was not very great.   After a time, however, it is apt to disappear, yielding place to obsessions properly so called.

In the cases in which we are particularly interested at this juncture, the serial story develops further to become a need or an impulse.   The patients feel a persistent need to go back to their story, to continue it by repeating the same chapter an indefinite number of times while making a very slow advance.   They are greatly annoyed if they are interrupted by being asked to perform some real action.   They are always absent-minded, because they are constantly thinking about their " story."   Sometimes they will make a peculiar gesture, will smile in a marked way, or will utter a few words in a low tone, these actions betraying their perpetual reverie.   It would take too long to enumerate the cases in which I have evidence of the existence of such interminable reveries.   I have published a few reports of the kind, and the other cases that have come under my notice resemble these.—Obviously Lydia's obsession with the thought of her beauty was gradually superinduced upon a reverie concerning her social successes.   " Nothing did me so much good as to tell myself stories about the ball where I was such a success.   In imagination I was there, and my triumphs caused me infinite delight.   I have never had any real interest in my life, except in these stories."—We are amazed to find that Rc. (m. 30) spends his whole time in fluttering the pages of the Paris Directory, and that he is furious if we try to take away from him a book which few people find engrossing.   The reason for his passion is that the names and addresses are merely the starting-point for imaginative excursions.   Each word sets him off upon one of his ambitious reveries.   " I fancy myself to be the leading man in this district, the king of this country. . . . When I walk about assuming regal airs, when I behave like some great personage, I feel myself to be better adapted, to be freer, to be free to do anything I like.   In general, I feel that I lack firm ground to stand on, and I need to strengthen my position by saying to myself that I am some one of great importance, some big mandarin, no matter who.   The Directory helps my imagination in these matters."

As we see in the account of the foregoing case, the content of the serial story may have a morbid character in relation to these depressed patients' need for excitation. Psychasthenics who are affected with psychological inadequacies of the sexual functions (which must not be confounded with physiological inadequacies of the same functions) have peculiar serial stories concerning their love tendencies. One will represent to himself that he is the victim of a huge, fat woman, a grossly vulgar woman, who climbs upon him, crushes him, and beats him. Many such patients will imagine that they are harshly and brutally ordered about by some one who imposes offensive tasks upon them and punishes them in a humiliating way.—Xg. (m., 42) is constantly picturing in his mind that a sordid person comes into the room where he is in bed with his wife. This person makes him get out of bed, forces him to prepare coffee at the stove and to serve it up, while the intruder has intercourse with the wife under her husband's eyes. The remarkable thing is that these stories, continually repeated, give the day-dreamer great delight, take him out of himself, and often culminate in voluptuous orgasms which the subject cannot procure in any other way. The patient seems to stimulate himself by the imaginative reproduction of a humiliation which awakens a tendency towards defence and arouses indignation. These tendencies stimulate the inadequate sexual tendencies. We have here a complex combination of erotomanias and impulses to reverie.

One stage further, and such reveries take the form of more or less real actions. The subject feels the need of fixing them in the written word. This is the starting-point of those numberless letters, those lucubrations which some patients spend the whole day in writing. " Before my husband comes back to see me, he writes me interminable letters as ardent as they are absurd. He feels a need to wind himself up, a need to spur himself." The celebrated case of Hélène Smith which Flournoy has recorded in his book, *Des Indes à la planète Mars* (1900), deals with a case in which the serial story took this form.

A remarkable instance may bridge the transition between impulses to devotion and literary or artistic impulses. Ih., a man of thirty-six, not very well educated, suffers from a mania which he himself recognises to be absurd but from which he cannot free himself. Almost every day, and sometimes several times a day, he composes letters addressed to the great people of the earth, to kings, ministers of state, generals. These letters are exhortations to kindliness and love. As soon as he reads in a newspaper that any one has received a severe sentence, he writes to the sovereign of the country to ask that the condemned should be pardoned. He is constantly writing to the tsar of Russia on behalf of the Siberian exiles.

He sends these letters by registered post, and says gloomily : " This will cost me a lot of money." He has no delusion in the strict sense of the term, so that his mania for letter-writing is not like that of one who has a claim to push, or who is suffering from delusions of persecution. The good fellow knows perfectly well that his letters are of no account, and that they will probably never reach the addressee. " After all, it is not for the tsar that I write, but for myself." Primarily, he opines that by these generous demonstrations he will atone for imaginary crimes of which his tender conscience accuses him. Next, he feels a childish vanity at the thought that he knows how to indite a letter to the tsar of Russia. " If I post these letters, it is because that makes them seem more serious to me, gives them reality."

An ardent and usually impulsive search for mental excitation is common. Many patients have, as Noémi says of herself, a " mania for intellectuals." They constantly aspire to get in touch with persons who have a reputation in art or letters. They fancy that they would get well at once if they could only escape from the humdrum environment of their family and associate with persons of talent. A great many women have a passion for luxury, intellectuality ; they detest practical life ; they would like to move in literary circles instead of associating with husband and children, who make them ill. Others have an itch for attending lectures, for seeing sights, for going to concerts.—" Unless I do this," says Pepita, " I get bored to death and fall sick." Those who have tasted the delight of posing on the stage, can never get over their regret for what they have lost. " In the ordinary world I titivate myself for three persons ; in the theatre I used to do it for thousands."

Reading is, for many, a need which can speedily become a dangerous mania. It is an easy kind of work, demanding very little effort, but enabling the reader to get out of real life, and facilitating reverie. When Pepita is reading, she gives free rein to her imagination, always fancying herself to be playing the part of the leading characters. Moreover, she does not hesitate to modify the story in order to give herself a more splendid part. It is quite common to find neuropaths who have an impulse " to gobble up the library."

Some of these patients, and by no means always the most intelligent among them, go yet farther, and engage in serious study. They will even undertake literary composition.— Emma fancies that it is her vocation to be an author ; she has a passion for perfecting little literary morsels, and even tries to write novels. " All sorts of familiar and outworn ideas come to me as discoveries and treasures. How delightful it is to describe, a storm, moonlight, love, anger ! I find in this a mysterious power which transforms me. Literature enchases my ideas."—Yd. forgets from time to time to devote himself to the education of his young friends, and writes a book. " This will be the great work of my life." And he brings to this work the same exclusive passion as to his homo-sexual amours.—Uj. (m., 42) spends several hours a day in writing strange, fantastic, and complicated literary pieces. He says : " For the time being, I am the only person who can understand them, but some day they will bring me immortal fame."

Sometimes a peculiar taste leads psychasthenics to the study of psychology and philosophy.—Kb. (m., 29) is drawn towards " the dissection of minds."—Uw. (m., 47) has a craze for philosophical disquisitions and for studies concerning what he terms " the technique of reasoning." We find in his writings a mania for perfection and for extreme scrupulousness. His technique of reasoning is obviously a system which he wishes to apply to himself in order that he may reason well, just as other investigators seek systems that will teach them how to breathe well. But some of his studies have a modicum of value.—There is no doubt that a good many writers who have attained a fair amount of reputation have been impelled to write by a morbid desire for excitation. In some of these neuropathic patients we can note an impulse towards musical composition, or even a more or less serious impulse towards scientific research.

We have already had occasion, when studying fatigue, to note that phobias are often defensive reactions through which the mind attempts to avoid exhaustion by inhibiting this or that action, either because it is really one which demands a great expenditure of energy, or else because it is wrongly considered a costly action. If I mistake not, a great many impulses are phenomena of the same kind. They are defensive and curative reactions of the mind, which is trying in this case, not to avoid exhaustion, but to develop energy and to acquire a higher tension by seeking out certain kinds of action which are really stimulating or are believed to be so.

4. WORTH OF IMPULSIVE ACTIONS.

The development of impulsive actions is regarded as a morbid phenomenon, and this view is correct, for such a development is the outcome of the diminution or suppression of reflective assent.   That is to say, it is due to a notable lowering of tension. People generally infer from this that the actions performed by the patient under the influence of an impulse must be absurd and dangerous, and that they cannot possibly be of any use to the doer. That is too hasty a conclusion, and one which demands closer examination.

Obviously, the judgment is correct as regards many of these actions. The varieties of intoxication, alcoholic and other, and over-eating, cannot fail to increase the disorder of health. Far from relieving depression, these actions increase it. The search for sexual excitation at any cost, the search for accommodating lovers who are unworthy of the seeker, exhausts these patients, leads them into sexual inversions and perversions, exposes them to all kinds of dangers, and brings them into extremely humiliating situations. Kleptomaniac practices are discovered in the end, and result in arrests, prosecutions, and disasters of all kinds, which are not likely to be helpful in the treatment of a woman suffering from depression. Domineering impulses, impulses to tease, to sulk, to be ill-natured, domestic scenes, weary and disgust the patients' associates. The result is that the patients are cold-shouldered, which they dread more than anything else in the world. The mania for loving and being loved is not understood, the woman who has this craze is regarded as forward and dangerous, as a person to be dreaded and avoided. The patient may do harm to himself in his sulking-fits, in the comedies he plays in order to attract sympathy and to make himself seem interesting. A man will bare his chest and abdomen and go on to the veranda to expose himself to an icy wind. He does this in order to punish his wife for having neglected him. He wants to show her that he will fall ill through her fault ; and in fact, he does succeed in giving himself an attack of diarrhoea which might just as well have been pneumonia. The people who, as the saying goes, " cut off their noses to spite their faces," are only sulking to an extreme degree. Girls will refuse to eat in order to alarm their parents, and will carry their sulking-fits so far as to induce anorexia and even tuberculosis. Pseudo-suicides, staged in order to attract attention, may have disastrous results. It is obvious, then, that there is a real element of danger in all these actions performed under impulse.

In other cases, the aim which the patients set before themselves is obviously unattainable. They try to do impossible actions, and along this route they can never achieve success and can never bring about a cure.—Uj. will never be able to make the whole world strait-laced " while reserving the secret garden for himself."—When Pepita draws a fancy portrait of the perfect lover, we know that she will never find such a person. These women want to conciliate their taste for risky adventures and their love for middle-class respectability. " I need to love madly, but I want to guard my domestic hearth which is respectable and solidly built. I am an old picture which cannot do without a frame." All very well, but in extant society these two wishes are incompatible, and it is obvious that attempts of the kind are foredoomed to failure.—Lox. (f., 50), when making a journey in war-time, was present at a dangerous explosion, and was subsequently transformed for several days. " Still," said her husband sadly, " I cannot every day furnish her with bombs which explode only a hundred yards away."

In other circumstances, the actions undertaken are merely very difficult ; they need attention, perseverance, and a great expenditure of energy.—" Love itself is an effort," says Héloise. " It is hard work to please, to make conquests and to keep what one has won. What I want is that the delight I feel shall dispel the sense of effort, but that rarely happens."—Thus our patients exhaust themselves in the search for the perfection of love.—Ib., a young woman of twenty-three, who has been carrying on five amorous intrigues at once, can no longer persist in them. " These calculations, these combinations, these continual falsehoods, have wearied me and got me into difficulties. In the end I have grown sick of them."

Women whose only aim is excitation in the successes of society life, devote enormous pains to their toilet, to their visits, to their at-homes. " If I make overwhelming efforts in order to please when I am on a visit or at a dinner-party, something goes wrong in my head. I can no longer follow the conversation, I feel that I have exhausted my powers and that it is doing me harm. I come home utterly worn out, and on the verge of a fit of hysterics."—Emile (m., 18), suffering from agoraphobia and from obsessive over-scrupulousness, no longer wishes to engage in any activity except reading. He devours huge tomes dealing with literary and historical topics ; he reads at meal-times and even after he has gone to bed. When any one tries to take away his books, he grows violent. Reading, which began as an easy and stimulating distraction, has become absorbing and exhausting. In a word, the expenditure necessary to satisfy the impulse is now greater than the advantage accruing, the net upshot being that the patient is exhausted instead of being benefited.

In some cases, the impossibility of resignation, the indefinite prolongation of effort although the circumstances are utterly unfavourable and although exhaustion has ensued, will actually induce delusions. The patient, who has always had an inclination to play a comedy, is obstinate in the continuance of his action, his affirmation, despite all opposition and even when the action is ill-adapted to outward circumstances.—Sophie continues to devote herself to her mother, to bring the mother pillows, to pad the corners of the furniture with cloths, although in reality she is in an asylum far away from her mother.— Ue. (f., 35), who seeks love in order to restore her mental level, masturbates while declaring that she is giving herself to chance-comers, and that by doing so she is saving the world. Tc. (m., 45), obsessed with the idea of love, is continually talking to the photograph of his inamorata, and imagines that she answers him out loud. Here we discern one of the most remarkable ways in which delusions and hallucinations may originate.

When we recall these inconveniences and dangers, we see that the doctor has good reason for regarding such impulses (which are supposed to be stimulating) as undesirable and dangerous, notwithstanding the patient's illusions on the subject. It is not difficult to discern, in the behaviour of persons prone to impulsive action, the characteristics which entail all these dangers. Such actions are ill adapted, and display features due to ignorance. The patient seems to hurl himself into the first act that can procure him a momentary pleasure, and does not worry about the consequences. The exaggeration of the action is manifest, and the patients will obstinately repeat actions which become absurd and dangerous through repetition and exaggeration.

The great inconvenience attaching to these impulses to search for excitation and happiness is their narrowness, their exclusiveness. One patient will expect to find happiness in drink or in theft, another that he will find happiness in the love of some particular person, and each of them is incapable of thinking of anything outside his own peculiar fancy. The exclusiveness is an outcome of the malady. A restriction of the field of consciousness does not exist in the personal functions of the hysteric alone ; it is also characteristic of the actions and efforts of all psychasthenics. Not one of them can engage in more than a single activity at a time : they expend all their energies upon one thing only; and when they are animated by an ambition, they cannot conceive the possibility of any other. Céline, who spends her life " waiting for the sound of the footsteps of lovers who will come up the stairs in search of me," is aware that for fifteen years she has not been able to think of anything else or to dream of any other aim in life.—Héloise, who has a passion for making subtle reflections concerning her feelings, is also fully aware of her exclusiveness. " In the abnormal state, patients like myself reduce everything to unity. I am afraid of only one illness, I am concerned about only one danger, I have only one passion. It is as if everything in the mind were darkened and indefinite, except at one point where all the light is concentrated. Owing to this unity, there is a complete lack of balance. It is as if a man were to try to run with only one leg ; it is like having only one eye. How

terrified the one-eyed person is at the thought of losing this
one eye, how keenly he feels its worth and its fragility ! One
thing has become everything, with the result that there is
constant anxiety, uneasiness, infinite pain punctuated by
occasional joys so intense that they grow painful and leave a
bad taste behind."

In fact, this exclusiveness leads to an exaggeration of effort
and to obstinacy. The action which, if performed in moderation, might perhaps be a tonic, is pushed too far, and is
indefinitely repeated until it gives rise to exhaustion. " I
know nothing of half-measures or half-affections. How can
I be content with half-measures when they are contrary to
my nature, which is one that finds doing things by halves,
or giving by halves, impossible. When I am well, I know
that I can get on for a time without some one of whom I am
fond. But, in this abnormal state of depression, I am incapable
of bearing the thought of even a momentary separation. My
disquietude makes my passion stronger. From moment to
moment I dread a catastrophe. I cling desperately ; I am
perpetually exhausted ; I lead a terrible life."—In a word,
we rediscover here the usual defects of the actions of depressed
persons ; their lack of reflection, their " attachments," their
incapacity for resignation and change, their manias for effort,
and their obstinacies. " People believe me to be energetic
because I never give in. I go on working indefinitely until I
am worn out, although it is obvious that I shall never attain
my end." The dangers attendant upon impulsive actions
are thus, in a measure, accidental. They are the outcome of
the ill-adapted way in which the actions are performed.

Still, even when we have realised these drawbacks and
dangers, we must not immediately infer that the patients'
impulses are utterly absurd and can never be of any use to
them. Such impulses would not be so common and would
not last so long if they had no value whatever. If we ourselves
are inclined to regard them as invariably absurd or dangerous,
this may be because we are placed in bad conditions for observation. The doctor does not notice the impulses except in
a patient who consults him specially on their account, that
is to say in a patient who has noticed that the impulses have
unfortunate consequences. In a word, the impulses only come

under our notice as medical practitioners when they have failed to have their proper effect. If the gratification of one of these impulses has a favourable effect and relieves the subject of his depression, he does not come to the doctor for advice, and we shall not see him at this particular time. The reader will remember that Madame V. ceased consulting me during the period that she was stealing in the large shops, and that she did not fall ill again until her thefts were interrupted.

In an earlier chapter we noted a curious circumstance in connexion with " groups of neuropaths." We saw that, around the patient who is recognised to be ill and therefore comes or is brought to consult a doctor, there are almost always in the same family two or three other persons affected with the same psychasthenic ailments, often seriously affected, although the illness has been overlooked. In many cases these people, who are really sick though not recognised to be so, are authoritarian persons, exacting, prone to tease their associates, with a mania for making scenes, and so on. Is it not a plausible theory that their authoritarian impulses satisfy them and raise their spirits sufficiently to mask, more or less completely, from others' eyes and from their own eyes, the depression from which they suffer. In order to grasp the real effect of certain impulses, we must study them in the patients who do not complain of them, and in whom, generally speaking, they exist without even the doctors being aware of the fact ; or we must examine the earlier effects of these impulses in our patients, before they became, as they now are, useless or injurious.

If we study the matter in this way, we are constrained to admit that a great number of the impulses we have been considering have had good effects for a time, that they have helped to raise the patient's spirits and to suppress or diminish his depression. In an earlier book I have recorded numerous instances of at least temporary relief, brought about by these actions which the patients perform impulsively.[1] I can now add additional observations of the same kind.

Ms. (f., 35), suffering from dromomania, would run thirty miles behind a carriage. For several months, while doing this from time to time, she was far more active, and her feelings were practically normal. When she felt overtired, she gave

---

[1] Les obsessions et la psychasthénie, 1903, vol. i, p. 543.

up the practice, and thereupon she began to suffer from bulimia, replacing one form of excitation by another. Overfeeding induced disorder of the stomach. When she was prevented from undertaking excessive physical exercise and from eating to excess, she passed into a condition of complete depression. A great many of the mothers whose authoritarianism and spitefulness I have described in the foregoing pages, fell sick when their daughters were taken out of their hands. They needed an outlet for their spleen, an object on which it could be concentrated, and they could only maintain their psychological tension if they had some one to torment.

In Mc. (f., 25), the thefts she had been practising in large shops are now regarded as the fruit of a morbid impulse, because, when she was prevented from practising them, the subjacent depression became manifest. A few years earlier the same patient was affected with an impulse to drink and to go on the loose, and this was regarded as simply immoral behaviour. But at that time, her depression was kept entirely in abeyance by the excitation. She was active and cheerful, and had no obvious mental disorder.—Len. (f., 35) only relapsed into melancholia and thoughts of suicide after her thefts had been prevented. She said: " My people would apparently prefer me to commit suicide ! "

We must not forget the remarkable case of Madame V. : how she had had two prolonged attacks of melancholia ; and how a third attack, when it was obviously coming on, was completely warded off for eight months by her kleptomaniac activities. The effect was marvellous, for throughout the summer the depression was to all appearance completely overcome. She was active, free from hesitation, and no longer suffered from constipation and insomnia. All her associates believed that she was cured. The excitation continued for a few days after her arrest, and Madame V. declared that she still had a wish to go on with her thefts. Ten days later her attitude had completely changed. Now, far from wanting to steal again, she was grievously ashamed at the thought of what she had done. Simultaneously she was once more extremely depressed, and the depression continued for three months after the cessation of the thefts. Obviously, then, the thefts had the remarkable power of interrupting the course of a paroxysm of melancholic depression, and of transforming the patient's body and mind for eight months.

Vc. (m., 43) is evidently a weakling. In youth he suffered from obsessive over-scrupulousness. He has always been a great gambler, saying : " Never in my life have I had any interest except in the emotion of gambling." But recently, after very heavy losses during a single night, he took fright, and, upon the urgent recommendations of his family, he completely renounced gambling. A few months later he began to suffer from various hypochondrial obsessions and from phobias. Are we not justified in presuming that the suppression of gambling was one of the causative factors of the mental disturbance ?

Nowadays, when sexual psychopathology is a renewed subject of study, I think it will be of interest to recall some characteristic cases of amorous impulses.—Wb. (m., 58) has always been successful in his love affairs. He was fond of coarse jokes, had a taste for Anacreontic verse, and flattered himself with being a modern Don Juan. But at length one of his adventures turned out ill, and made him feel that at his age it was advisable to sober down. The disturbance brought about by this disappointment and by the consequent change in his habits was enormous. Not only did Wb. entirely lose his interest in sexual concerns, in coarse jests, and in salacious poetry ; but his will powers were completely paralysed, he lost all belief, and became utterly inert. For twenty months he remained in a condition of profound depression.— The case of Pya. is analogous, although here the lover's tastes were of a lower character. A man of forty-five, unmarried, fairly well off, and not having to work for his living, all his interests throughout life had been concentrated on easy conquests. As I have already remarked, it was from this source alone that he derived his psychological excitation. After a tiring journey, and when suffering from a fear lest he should have sustained a genital infection, he found himself completely impotent in his relationships with his mistress. At first the depression related solely to the sexual functions. Pya., believing himself to be impotent and behaving as such, completely lost interest in women, in intrigue, in women's dress, in the smutty photographs which had been his chief delight since youth. But the depression speedily extended its scope. All his other interests and all his other activities became involved. At length an absolute inertia ensued, with sentiments of incapacity and suicidal longings. " I have never had any other joy, any other happiness. Now that this has been suppressed there is nothing left for me in the world ! " —Bsi. (m., 41), after the mistress who had kept him in good spirits and had made him work had left him, likewise exclaimed : " Alone ! alone ! alone ! there is no longer any one for me in the world. I live in a void ! "—We notice in all these patients who have lost their stimulating tendency, that there ensues a profound depression as if they had no longer any reason for living. This is because that particular stimulant was the only one which kept their vitality going.

After being ill for twenty months, Wb. showed he was on the mend by casually remarking that a woman was pretty and well-dressed. In Pya. the gradual restoration of the sexual functions was in like manner the starting-point of the cure. I consider these facts of so much importance that I want to illustrate them by additional observations.

The psychologist cannot but be interested in Pepita's story. She has a clear memory of all that has happened to her. She regrets her losses of jewellery and money, and is sorry that she has caused her family so much suffering. But she has a satisfactory explanation of her behaviour. " What was I to do ? My last adventure took me rather far afield, and I agree that it did not turn out very well. But before that, I had plenty of adventures of which the memory is delightful. I suffer terribly in the monotonous quietude of ordinary respectable life. The hours seem long and gloomy. I become horribly ill unless I kick over the traces a little. What is the history of my life ? All my serious nervous disorders came on during the periods when I was behaving ' properly,' and I could only get well by doing the other thing. At home I lived most respectably, most decorously ; but really I have a taste for debauchery ; I love the atmosphere of vice, it intoxicates me and makes me well again. I like to live several lives at once ; one life is too monotonous for me. If it were only possible, I should like to be sometimes a man and sometimes a woman. Since I cannot manage that, I change my environment, my name, all the external circumstances of my life. I contemplate the strange existence of people who

amuse themselves, who engage in conspiracies, who steal ;
I mingle in their activities. Besides, I think that I have been
able to do fine things. I wanted to cure this young fellow,
to raise his spirits, to find him a position. Yes, I, too, have
a taste for uplifting fallen angels ; it was a distraction at any
rate. If I did not lift him up, at least I raised my own
spirits, for I have never been so well as I was during that
adventure, while since it came to an end I have been ill all
the time." Her amorous adventures were horribly dangerous,
no doubt, and it was my duty as medical adviser to guard
against their recurrence. But if we adopt a purely scientific
standpoint and do not concern ourselves about moral canons,
we are obliged to admit that during the eighteen months of
this adventure, when for a considerable part of the time she
was leading a double life, Pepita was perfectly well ; whereas
before it began she had been almost continually ill and under
restraint in asylums, and whereas since the end of the adventure
she has been wretchedly ill once more. We see also that even
now she gets better for a time when she entertains the hope
of resuming her adventures.

Ib. (f., 23) is to-day in a condition of exhaustion, after a
period in which her love affairs have been excessive and
complicated. She had five lovers at the same time, and not
one of them was to be allowed to know of the other's existence. She found it necessary to give up these difficult intrigues,
" because they were becoming too much involved, and in the
end they were more fatiguing than amusing." Still, the
intrigues kept her going for more than a year. " These little
incidents helped me to live, and I can hardly say that I have
been alive since I had to give them up."—Céline's reveries
concerning marriage and concerning the betrothed whose
steps she used to listen for on the staircase gave her courage
to live ; but when, in order to cure herself of the practice of
continual masturbation, she decided to abandon her fantasies,
when she declared to herself that at the age of twenty-nine
it was time to renounce the thought of love, she became far
more depressed, practically desperate, and it was necessary
to strive against this renouncement.—Yd. (m., 33) leads a
preposterous life with a number of scamps whom he wishes
to make into gentlemen. Unquestionably the life was out-
rageous. Nevertheless we have had to care for him medically

since the time when his best-loved intimate deserted him.
For more than a year, his cohabitation with this youth enabled
him to work hard and to believe himself cured. The various
fugues we have described seem to have checked in him a com-
mencing depression, for, as soon as they were interdicted, he
became far more ill and had to spend several months in an
asylum.

The case of Xc. (f., 37) is extremely interesting. Since
early youth she has suffered from grave depression and has
been affected with obsessive over-scrupulousness. When she
was twenty-five years of age her mother became seriously
ill, and Xc. had to care for her. Little by little, the young
woman acquired a passion for the new duties, thinking only
of her mother, caring for her by day and by night with an
obvious excess of devotion. To all seeming, this passion for
self-immolation distracted her mind from her obsessions for
nearly two years. When the mother died, Xc., at a loose
end once more, relapsed into abulia and over-scrupulousness,
with insomnia, emaciation, etc. A year latter she met a young
woman who was intelligent and good, but of an amorous
nature and perverted. This woman seduced Xc., and taught
her to appreciate the joys of Lesbian love. Notwithstanding
the almost insuperable difficulties arising out of the indignation
of the parents and the hostility of public opinion in a little
country town, the two women set up house together. What
was the result? For three years, Xc. was perfectly well,
and quite free from nervous and mental disorders. To-day,
Xc. has renounced her immoral relationship and has broken
off the association. It may be that religious influences had
their part in causing this rupture, or perhaps excesses and
fatigue destroyed the charm of the love affair. However
this may be, she has once more become inert and subject to
obsessions. Indeed, she has a new one as well as the others,
for she is now affected with agoraphobia. If, at the moment
when she first met the friend with whom she subsequently
lived for three years, Xc. had consulted a doctor on account
of her psychasthenic disorders, and if that doctor had prescribed a treatment which had cured her for three years,
every one would proclaim this a triumph of medical skill.
Throughout the present work I have maintained that a cure
for at least a year in which there was no relapse was a proof

that a method of treatment was extremely valuable. We will say nothing about moral values ; but how can we ignore the medical value of the perverted love which transformed this young woman for three years.

Héloise has only been regarded as ill for two years, and it is simply during this period that her amatory impulses have been considered morbid. But she tells us that for fifteen years she has been subject to love passions of the same kind. " I have always been addicted to love adventures, except during the times when I was pregnant and when I was suckling my children." What does this mean ? During the exceptional periods, during the times of pregnancy and lactation ; there was going on, as we have observed in a hundred other cases, a natural physiological excitation which dispelled every inclination to depression. But at all other times this woman needed a peculiar form of mental excitation in order to keep up her psychological tension to an adequate level. Her impulse towards amorous adventures appeared in regular fashion as a defensive reaction. " During the periods when I was living in an atmosphere of tender and respectable affection, I radiated happiness, I was alive and could breathe life into others. Now I am merely a dead woman who can speak and weep. I was cured of all my troubles when I was in love. Think of the muco-membranous enteritis from which I suffer. I might be having as many as twenty-five loose motions charged with mucus every day. The whole trouble would pass off in five minutes and my bowel would digest perfectly for a fortnight if only I should receive a sweet letter from my lover. This has actually happened." A few social successes suffice to fill her with enthusiasm and restores her for the time. " What a lot of details there are to arrange ! So many people to introduce, so many mistakes to avoid, so many compliments to pay. One has to say this to the person on one's right, and avoid saying that to the person on one's left ; red wine for one guest, white wine for another ; brandy for this one, a special liqueur for that one ; to remember which kind of cigarettes particular people like—how is it possible to be ill when one has all these things to do ? " The cynical observer may say that these are trifles, but, however that may be, after this party of hers she slept soundly, a thing she had not done for months ; and she had no complaints to make of her health for the next week. " If it happens that some really intelligent man seems to be interested in me, my eyes sparkle so much that I positively dazzle people who look at me. You may hardly believe it, but this is the best medicine for me."

The ardent pursuit of social successes, vanity concerning her beauty, childish coquetry, seem quite out of place to-day for Lydia in her simple little household ; and we share her own astonishment at her perpetual obsession with this thought of her beauty. But when she was still quite young, such behaviour was regarded as charming, and for years brought her much admiration. " I was not really any stronger when I was young than I am now, and yet I could do masses of things then which I am no longer able to do. I went for walks, skated, went out to dinner and to lots of dances. I was surrounded by men who courted me. I never asked if I was pretty, for every one told me I was without my asking. Even in those days if I thought that I had had less success than usual at a dance I became ill, and I could hardly drag one leg after another until the next dance came, then I picked up once more. If you are to live your life and not simply look on at life you need success, and a woman must succeed as best she can."

The foregoing conclusions regarding the influence of impulsive actions may be summarised by recalling earlier studies concerning the effects of acting on impulse. Happy transformations of the same kind were noted long ago in the case of patients who yielded to their impulses. Magnan used to lay stress upon the characteristic condition of satisfaction which ensued upon the carrying out of an impulse. He gave rather a vague description of this condition of satisfaction, and even to-day it has not always been clearly understood. Pitres and Régis point out that in impulsive persons, after a crisis, what we notice is not so much joy as a sort of appeasement ; they are simply satisfied because they are no longer tormented by a distressing agitation.[1] In my book on obsessions I shared the opinion of these authors, and expressed my dissent from Magnan saying : " Is the patient really happy ? He experiences a very natural relief when the distressing crisis is over, but he is not proud of himself, and is displeased at having

[1] Pitres et Régis, Rapport sur les obsessions au Congrès de Médecine de Moscou, 1897, p. 54.

again yielded to an impulse which he regards as foolish. The patients are by no means pleased with themselves at the close of an impulsive crisis ; they are fatigued and ashamed." [1] In certain cases, I could only detect marked satisfaction when the patient, through yielding to an impulse, was enabled to escape great anxiety or suffering.[2]

To-day I feel that these criticisms were excessive, and that there is a great deal of truth in what Magnan said. Owing to a lack of precision in the descriptions, we were not considering the same patients or the same phenomena. The state of satisfaction to which he refers does not appear invariably after yielding to impulse ; but it appears after yielding to impulses of a particular kind, those which I have termed impulses in which excitation is sought. Furthermore, the satisfaction does not in every case immediately follow the performance of the act ; and, indeed, it is usually absent when the impulses are intense and continual. Precisely because the feeling of satisfaction has not ensued, the patient is led to repeat the action again and again. But the feeling of satisfaction is sometimes peculiarly conspicuous when the action has been successful, and it is at this very moment that the impulse ceases to be felt. Among the instances I have just been describing, I may recall that of the patient who stimulated himself by long walks and by fugues ; whose sadness and incapacity vanished after he had been walking for several hours ; who then declared that the night was a beautiful one, that the country was lovely, and who thereupon felt inclined for hard work. I agree with Pitres and Régis that such a feeling may be mingled with shame at the thought of what has just been done. This complex condition could be noted in Oc., who treated his acquaintances at the public-house with money he had stolen from his employer ; and also in Madame V., who was caught in the act of stealing in a shop. But none the less in both these patients the satisfaction was extreme. The delight felt is connected with the sense that individuality has been restored and that relationships with reality have been reestablished ; it is analogous to that which occurs in hysterics when complete somnambulism has been induced. The reader will remember that at this instant they declared that the light seemed brighter and that

---

[1] Les obsessions et la psychasthénie, second edition, 1908, vol. i, p. 54.
[2] Ibid., vol. i, p. 264.

things were more real than before. Such observations could be indefinitely multiplied, and they have considerable interest. They show us that a great many people may be extremely feeble, and may yet maintain their mental health thanks to the performance of more or less reasonable and appropriate actions which play the part of stimulants. They show us that these persons fall sick as soon as the possibility of this stimulation vanishes. Overfeeding, long walks, sports of various kinds, debauchery, gambling, the exercise of power, the search for love, intrigues of all kinds, the pursuit of success, and likewise literary and scientific work, keep up a great many people's spirits and save them from depression. The pursuit of these excitations seems to us perfectly natural in persons who maintain a normal psychological tension ; that is to say, it seems natural when it succeeds. We only describe it as a morbid impulse when it is inadequate, when it is unsuccessful. The psychologist has no right to despise these impulses of psychasthenics because in actual fact they have become wrong-headed and absurd. Obviously, he must not encourage them when they have assumed so dangerous a form. He will not think of sending Pepita back into the arms of her hooligan, or of encouraging Madame V. to go on stealing. Still, it is his business to find out what was the good element, however transient, in these impulses. He must learn what made them useful, so that, if possible, he can continue to turn these useful factors to good account.

5. Problem of Excitation by Action.

We cannot entirely dispense with theories which give us a general idea of phenomena, which enable us to group them if not to understand them, and which guide us in future experiences. In this connexion we have to consider three problems :

1. What is the difference, if not in the content, at least in the performance, as between actions which induce impoverishment and depression, and actions which induce enrichment and excitation ? What are the characteristics of stimulant actions ?

2. How can we picture to ourselves the mechanism of excitation produced by acts of this stimulant character ?

3. What are the conditions which can facilitate the production of these stimulant actions ?

1. *The Characteristics of Stimulant Actions.* The foregoing phenomena are remarkable, for we have devoted a considerable time to the study of the precisely opposite phenomena. We have seen that in these easily depressed individuals, actions, often the very same actions, owing to the efforts and the expenditure they necessitate, were almost invariably the starting-point of depressions. How is it possible that the performance of these difficult, tedious, and costly actions can now become the origin of an excitation ? I need not lay any stress upon the superficial differences to which we might be inclined to attribute undue importance. We might say that the depressing actions are difficult in themselves, or difficult relatively to the subject, to his faculties, his habits ; and we might contend that stimulant actions are those which can be easily and successfully performed at little cost. Sometimes, this statement seems to apply, but its validity is no more than apparent. When we see a woman become depressed and fall seriously ill because she has had to receive into her flat some furniture which she has herself ordered, and yet that this same woman is stimulated to good effect because she spends the whole night caring for children during a shipwreck, we must realise that we are not entitled to say much about the difficulty of an action as being the cause of depression. Besides, it is obvious that most of the actions performed by our patients as the outcome of stimulant impulses (such actions as fugues, thefts, and intrigues) are extremely complicated and difficult. Another point which might be made is that actions which are often repeated, and are continued for a long time, are inconvenient, and are much less likely to be beneficial than actions rapidly performed. It is true that long-continued actions may often prove exhausting. Still, we cannot generalise here. Let us recall the adventures and intrigues of Pepita which lasted for two years, demanding an almost incalculable amount of patience and perseverance ; and let us bear in mind that in her case these prolonged and arduous labours had a remarkably beneficial stimulant influence.

I think it will be better to bring into relief certain more intimate characteristics which, if I mistake not, can be detected in all the cases we have been considering. In contrast with depressing actions, which from many points of view are abortive and inadequate actions, the actions which prove stimulating are complete and successful actions.

First of all, they are objectively satisfactory and successful actions, which have definitely induced in the outer world the modifications which the doer required at that moment. A shy person tries to speak, but he is really unable to speak, and it is precisely because he does not succeed in speaking that he has a crisis of shyness. On the other hand, we see that in the cases where actions prove stimulating, the social action was fully performed.—Lydia actually did go to the ball, and when there she had a conspicuous success.—Héloise did not merely try to arrange for her great dinner party, but organised it admirably and successfully.—Oc. did in actual fact take money from his employer's till, and did actually use it in order to treat workmen at the public-house ; he played the part of a vulgar Amphitryon, but he played the part very well.—Tt. does really drive his motor car, and drives it successfully.—The actions necessitated by the house-moving are successfully performed, and after the move, the furniture is successfully installed in the new flat. But in earlier cases, where a house-moving has been described as a cause of depression, the patient did not organise anything, did not feel at home in the new flat, and after the lapse of six months still found everything unfamiliar. In struggles which have proved stimulating, the subjects have battled seriously and courageously.—In the shipwreck, Wo. rendered valuable assistance to her companions in misfortune.—When discussing crises of depression brought on by the death of parents, I insisted upon the important fact that the patients, Irène in especial, did not do any of the actions necessitated by the death of the father or the mother. Irène did not manage the little household, did not watch over her father, would not even put on mourning.—On the other hand, when the death of the parents has had a stimulating effect, the conditions were the very reverse of this.—Justine, as she herself said, set the whole place in order and worked very hard after her mother's death.—Claire, after her father's death, organised everything and was a great consolation to her mother.—We see the same thing in connexion with engagements and marriages. The depressed individuals were those who were incapable of deciding, of making things ready, of performing the sexual act ; the people who were stimulated were people who made decisions, who got their new household in order, who were fully able to perform the sexual act.—I need hardly dwell upon the same characteristics in the case of amorous adventures. We have seen that those who were stimulated by such adventures were persons who displayed in them boldness, perseverance, amazing ability. For two years, Pepita was engaged in the most complicated intrigues without her family's knowing anything about it ; and in order to deceive her associates, she displayed a skill which would have done credit to a diplomat. In all these instances, the action which proved stimulating was materially completed, and successfully performed. This is the first essential point we have to bear in mind.

In the second place, the success of the stimulating action is also a social success. Most of these actions have had witnesses who have manifested approbation. That was the case at the dinner parties and dances, in the distribution of stolen objects, in the treating of comrades at the public-house, in the cases of devotion, in the religious ceremonies, and in the literary performances. In other instances, success was proved by the overthrowing of an adversary. The victim of the authoritarian, or the vanquished lover, testified to success by submission.

Finally, it is important to note the great psychological difference in the state of mind of the depressed subject as compared with that of the simulated subject. In the actions of depressed persons, as I have frequently shown, the tendencies are thwarted and checked at an inferior stage of activation. They are merely half-formed wishes, efforts or actions which are not animated by interest ; they represent a mere playing at action. They do not succeed in arousing the feelings really appropriate to action ; the sense of personality, reality, unity, freedom. They leave in the mind a mass of sentiments of incompleteness. Even if to the onlookers his action has seemed perfectly adequate, the subject is far from satisfied with it. He complains that nothing has been finished, nothing has been liquidated ; that he has not made up his mind, that he has not achieved any of the satisfactions or experienced any of the joys which crown a completed action. The psychoanalysts, in especial, have pointed this out in connexion with sexual acts which are not accompanied by a feeling of enjoyment and are not followed by a true release of tension. In this respect I agree that they are often right, and it is to their credit that they have drawn attention to a matter which has not previously been described with any precision. But we should make a mistake if we were to think that this incompleteness is peculiar to sexual actions. Even in the adventures which accompany the actions, if these adventures are not successful, we find the same characteristics. " Just now I can achieve nothing ; I can neither live respectably nor go on the loose. Everything in me seems unfinished, and I do not succeed in being either a courtesan or a respectable mother of a family. . . . I have all the tedium of the unfinished and none of the joys of the finished. . . . It is a hotch-potch which contains everything no doubt, but contains nothing perfect, for it is only made up of fragments."—We find the same characteristics in all actions which prove depressing, whatever their kind. " I do everything by halves only, and nothing can be more tiring than to do things by halves." It is, in fact, in connexion with such half-finished actions, that there ensue fatigues, agitations, hesitations, fresh beginnings, retrogressions, " attachments."

On the other hand, stimulating actions are those which are complete, are perfect from every point of view, even if they are performed by subjects who are not accustomed to act in this way, and who are surprised at being able to do so. Such actions are finished, definitive, and are accompanied by satisfaction and pleasure. We see the same characteristics alike in sexual acts and in stimulating adventures.—" I suppose," says Pepita, " that I have the temperament of a street-walker ; but what am I to do ? I felt uneasy and wretched at home ; I was out of place there and had no pleasure in anything. On the other hand, I felt perfectly at home in a boozing-ken, and enjoyed myself there immensely."— " It was certainly my very self that stole, " said Madame V. " Never before had I felt so full of activity and resolution."— Religious activities are only stimulating in persons who engage in them with faith, who have full conviction. The intellectual work which proves stimulant is work accompanied by feelings of clarity, certitude, and satisfaction.

It is in connexion with these phenomena that our patients are apt to employ the word " emotion," but they use it in a rather vague way.—" All true emotion," says Claire, " does me good when it has been really felt." The word " emotion " here signifies the characteristic feeling aroused by a tendency in exercise. What Claire really wants to say is : " I feel stimulated when I realise that a religious action, or an act of love, is performed by me completely and correctly."— Noémi even distinguishes the emotions " which miss fire " from the emotions " which hit the bull's-eye." She says ; " to play the piano in public strikes chill to the heart ; it needs an enormous effort ; but when I succeed in doing it, it raises my spirits immensely and fills me with joy."—In a word, an essential characteristic of these stimulating actions is that they are psychologically complete, that they are accompanied by all the sentiments typical of joy.

These observations may be summarised very simply. Excitation is the outcome of successful actions ; of actions that are successful physically, socially, and psychologically ; of actions that have been carried to their final conclusion without being checked by exhaustion. On the other hand, we see exhaustion make its appearance in the course of other actions, giving them from the very beginning, or at a later stage during their performance, the characteristic of inadequate tension. When this happens, the actions are followed by more or less depression. Nothing succeeds like success, and failure breeds failure.

2. *The Mechanism of Stimulant Actions.* I need hardly remind the reader that it is difficult to explain all these phenomena ; they cannot be crudely interpreted, or grouped in accordance with purely conventional theories.

Some of the foregoing observations may perhaps be connected with the theories which I have already discussed, the theories concerning traumatic memories ; the theories of *liquidation* and *discharge.* Useful liquidations may take the form of confessions, religious absolution, reconciliations, victories, various definitive actions like marriage, entering into a business partnership, and so on. Merely to clear up the litter on one's desk, to arrange one's affairs and one's papers, facilitates or renders needless a number of subsequent actions. If we engage a good servant, or get the services of a useful helper, or accept valuable guidance from another, we shall greatly simplify our subsequent life. It is probable that economies of this kind afford a partial explanation of the enrichment we can observe in our patients after a well-performed action.

In the second place, a complete action, although for the time being it involves expenditure, may subsequently lead to an increase of energy ; it may be like a good investment which brings a large return in the way of dividends. To eat involves fatigue, and so does the act of digestion ; nevertheless the taking of food provides us with new energies. Lagrange is one of the few authors who have a real grasp of such problems. In his book on mecanotherapy, he makes similar reflections concerning sleep. He apparently adopts the view which I put forward long ago, that sleep is a form of action, is a difficult action, which demands an expenditure of energy, an investment of funds. " It appears that in order to go to sleep we must have at our disposal a certain amount of available energy. Sometimes a moderate excitation of the nervous system induces sleep, which may be brought about by a cold douche and electrification." [1] Nevertheless sleep enables us to recuperate our energies. " He who withdraws from this reserve capital a moderate amount, and utilises it in order to win a good night's sleep, has made an advantageous speculation, inasmuch as by a trifling expenditure he has increased his general fund of energy, for sleep is the supreme restorer of energy."

An act well performed to the last degree of tension sets new tendencies to work, and probably entails the activity of additional bodily organs, whereby we are subsequently enabled, not only to repeat the same action at less cost, but even to acquire new capacities and more energy. When the owners of a factory expend a large sum of money in buying new machinery or in providing a new furnace, they are likely, ere long, to win back a great deal more than they have spent. It is probable that an act well performed will thus be the starting-point for the acquisition of considerable profit in the long run.

In the same chapter as that in which we discussed liquidation, we referred to the theory of the discharge, which likewise

---

[1] Langrange, Les mouvements méthodiques et la " mécanothérapie," 1899, p. 438.

finds numerous applications in this connexion. In persons who are well balanced, I said, there must be a definite relationship between the amount of available energy and the psychological tension. It is undesirable to retain a large quantity of energy when the tension has been lowered, for this gives rise to agitation and disorder. When the tension is low, it may be well to dissipate in one way or another a considerable amount of energy, so that a proper balance can be reestablished between the quantity of energy and the psychological tension. Such a discharge may be secured by a great many stimulant actions, such as those we have been considering. The discharge may take the form of intellectual work, going in for an examination, occupational activities ; or it may take the form of going to dances and evening parties, or that of all kinds of adventures. When we see in any one an impulse to seek pain, or to engage in debauchery of one kind or another, we suspect that the patient is trying to rid himself of an excess of energy, as if by a convulsive crisis ; and we hope that he may recover tranquillity and self-control thanks to the consequent enfeeblement.

I feel however, that we should exaggerate greatly if we were to explain all the phenomena as the phenomena of such a discharge. When I think of a great many stimulant actions, such as religious exercises, acts of faith, decisions, distress at the death of near ones and dear ones, amorous contemplations like those of Bul. who stares at a young man passing by, acts of command, acts of depreciation or teasing, triumphs, intellectual work, reveries, etc., it seems to me that in these there is very little expenditure of movement properly so called, and that we are hardly entitled to speak of them as discharges. Besides, before we can say that there has been a discharge, there must have been, to begin with, an excess of energy and of agitation ; and, after the action, there must be a manifest enfeeblement, like that which we see after debilitating illnesses or convulsive crises. Now, unquestionably, we cannot detect such characteristics in all the cases in which the action has been stimulant.

I think, then, that we must supplement the foregoing theories by two other conceptions which will perhaps be found important in the future, that of *psychological mobilisation* and that of *psychological irradiation*. The former of the two conceptions may be placed under the patronage of William

James, for it has been inspired by his interesting essay, *The Energies of Men*. There can be no doubt that, in the activities of daily life, human beings do not expend all the energies they possess, for they keep a large amount of energy in reserve. Under the pressure of unforeseen happenings, not only the normal individual, but even an extremely depressed patient, will be found capable of a quite unexpected activity. He is able to call up his reserves. The amount of these available reserves varies much from person to person. It is probable that some people have very little reserve energy; and that others have too much, because they use too small a proportion of their strength. At present, it is far from easy to distinguish, in practice, between these two categories of persons.

The real activity, the quantity, and above all the tension of the action, do not depend upon the total energy of the individual, but upon his available energy, upon the amount which at that particular moment can be expended, can be put into circulation.[1] In this connexion, we may return to our previous simile. The work performed in an industrial enterprise does not depend only upon its total capital, but also upon its circulating capital, upon the liquid cash. The enterprise may have large sums in the form of unmobilised reserves; in buildings, machinery, investments, outstanding credits which are not easy to collect. Yet, at a given moment, it may have very little available cash; and it may even, for considerable periods, find itself financially embarrassed, and be obliged to refrain from expenditure which might be most advantageous. Now, William James points out that neuropaths are often in a similar position. They have considerable reserves; but these reserves are not fluid, and for practical purposes at the particular time when the patients come under our observation the amount of their available energies is insufficient, for the bulk of their forces cannot be mobilised at this particular moment.

In such cases, it is very important to restore the power of mobilising the reserves, and a serious happening which shakes the invalid out of himself may do him a great deal of good. Once more, in the case of the factory, some accident like a fire or an urgent call may make it necessary to have recourse to the insurance company, to open a special fund, to call in

[1] Cf. Lagrange, op. cit., p. 439.

money that is owing ; and it is likely enough that the reserves of money thus mobilised will amount to a larger sum than that necessary to cover the immediate demands made by this special emergency. The money thus put into circulation will therefore do something more than repair the effects of the accident ; it will lubricate the whole machinery of the undertaking, and may restore prosperity. The feeling of imminent danger, what we call a strong emotion, may have the same effect upon the mind. It may compel us to perform energetic actions which cannot be achieved without calling up reserves of capital, without mobilising latent energies. Thanks to this change in the distribution of our energies, all our activities will be promptly transformed. It is because of the notable, the stimulant, part thus played by action, that patients so often seek to magnify the importance of what they are doing ; to increase, by various artifices, the effect of the action upon their emotions. Hence the mania for making solemn engagements, for making vows; hence the fondness for mystification, for the occult, for the melodramatic aspects of activity. We have often noted these peculiarities in depressed persons. The patients are trying to mobilise their reserves and to profit by the use of these latent energies.

It is essential that the psychological tension should be simultaneously raised, for otherwise this mobilisation of energy will only produce agitation. An energetic action should not only put at our disposal a larger amount of energy ; but it should also, in various ways, lead the whole mind to do this work at a higher tension. We have within us mechanisms or tendencies whose purpose it is to raise or lower tension as circumstances may demand. When we are resting, when we relax ourselves among friends, when we go to sleep, our tension is lowered. On the other hand, when we begin an action, when we have to put on our company manners, when we are preparing for a struggle, or simply when we wake up, our tension increases. An important action, and especially a successful action, stimulates the automatic mechanism whereby the tension is raised.

In all the cases we have been considering we can note many phenomena which can be ranged under this head. Persons who have performed a successful theft, the man who treats his friends in the public-house, those who have been able to make others obey them or have merely been able to make others suffer, those who have been paid a compliment, assume the air of a conqueror and maintain this attitude for a time while performing other actions.   The fact is so obvious that many of the patients note it themselves.—" A compliment paid me by the general," says Ba. (m., 27), " sets me on the go like a horse that is spurred ; I become more energetic for several days, feeling myself to be a man of whom the general thinks well."—Zob. (f., 50) says : " What I need is that my daughter should be continually saying to me : ' You are the most adorable of women, and everyone is passionately devoted to you.' This makes me feel thoroughly satisfied with myself, like a woman who is passionately loved, instead of feeling utterly flattened out like a woman who is crushed by contempt."—For Len. (f., 38), who has read a great many detective stories and who congratulates herself upon her cleverness, a successful theft is a stimulant.   " The dread of being caught in the act, the fight with danger, the pricks of conscience, and then the triumph—all this makes me feel enormously better, makes my eyes sparkle, and the effect lasts for a long time."—" It is really very surprising," says Kv. (m., 36), " I am, generally speaking, so much exhausted that I cannot endure the fatigue of the sexual act.   When I have intercourse with my wife, not only does the act give me no pleasure, but I am ill for a fortnight afterwards.   Well now, I have just had a little adventure with my sister-in-law. You would have thought that this, too, would have been most fatiguing, for I experienced a very powerful voluptuous sensation.   Why has it completely cured me of my wretchedness ?   I suppose, because I made a conquest."—A great many women who are exhausted by intercourse with their husbands (which is rendered incomplete by vaginismus, and is followed by hysterical fits), can have normal and restorative intercourse with their lovers.—A simple sense of gaiety may have similar effects.—" It is very remarkable," says Ed. (f., 60) ; " the young woman made me laugh after dinner, and I slept well that night, the first time for months." —Bp. (f., 27) suffers from depression taking the form of doubt.   She feels that everything is covered with a veil ; the passing of time fills her with dread.   While in this condition she meets a young man who tells her a funny story.   She listens, with a considerable effort of attention. Grasping the point, she bursts out laughing. " From that moment, my troubles were over ; I was transformed. One cannot at the same moment be laughing with delight and have a dread of life."—In all these cases, the tension necessitated by the action has induced a general condition of tension which has persisted for a considerable time. We may speak of this as " psychological induction " or a " psychological irradiation," and we may contrast it with the phenomenon of derivation which we have studied in connexion with depression.

This interpretation is not absolutely opposed to the foregoing theory of the discharge, and is perhaps merely another aspect of the same theory. The discharge may not be simply a loss of energy ; for it may also be a putting into circulation of forces in a way which favours a new distribution, and, in especial, favours the transformation of part of the energy into tension. When there is a great deal of expenditure, there may simultaneously occur favourable investments. This explains why it is that, after the violent movements of the convulsive paroxysm, and after exhausting exercise, we may note, in certain patients, not merely a disappearance of agitation, but an actual increase of psychological tension. If, some day or other, I am able to publish my lectures delivered at the College of France, I shall be in a position to discuss these problems with more precision. All that I can hope to do here is to give a hint or two which may be useful guides to research and to attempts at treatment.

3. *The Conditions which can facilitate the Production of Stimulant Actions.* This matter is so important that I shall devote a separate section to its consideration.

6. CONDITIONS OF STIMULANT ACTION.

How is it that these patients are able to perform certain actions completely, and with a tension able to raise their spirits as a whole, when for a long time they have been depressed persons unable to perform any action of this kind, and when, generally speaking, they have been checked by exhaustion long before the action was completed ?

A primary condition is, obviously, the existence, within

the mind, of latent energies able to come into play under certain conditions. It is probable that the chief difference between simple psychasthenics and asthenic dements is that the former are not, and that the latter are, utterly depleted of their reserves. But the matter that we have to study is, what are the special conditions which facilitate the activation of these latent energies ? As regards this problem, just as regards the one I have recently been discussing, I can only offer a few brief reflections.

The stimulating circumstances which induce an action of high tension would seem to be circumstances which are spoken of as " serious "; important needs, dangers threatening our own existence or the existence of persons dear to us, or pecuniary hazards. We have seen many examples of this. I think that the facts may be explained as follows. Reserves of energy are especially localised in the deep-seated and elemental tendencies, in those whose function it is in case of urgent need to safeguard the life of the individual or the life of the species. In ordinary circumstances, such tendencies scarcely come into play, for we seldom feel ourselves to be in danger of death, and we rarely call upon our most important reserves unless life is in imminent danger. But when these tendencies are awakened, they promptly place at our disposal a very large amount of energy. That is why all such " serious actions " are so stimulating. That is why, in many cases, " trifling actions " induce disturbances, such as abulia, and give rise to derivation ; whereas " serious actions " induce progress by giving rise to tension, and lead to irradiation. I have already given a good many examples of these phenomena. It will suffice to recall that many patients have been stimulated by a great danger to themselves or to their children.

Besides these reserves which may be called general, there are special reserves peculiar to certain persons who have a marked development of this or that tendency in virtue of a sort of education, and who have made a practice of appealing to this tendency in case of need. The women whom we have been describing know that they have always had their spirits raised by devotion, by adventures, by social successes, or by love. " There are not many levers in this world," said one of them. " I know three : fame, money, and love. Fame and money are reserved for men, who alone are able to reach an exalted position, or to earn a great deal of money ; women stand on a lower plane, and have comparatively little creative power. For most women, at any rate, nothing is left but love : parental and filial love, conjugal love, and love unqualified. For my part, I have always cured myself of all my troubles by seeking a lover, and I cannot think of any other remedy." Thus, when the favour of circumstance awakens such tendencies, an action can be completely performed, with due effect upon the whole mind.

Here we encounter a great difficulty. In an earlier chapter we saw that such an appeal to deep-seated tendencies was very dangerous. An appeal of that kind gives to the perception of a situation what psychoanalysts call its " affective charge " ; what we have regarded as an excess of energy, an energy disproportional to the tension ; this is the starting-point of traumatic memories, obsessions, " attachments " of all kinds. To avoid such dangers, and to make things work out in a different way, the action must be differently performed. Instead of being an incomplete action performed at low tension, instead of being an " attachment " which will leave a moiety of the mobilised forces unoccupied, the action must be complete, must be performed at high tension, must control the forces utilised, and must carry back to reserve after the triumph any surplus of unutilised forces. In a word, it is not sufficient that a powerful tendency shall have been awakened and that a large quantity of energy shall have been mobilised ; it is further essential that the environing circumstances shall, in their totality, be sufficiently favourable to enable the action to be carried to its term.

We are ill informed as to the nature of these favourable conditions, but it is reasonable to suppose that the moment at which the stimulation to action occurs must play a part here. Except in the case of very young patients, and in those whose depression is only moderate, stimulant actions do not, in most instances, manifest themselves until several weeks or months after the first onset of the depression. It would seem that a certain time must elapse for the reparation of the forces exhausted by fatigue or emotion. But we must not delude ourselves, and we must recognise that we know very little about the laws which regulate the duration of these reparative processes.   Except in the case of patients who are already well on in years, and who have had numerous crises superimposed, as it were, one upon another, we cannot predict with any sort of precision the duration of the reparatory period.   It seems probable, however, that in a great many cases the morbid symptoms continue beyond the expiration of the time really indispensable for repair.   We often see our patients get the better of their depression, thanks to fortuitous stimulant circumstances, when, but for these circumstances, they would probably have remained far longer in a state of depression.

Apart from this question of the need for a definite lapse of time after the onset of depression, we note that there are special periods, varying from case to case, in which stimulation finds the subject favourably disposed.   In certain persons, stimulation can only be successful in the afternoon or the evening.   In some women, stimulation is only successful during the days just before menstruation ; and in others during the days just after menstruation.   " How could my mother have been so stupid as to talk to me about a proposal of marriage on the very day after I had finished being unwell ! " The circumstances preceding the event must also be taken into account.   The subject should have been resting for some time ; should be in a good humour ; should be prepared by having had a good meal which is being well digested, and by little preliminary successes.   It would take too long to give details here, but the reader must not fail to recognise the importance of such matters.

Special stress must be laid upon another circumstance which I regard as of extreme importance.   The stimulant circumstances must develop slowly enough to leave the patient the time requisite for an unhurried reaction.   I have already referred again and again to the fact that, in psychasthenics, slowness is an essential characteristic of action.   (I am referring, of course, to their complete actions, and not to the various agitations from which they suffer.)   In them the rhythm of action differs from that of their associates, and this slowness of theirs gives rise to a great many disharmonies. Many of the manifestations of impotence and many of the emotional derivations that occur in psychopaths, result from the fact that, as the patients themselves say, " the others go too quickly, and it is impossible for me to hurry so as to catch them up." In an earlier work [1] I have studied the remarkable symptoms induced in these patients by the simplest events when they happen with undue speed. On the other hand, when the circumstances awaken the tendency gradually, and leave plenty of time for its development, the act may reach a degree of tension which we had imagined the subject to be incapable of displaying. But what we have to recognise is that in such patients the preparation for action often lasts an enormous time, so that we shall frequently be surprised by the apparently sudden performance of an action which has been developing in the depths for several weeks past. This matter is of considerable therapeutic importance, and I shall return to it.

Another important condition is the feeling that the act is a necessary one ; the feeling that attaches to the gravity, to the significance, of the action.—" When I absolutely have to do something, it is good for me. I lack strength to force myself to do anything, and what I need is that outside circumstances should compel me."—That is why these patients nearly always do things late, at the eleventh hour, and when necessity urges them to act. The feeling of necessity gives birth to effort, and the importance of this is very great. I regard effort as the complication of the activation of a tendency by the mobilisation of kindred tendencies which add their energies to the energy of the primary tendency. Moral tendencies, the desire to demonstrate one's freedom, to exhibit one's individuality, the dread of humiliation, and even more elementary tendencies such as ambition, love, and fear, will thus be superadded to a comparatively weak tendency, such as the tendency to say something or to write a letter.

Efforts always demand a great expenditure of energy. It is remarkable to note how, in the foregoing cases, and in some others which I shall describe, they nevertheless play a great part in excitation.—Byc. (m., 50), suffering from extreme abulia, who will spend hours in front of the mirror combing his beard and unable to finish dressing, and who is incompetent to come to the most trifling practical decision, will nevertheless show a remarkable amount of commercial and industrial activity in difficult circumstances. " I cannot do anything

---

[1] Les obsessions et la psychasthénie, 1903, vol. i, p. 540.

effective unless I make a great effort ; I need to have considerable obstacles to overcome ; I find it comparatively easy to
do difficult things, but difficult to do easy things." It is a
remarkable fact that this man can only succeed in acting
when the action has been pondered long beforehand during
a period when he seemed to be inert, and when, at the last
moment, he has found himself in a bustling and lively
entourage.—Wkx. (m., 28), who is ordinarily incapable of
acting, behaved very well when he was in the army ; and
during the war he showed considerable energy and endurance.
The reason he gave was : " At that time I had to make efforts,
and it did me a great deal of good."—" When I am really
compelled to act," said Anna, " it is frightfully difficult,
but my whole personality is changed. The difficulty gives
me a proof of myself, of my own existence, and this is the only
thing which can make me really live."—In the case of Simone
(f., 26), we see the remarkable effect of excitation through
effort. This patient, when she is in a state of depression, has
manias of recrimination against all and sundry, and is affected
with ideas of persecution. " It is very remarkable," she
says. " When I make an effort to speak to people whom I
detest, their faces seem to change, just as if they were puppets
and I were pulling a string. First of all their faces are
disagreeable, and then they have a charming expression."—
Such a transformation of the social sentiment through the
excitation connected with effort is most characteristic.
Improvement through making an effort to take a long walk,
an effort to drive a motor, the effort needed to care for a
child or a sick person, is often conspicuous.

But effort does not invariably produce good effects. A
great many patients have occasion to lament their unceasing
and fruitless efforts.—" I need to make a great effort for the
most trifling actions, even if I merely want to see anything
distinctly. It is so exhausting. I have to begin over and
over again, and never succeed in finishing what I do."—" It
is wretched to live always on the stretch, and still to slip
back unfailingly into ridiculous obsessions."—Precisely because
an effort has been made, and might have been expected to
have good results, these patients are continually repeating the
effort in season and out of season, until they become affected
with a mania of effort, a morbid impulse to effort. But is

not this the common fate of all stimulant actions ? Are they not all liable to degenerate into sterile impulses when they are repeated an indefinite number of times without due precautions ? If effort is to be fruitful, it must be moderate, and it must be made in the favourable circumstances we have just been studying. As a method of excitation, it is delicate, but sometimes its effects are remarkable.

Finally, one of the circumstances which plays a very important part as a factor of the success of an action, is the presence of particular persons and the part played by these. The action exercised by individuals one upon the other, a matter we are continually studying, is extremely complex. We have already seen that one form of this action is the order, and that another is the suggestion. We have also studied yet another form of this action of individuals upon one another in connexion with the persons whose mere presence is depressing to others, and necessitates from those others a great expenditure of energy. This has enabled us to understand the cause of what is known as antipathy. Now, conversely, we have to recognise that there are stimulant personalities ; that there are persons whose presence and words favour complete action, and enable the actions of others to be performed at a degree of tension which is irradiated throughout the whole mind of the doer. This is the converse phenomenon to antipathy, the phenomenon termed sympathy. Herein we discern the famous " personal magnetism," the " current of mental energy," of which the American advocates of the Mind Cure are never weary of speaking.

We find another person " sympathetic " when he is not " costly " to us ; when his presence and his words do not necessitate on our part a great and fruitless expenditure of mental energy. But there is more in sympathy than that. Some individuals do not exercise this purely negative influence ; they positively transform us by increasing our powers of action. They know how to show us that we have an interest in performing some particular action, and they can teach us how to energise it by powerful tendencies. They can help us to act while concealing the fact that they are helping us, while allowing us to believe that we are doing the whole thing, and even appearing to believe this themselves. They seem to obey us, and call us their master, although this alleged master does not really know how to command. They place themselves at a lower level than us ; even while showing us that they are of great worth, and that they are at a higher level than a good many others. This, of course, subtly flatters our self-esteem. They are competent, by skilful and masked praises, to induce in us mental attitudes of confidence and pride. They convince us of their loyalty, and that it will be unchangeable even though we can give them nothing in exchange ; for they make us feel sure that they love us for our own sakes and that they cannot change. These are the persons whom we find truly and enormously sympathetic.

It is not difficult to recognise the characteristics which make them sympathetic. Alike from the psychological and from the social outlook, they are strong and wealthy persons, who can thus diffuse fortune around them because they possess a great deal more than will suffice for their own needs. Such persons provide the invalid with " a padded entourage which prevents him bruising himself against sharp angles " ; they even enable him to accomplish on his own account marvels which transform him, and gradually render him stronger, make him " unbreakable." When we are beginning our study of mental disorders, we may be surprised to meet so many persons who are perpetually talking about love, and who are always craving for the same thing expressed in a hundred different ways—who " want to be loved." When we think of the part played by sympathetic persons in relation to weaklings, we can understand how natural it is that it should be the dream of all these weaklings to discover such resources in their neighbourhood, and how it is that this insatiable desire should so often degenerate into a morbid impulse. But the fact that so disastrous a transformation may occur, does not obviate the fact that there is a deep reason underlying their search ; nor does it annul the essential importance of a sympathetic and devoted group of associates in such cases.

These reflections belong to the domain of philosophy rather than to that of pure science, but we will try to draw from them practical indications. The doctor must realise that certain patients, although extremely depressed, are still capable of performing a few energetic actions ; and that these actions, far from exhausting the mind through the expenditure they entail, may lead to a fruitful discharge, and may even bring about a new distribution of energies and give rise to a higher tension. Such fortunate actions would seem to be those which have been performed completely, have been carried out with real success, and which, for a time at least, have been characterised by a considerable tension. They occur when special happenings awaken deep-seated tendencies, tendencies that are highly charged ; and when circumstances are favourable to the complete activation of these tendencies.

7. Useful Actions.

Attempts at treatment made by myself for a good many years may now be considered in connexion with the foregoing studies. In order to expound them, I must first examine three problems.

1. What are the actions which it is desirable to make these patients perform ?

2. In what way ought the actions to be performed ?

3. What, in the cases that have come under my notice, have been the most obvious modifications, immediate and remote, determined by these actions in the subject's state of depression ?

First, then, what kinds of action are desirable ? When we have to do with a patient who, as is most often the case, is simultaneously depressed and agitated, with one who is making confused attempts to perform all sorts of actions impulsively and is nevertheless unable to do any of them properly, we shall often find it useful to canalise the patient's activities and to make him concentrate his efforts upon some particular action. In some cases the choice of this action is more important than it is in others.—In this connexion I shall classify my observations under three heads. First, cases in which a particular action seems more useful than in others, and is chosen by preference. Secondly, cases in which the action is less specific, and in which we are concerned rather with a group of actions of a similar kind, connected with a particular tendency whose development seems essential. Thirdly, cases in which the nature of the act to be performed does not seem to be of much importance, and in which action is the main thing, of whatever kind and however performed.

When the whole illness is dependent upon the absence or inadequacy of a particular action, obviously the performance of this action is what we need to secure. Here we are concerned with troubles of the kind we have classified as " attachments." These attachments exhibit themselves in two different forms, according as the disturbing event is still real and extant, or exists only in the past and in the patient's memory. In the first case, we have to do with an act of reflective assent, or with an effort which the subject is unable to make, with incapacity to make a decision or to do a particular piece of work. In the second place, we are concerned with an inadequacy of triumph in a subject who is unable to achieve a liquidation. In both these classes of cases we have shown that the best treatment is to bring the subject to the performance of the necessary action, for this promptly puts an end to the indefinite persistence of difficult and costly efforts, and enables a great economy of energy to be effected. I may add, now, that the accomplishment of such an act, through the sense of satisfaction that is induced by overcoming a difficulty, and through a well-marked psychological irradiation, also contributes greatly to raise the tension.

In order to achieve these results, we must have a clear notion of the action which is to be performed. The more definite the doctor's ideas upon this subject, the more likely is it that he will be able to make the patient perform the necessary action. We have already studied this problem in Irène's case ; we come into contact with it again in connexion with certain other cases with which I have dealt in the foregoing chapter. The notes of these cases must now be supplemented from this point of view.

Zoé (f., 23), a neuropath by hereditary predisposition, has already suffered several times from depression, with various forms of mania. For fifteen years she has been her brother's confidant in a love adventure of his which has been equally absurd and unfortunate. For her brother she was at once guide and consoler ; but as far as she herself is concerned, this affair has inspired her with a supreme contempt for love sentiments, and with a great fear of them, seeing that they can lead to so much impropriety and so much suffering. She has definitely made up her mind that she will have nothing to do with such sentiments in her own case. In a word, her brother's confidences had drawn her attention to the love sentiment and had made it a more difficult matter for her to experience anything of the kind herself. On several occasions, proposals of marriage induced in her nervous symptoms, sadness, and phobias ; and the rejection of the proposals was followed by a cure. In one of these crises, which took rather a grave form, and whose true cause was not acknowledged, the patient was subjected to the treatment then fashionable of cauterisation of small areas in the interior of the nasal cavity. This treatment was followed by wonderful improvement. If this doctor had paid a little more attention to what his patient was thinking about, he would have learned that, at the time when the improvement took place, a suitor whose proposals for her hand had been a great worry to her and for whom she had no liking at all, had just been definitively rejected by her family. Had he known of these facts, the doctor would not, perhaps, have attributed the cure to his cauterisation.

When she was twenty-three, she met a young man who made a stronger impression on her feelings, and she realised with terror that if she let herself go she would soon be ardently in love with him. Her family would have approved this marriage, and in fact wished it to take place. The actual proposal of marriage was made under unfavourable conditions, and rather tardily perhaps. " I should have received it better if it had come sooner. If I am allowed to hesitate, I am lost." However this may be, when the proposal came, Zoé found it necessary to make a decision. Yet she was unable to accept or to refuse. She did not know what attitude to adopt towards this suitor. She was hesitant and irritable ; and then, when the suitor withdrew for a time, she was in despair. Now, doubt, indecision, and abulia became extreme. Phobias and criminal obsessions of various kinds developed. It would be needless to describe this psychasthenic condition, which speedily became grave. When I saw the patient eight months after the beginning of the crisis, she was extremely ill, both physically and mentally. I regard these disturbances in their totality as constituting a typical case of " attachment."

The evolution of mental life had been arrested by an obstacle which had proved insuperable, one against which all her energies broke in vain. The therapeutic problem was simple enough. It was necessary to overcome the obstacle, to lead the patient to take the necessary action. This action was the discovery of a solution which could conciliate her horror and contempt for an irregular and unfortunate love, with the wish for a correct and fortunate love. What she needed was simply a discussion, a comparison of motives, and a conclusion. In a word, reflective assent. This was the direction in which I guided the patient, and the results were demonstrative. I shall return to the matter in due course.

I may associate with this case, a number of similar cases in which the action to be performed was equally precise.— Newy (f., 48), whose case has already been considered in connexion with the sexual theories of psychoanalysis, had apparently overcome an obstacle similar to the one which blocked Zoé's progress. Newy had been married for eighteen months, and had become pregnant. How had these things come about ? The young woman, who had always been infirm of will, had lived with her mother and her sister all her life. " I felt that they were above me," she said, " and that they decided everything for me." When her marriage took her away from these guides, she suffered from tics, and scruples. She had allowed herself to be pushed into the marriage " without reflecting, and without accepting anything. Everything happened as if in a dream, as if the person concerned in the matter were not myself. I took no pleasure in anything, had no interest in anything. I received my betrothal presents without looking at them, and without really understanding that they were mine." Since the marriage, the troubles have grown worse. The patient stays at home, inert and agitated. She says : " I can do absolutely nothing. I cannot even sit down and rest. I feel crazy at the thought of the most trifling action. As soon as I try to begin it, everything in me gets stiff, and I have to stop. If I go on trying, I burst into tears. I cannot do anything in this house, which is not my own house. I do not know whether I love my husband or not, whether he is going to stay with me or to go away from me at once, or whether I am going somewhere or nowhere, for I am obsessed by the idea of leaving everything."

I need hardly say that the sexual act is unsatisfactory. This woman who, before marriage, was addicted to masturbation and found it pleasurable, has become frigid, and submits to sexual intercourse with complete indifference. As I have noticed in other and like cases, she has neither sexual shame nor sexual desire. All the same, she has become pregnant. Nevertheless, as I pointed out when discussing the sexual theory of the neuroses, we must not jump to the conclusion that all her troubles arose out of her sexual frigidity. This latter is only a particular aspect of a general disturbance of her sentiments and all her actions. " Nothing seems really of importance, nothing exists for me, not even my mother or my sister, and I no longer care for them." I have already referred to the remarkable change in the sentiment of ownership. " I do not feel able, as do other young wives, to say to myself, that everything is so attractive in my new house, or that I have pretty furniture. For nothing is mine. The husband is not mine ; the things in the house are not mine ; nothing given to me since my betrothal is mine. I want to wear the old dresses which I had before I was married, for these really seem to me to be my own clothes." This patient has already been treated in various ways. More especially, she has twice been isolated in a sanatorium without any other result than an increase in her agitation. We may regard the whole illness as an " attachment " akin to that of Zoé. She has not accepted the husband ; she has not adapted herself to conjugal life, to the joint life in a specialised environment. The disturbances also depend upon the inadequacy of these actions, and upon the fruitless efforts she makes to perform them. What is requisite is, either that the marriage should be dissolved, for then these efforts will cease ; or else, which seems to me possible and certainly in this case more desirable, that the patient should be helped to achieve the complete performance of the actions which she has not yet succeeded in performing. Though this latter may be difficult, the attempt ought to have remarkable results.

We often observe the onset of phobias or strange obsessions shortly after marriage. Some instances of this have just been considered. The differences between the various cases are apparent merely. The fundamental trouble is always a depression, exhibited now in one way and now in another, but invariably related to a thwarting of the acceptance of the sexual partner, or to a difficulty that is experienced in achieving that acceptance.

The same problem may arise in different circumstances. What happened to Irène can be regarded as a typical " attachment." This young woman had lived for some time with a woman friend of whom she was extremely fond. One day she was stupefied when her friend accused her of making love to an elderly man. After some scenes between the two friends, Irène had to leave the house. She was able to exculpate herself fully from the charge, but, she says: " I did not succeed in confounding my accuser, in humiliating her, in revenging myself upon her." For eighteen months after this incident, Irène remained ill, suffering from abulia, from invincible inertia, unable to sleep and equally unable to work, tormented from moment to moment by obsessions concerning the affair, by impulses to seek out the quondam friend, to make a scene in her house, to confound her, to avenge herself and so on. Although nobody accused her, and although every one was perfectly satisfied that the whole trouble had arisen out of her friend's morbid jealousy, she could not " liquidate the situation," and she was interminably confronted by the same event without being able to get beyond it. Here we have a typical instance of the liquidation which the doctor must often enable the patient to achieve if nervous exhaustion (which may become extremely serious when prolonged) is to be relieved.

In certain cases, the patients become " attached " to a moral problem, to a judgment which they have to make if their mental activity is to continue, a judgment which they are unable to make. An intelligent person cannot act without understanding, without believing, certain things. When he cannot either understand or believe these things, he can, of course, continue his elementary life, and even a part of his social life, but he remains perplexed, thwarted in his attempt to find an intelligent explanation such as all cultivated persons continually need to give themselves concerning their own lives and their own actions. Thus the whole behaviour of one in this condition is disordered.

In my first book, though it was a long one and perhaps unduly long, I was too summary in my treatment of obsessions.

I tried to show that the fact of having obsessions depended upon mental depression and upon subjacent sentiments of completeness. That is true, for were it not for this inadequacy, the subject would not remain "attached" to the various difficulties of life. Even so, however, we have to recognise that the various obsessions differ greatly one from another in their psychological mechanism. I have now to refer to special obsessions which are "attachments" to certain problems with which the subject is faced ; just as certain abulias or certain phobias are related to a check in face of a difficulty of social life.—Lydia, whose environment has been changed, and who finds the new circumstances of her married life humiliating, is unable to understand her new life and no longer understands herself. She is checked in face of the problem of her personal worth, and cannot find any solution. This insoluble problem has, in her, been symbolised in the form of strange obsessions with the thought of her own beauty.—Lise is continually thinking about the problem of her individual responsibility ; and in her obsession she gives this problem a symbolic form when she is perpetually trying to discover whether, in the next world, she will be responsible for her uncle's soul, or whether her children will have to pay for her misdeeds.—Jd. (f., 19)—and a good many other patients, for the phenomenon is common in young people— finds herself jostling against the moral problems which arise in connexion with the development of the sexual tendencies. These problems having once been raised in the mind, the subject, owing to her condition of depression, is equally unable to solve them and to give up thinking about them. The result is that for years she has exhausted herself in sterile meditation which has demanded an enormous expenditure of energy.

No doubt the doctor may notice that his patients are too much exhausted to be able to face their difficulties. He may be compelled, either to give them a preliminary rest, or else to restore their mental energies by a process of general education. But whichever course he adopts, the time will come when he will have to make the patient face the obstacle, when he must help the patient get the cart out of the rut in which it has been stuck, that it may resume its course along the road of life.

Far more often, the inadequate actions are more numerous' or are recurrent. It is not simply requisite to help the patient to perform an action once for all. We need to reestablish a tendency, and to teach the subject how to perform a particular kind of action again and again. For instance, in patients suffering from phobias, the anxieties which appear to supervene in specific circumstances are usually the outcome of the inadequacy of the actions which ought to be properly performed in these circumstances.

In a great many neuroses, disturbances of certain elementary psychological functions play their part as factors.— Sb. (f., 27) has for years been affected by a strange phobia accompanied by obsessive ideas tantamount to delusions. She is continually depressed by the dread that she has accidentally swallowed some large object near which she has just passed. It may not simply be an apple or an orange she has seen upon the table ; but perhaps a great carven apple of wood on the staircase, a large cushion, or even some big article of furniture on which her eyes have rested for a moment. Although she keeps on saying to herself that the idea is absurd, she is crazed and suffocated by the thought, and suffers from intense anxiety for hours. It is easy to note that, even apart from these crises, the patient swallows with difficulty, gulping down air with her food ; and we observe that she breathes badly. The most trifling emotion suffices to disorganise these inadequate functions, and brings on crises of aerophagia. Distension of the stomach with air, and a consequent interference with breathing, play a part in the obsession. I am inclined to try whether the restoration of these elementary activities, and the treatment of the aerophagia, may not have a happy effect in dispelling the phobia. Such treatment by action belongs to the domain of gymnastics, and especially to the domain of respiratory gymnastics, whose importance has already been discussed.

In many instances, it is easy to ascertain that disorders of sleep play a considerable part in causing the disease. Sometimes, even, we can perceive that such a trouble is the main cause of the exhaustion of the nervous energy. Now, we know that sleep is a form of action, and that this action, just like others, may undergo depression and may be affected by derivative troubles. We are, therefore, naturally inclined to attempt a direct modification of the action of sleep ; but, unfortunately, we find this very difficult. In most of my cases, where I have been able to improve sleep, I have done so indirectly by stimulating some other tendency.—Zob. (f., 50) could sleep all through the night if, on the previous evening, she had had an excitation, if she had been to the theatre or to an evening party.—Ig. (m., 30) can sleep well enough if during the evening he has had one of those violent scenes in which he delights, if he has been affected with strong emotions and has had a weeping fit.—Ed. (f., 60) can sleep if she has been made to laugh in the evening.—Nebo (m., 40) cannot sleep unless he has been able to do some work during the day.—In other cases, however, I think that a direct education of sleep has been useful.—Lib. (f., 44) is learning how to check her continual reveries and to get herself ready for sleep.—Dn. (f., 30) has been taught how to control the agitation and the screaming fits which used to supervene when she was about to go to sleep.—Kx. (f., 26), who used to spend the whole night in a vague condition of drowsiness, has been benefited by a practice which takes the form of resisting this drowsiness, getting out of bed, and then lying down again in order to go to sleep properly.—There is certainly a muscular attitude appropriate to sleep, a definite resolution to sleep, a relaxation of muscular vigilance which can be voluntarily sought and which is a preparatory stage to sleep. The search for " the action of sleep " is not the pursuit of a chimera.

Just as they do not know how to sleep, these individuals do not know how to rest. They are perpetually at work, or else in a state of agitation ; they are always stiff, on the stretch, and can never relax. Rest is a form of action, just like sleep, something we must learn how to do. It comprises special movements and attitudes, both physical and mental Depressions and forms of impotence may arise in connexion with this action, as in connexion with all other actions. " I do not even know how to sit down in an armchair ; I am always sitting on the edge, and can never sit right into the chair. . . . I do not know how to loaf. I do not know how to look on." Distraction, sportiveness, and loafing, are all part of the action of repose. These patients do not know how to play, how to be distracted. Rather late in the day

they come to recognise that, at an age in life when one sometimes needs relaxation of tension, they have tried to live too
austere a life, one of perpetual labour. These actions of
rest can be taught. The voluntary search for attitudes of
repose, of relaxation of tension, of play, is a salutary preparation for repose itself. It is in this way that the methods of
treatment we have been discussing, the methods of treatment
by rest and by physiological economy, are connected with
what we are now considering, treatment by action.

Doctors hardly realise how many nervous symptoms may
be occasioned by disturbances of the urinary function.—
Vor. (f., 45), when she applies for treatment, has the aspect
of one suffering from agoraphobia. She becomes intensely
anxious at the thought of going out into the street, and of
going to visit anybody. This anxiety has originated in a
woman who is obviously an uneasy and over-scrupulous
person. It came on as a sequel to an eczema of the external
genital organs, and of the extreme cleanliness which was
requisite in connexion with the urinary function in order to
cure this eczema. The necessity for constantly watching
over the function (one to which an excess of attention is
always dangerous) led her to feel an almost continual desire
to pass water, and to be always troubled by a feeling of
incomplete satisfaction with the act of urination. The result
was that she was passing water at every moment. She would
go to the lavatory dozens of times in succession before getting
into bed, for fear of having an accident. And she was afraid
of getting out of reach of this place of refuge even for a moment.
Her whole thoughts were concentrated upon the matter,
and she became exhausted by the precautions she had to
take.—Ub. (m., 44) had a strong impression made upon him
in youth by the painful treatment of a prolonged attack of
gonorrhoea, and since then he has always remained uneasy
concerning the urinary function. Having been exhausted by
family quarrels, and having had an unfortunate impression
made upon his mind at a medical consultation which was not
very discreetly conducted, he became affected with obsessions
and phobias. He is obliged to recognise that he has no real
disorder of the urinary function. But he says to himself:
" I am certainly going to become affected with spasms of the
urethra, which will necessitate extremely painful treatment

by the passing of a catheter. I would rather die than have to endure that sort of thing all through life." These troubles have made it impossible for him to do any work. Night and day he thinks about his urinary function, trying to pass water every moment, and feeling real or imaginary spasms in the pelvis. He is utterly crazed by these anxieties. The condition is getting steadily worse, although the patient has already been under treatment in a sanatorium for six months. —In these two cases, the trouble has definitely arisen out of the urinary function, which in both patients is physiologically normal. But the psychological aspects of urination, which are far more important than people are apt to suppose, have been utterly disorganised. Shall we not do well to attempt the reeducation of this function and the reestablishment of normal urination, and then to study the modification which a restoration of functions induces in the other mental functions?

We should make a mistake were we to exaggerate the importance of sexual disturbances, but we must not overlook their great significance in the neuroses. It cannot be denied that, in many instances, a change, a depression, if not in the physiological elements, at any rate in the psychological elements of these functions, may give rise to a great many other neuropathic disorders. In this connexion, we may bear in mind that many young husbands, for one reason or another, prove temporarily impotent on the wedding night. Subsequently, emotion, dread of failure, and sometimes unwise advice, make the reestablishment of normal sexual functioning difficult, and create a true psychological impotence. This, in its turn, may give rise to the most varied neuropathic disorders. Similar troubles often arise in newly married women, although they are less often noted. They manifest themselves as vaginismus, or frigidity, and often play an important part in the depressions that are apt to ensue in early married life.

Still more serious are the matrimonial inadequacies which result from a thwarting in the psychological development of the sexual function, where this takes the form of an arrest at the stage of solitary masturbation, or an arrest at the stage of homosexuality.—Ae. (m., 27), sexually inadequate and psychasthenic, married at the age of twenty-five. During the two years that have elapsed since his marriage, his behaviour towards his wife has been very remarkable. When he is with her before witnesses, he pretends to be greatly interested in her; he is gallant, and even too free in his proffers of affection, being quite aware that in public he cannot go to extremities, and being proud to assume the air of a conqueror. At the same time he adopts towards her a superior and domineering attitude, pretending to treat her as a baby, and demanding from her constant tokens of admiration and submission. But when he is alone with her, the whole scene is changed. His attitude is embarrassed and timid. He is afraid to speak to her. He is careful to avoid letting her know anything of his tastes and sentiments, as if he dreaded intimacy. He seeks every possible excuse for keeping at a distance from her. If he is compelled to come near her, he will actually put on gloves before touching her; and his sketchy caresses, which lead nowhere, speedily become transformed into blows and pinches. He displays an almost incredible shamefacedness. He cannot bear her to touch him, and seems terrified at the thought that she might see any part of his body. Furthermore, he is constantly declaiming about the rules of religion and morality which regulate relationships between husband and wife. The husband is becoming more and more abulic and uneasy, and the wife now suffers from hysterical symptoms.

We know, of course, that it is often dangerous to urge people like this to perform the sexual act. I have myself seen very serious symptoms, and even a prolonged attack of mental disorder, arise after imprudent attempts of the kind. It is none the less true that the doctor must come to a decision here. He must either adopt treatment by economising the energies, and must separate the young couple so that they may not continually squander their forces in fruitless efforts; or else he must adopt treatment by excitation, and must induce the husband to perform a complete sexual act which will cure both husband and wife. More often than might be imagined, if the doctor is assisted in his endeavours by the wife, and if the latter is intelligent, treatment by excitation is practical enough, and will have a fortunate result.

The so-called sexual inverts are usually depressed persons in whom the sexual function has been arrested at an elementary stage of development. They are timid; they are sexual abulics who are afraid of the opposite sex, seeing that approaches to sexual intimacy are a complicated matter.—Xc. (f., 37), whose case I hope to relate in full some day, says justly : " I am twenty years behind."—More often than might be supposed, these patients can be educated, and thus relieved.

The psychological sexual functions can be altered in another way, not primitively by an inadequate development, but secondarily by a regression due to mental depression. A great many persons who have had normal sexual relationships, attended by adequate voluptuous sensations, become frigid and impotent when they are ill, or may regress into the practice of masturbation. This reduced form of the sexual act, a less costly form, then plays the part of a transient stimulant.—Bb. (f., 26), suffering from phobias and mental manias, is obliged to seek self-stimulation in this way when she wants " to be able to walk without continually counting her footsteps."—Conversely, we are familiar with the interesting cases of Wb. and Pya, men who have all their lives used the sexual act as a stimulant, and who fall into depression when the stimulant is no longer available. In these latter cases I was led to undertake for the patients the education of the sexual act ; and the result of this treatment, which I shall consider more fully later, were, I think, very remarkable. Though I do not agree with the psychoanalysts that the entering into sexual relationships always constitutes an ideal form of treatment, I am constrained to admit that sexual intercourse, when practised with due moderation and prudence, has shown itself extremely valuable in many of these cases. The doctor must not ignore its therapeutic value.

When the patients are suffering from one of the affections which are somewhat vaguely classed under the name of phobia of contact, we can easily discover that, underlying such a delusion or phobia, there is present an abulia, bearing more or less definitely upon this or that action.—Cc. (m., 55), who throughout life has been interested in horseback riding and in the care of race-horses, having had a disappointment in this field of sport, ceases to concern himself about horses and stables. He rationalises the renouncement as due to a dread of horse-dung. Then, reversing the terms as these patients often do, he extends his dread of contamination to all objects with which he may come into contact.—Df. (f., 22) explains all her impotence and inertia as due to the dread of cancer ; but her main trouble is her incapacity to attend to her household affairs after a change of domicile, her lack of power to adapt herself to life in new surroundings.—Similar explanations can be found in many other cases of the phobia of contact, especially in women.   Abulia in household life often underlies phobia of contact.   The actions we must seek to make the patient perform are obvious in such cases.

A great many neuroses have the aspect of occupational neuroses. We are all familiar with occupational obsessions, phobias, and tics. I have given several instances of the kind in the present work. Here are some more.—Ec. (m., 40) thinks that he is compelled to abandon his profession of dentist, in which he has been successful, because " the most terrible things will happen if I should prove unable to resist the impulse to take liberties with my female patients."— Fd. (m., 35) a chemist, made a serious mistake one day in compounding a draught. Happily the mistake had no ill results, but he was terrified at his momentary lapse of attention, and there ensued an obsessive over-scrupulousness which has made him abandon his occupation for the past year.—Nebo. (m., 40) after one or two unfortunate ventures in his business, found himself so terribly agitated whenever he went into his shop that he retired, and went to live in the country, until he grew worse there.—If we have occasion to note in such patients that the arrest of occupational tendencies continues to function as the chief cause of the general depression, we shall ask ourselves whether we should not rather try to reestablish occupational activity.   Retirement from business, or simply a very prolonged holiday, may be extremely dangerous.   A good many men whose occupational activity has been the only thing keeping up their psychological tension, are incapable of finding sources of excitation in any other activities.   We shall often find it desirable to make them resume the occupation which has kept them in good mental health for many years.

Among the actions that we have to advise in the hope of securing excitation, the most frequent are social actions. Claustrophobia, agoraphobia, erythrophobia, dysmorphobia, the numberless neuroses (often ill understood) which are varieties of morbid timidity or social abulia, must often be treated by exercising the patient in social activity. A great many of these patients must be compelled to pay visits ; " to remain in a room where there are two or three persons, without trying to run away like a madman " ; to travel in a railway compartment where there are some men, although " one shows by incessant blushing the longing that torments one, and although one utters nervous giggles which are provocations " ; " to take one's proper place in a church and not to hide behind a pillar, although one is defiling the ceremony by one's presence " ; to speak directly to people, " although one is making them feel ill by one's breath " ; to give orders to a servant, " although it makes one's heart almost stop beating " ; to make purchases in a shop, " although one would rather go into a cage filled with lions than to speak to the saleswoman " ; to go through a street where there are no chemists' shops, " although this is a terribly dangerous thing to do " ; etc. Sometimes the social actions we must make the patient perform, are of a higher grade. Many must be taught to speak, to listen, to hear a joke without growing angry, to take part in a discussion without getting heated. We must make the patients express their thoughts, and put forward their own side of a question in such a way as to avoid the petty failures which distress them so much and which are apt to be the starting-point of their phobias and obsessions.

These disturbances of social activity sometimes, in psychasthenics, assume very remarkable forms.—Ge. (m., 40) has been placed under restraint on account of a remarkable delusion. His family regarded it as a delusion of persecution. When he is alone, or believes himself to be alone, he sits quietly in his armchair smoking cigarettes or reading a novel, and behaves rationally enough. But as soon as any one comes near him, he jumps up, gesticulates, makes faces, tries to run away, strikes the furniture, breaks the windowpanes and cries out : " You are going to make me ill ; you are going to bring on a crisis, to make me mad ; you are dominating me, do not come near me. I shall have a terrible attack of delusions if any one speaks to me or makes me go out. Do leave me by myself." This comedy has been played again and again all through the last two years. The patient has always been a typical psychasthenic. After a little more fatigue than usual and some failures in his profession, he became affected with an exaggerated form of psychasthenic depression, his obsessions of shamefacedness and his social terrors being then aggravated to become delusions. In his case the social activity of seeing people and of talking to them is primarily disordered. The only way in which he can be cured will be by restoring the activity of this social function.

In such a case as the foregoing, what we have to do is to reestablish social relationships of any and every kind. In less serious cases, there is some specific form of social relationship whose restoration must be achieved. I have repeatedly pointed out that psychasthenics are not fond of rubbing shoulders with their equals. They seek their lovers or their friends from among persons classed as their inferiors in fortune, station, or education. Lads or grown men will not talk to or play with people of the same age as themselves, but only with young children. Conversely, girls and young women may only find themselves at ease with persons much older than themselves. In either case, what the patient is looking out for is an easy social situation; one in which docility, admiration, and indulgence can be easily secured; one in which unfailing consideration will be exhibited towards him. Whoever attempts the social education of timid or shy persons must constantly be warring against this tendency.

In certain circumstances a remarkable manifestation of " social " activity is to be found in the actions which the patient has to make quite alone, in isolation. Without entering here into the psychological study of isolated action, though this is a most interesting matter, I shall remind the reader that in beings of a non-social type the activity of an isolated individual would not have any characteristics peculiar to isolation. A special form of activity characteristic of isolation can exist only as a contrast to social activity. In virtue of this very fact, therefore, it is itself a form of social activity. That is why this kind of activity is so often disordered in extremely shy persons, in persons whose ordinary social activities are disturbed. There are cases in which we have to educate the power of isolated action, just as we have sometimes to educate the power of ordinary social activity.—Wkx. (m., 29), who has always lived with his family, who is invariably

accompanied by some one, and can never be left alone, suffers
from crises of psycholepsy, with a sense of strangeness, aloofness, and impending death, whenever he tries to perform
an action in isolation. For him, the most useful form of
effort is that he should undertake actions quite by himself,
and even take little journeys alone.—Many women who are
obsessed by the wish to be loved, exhibit a hopeless " attachment" on somebody because they feel themselves incapable
of performing any action when they are alone. Ought we not
to compel such persons to act, to go out alone, to have individual
tastes and to satisfy them, without continually worrying
themselves about what some one else may think of what they
are doing ? The restoration of the power of isolated activity
is often a sign of a recovery of mental tension. Zoé (f., 26)
has noted this in her own case. When she was at her worst,
she felt terrified whenever she was alone, and she was constantly
trying to lean upon some one else. Since she has begun to
get better, she has found that she can derive a certain advantage
from being alone, that it rests her to be by herself for a time.

In some instances our patients indicate that they are
suffering from a check in one of the mental functions, in some
particular category of perceptions, in some form of belief or
of reasoning. Here, likewise, the action we have to encourage
is obvious enough. I have often found it useful in the treatment of patients suffering from depersonalisation to direct
their attention to their tactile and muscular sensations, just
as if they were suffering from hysterical anaesthesia, although
in these particular cases there is no definite sign of anaesthesia.
I have treated three patients in this way with especially encouraging results.—Hd. (m., 42) is suffering from a peculiar
form of depersonalisation, which appears to relate especially
to his own utterances, and even more markedly to the hearing
of his own utterances. He knows full well that it is himself
who is walking or eating, that it is himself who feels a touch
or a pin-prick ; he will even admit that it is himself who sees
and hears when other people move and speak. But he is
tortured by the obsession that his own words have escaped him,
that it is no longer himself who is speaking, that the words
which issue from his mouth are no longer his own. He has
no delusions. Theoretically he is well aware that the words
which issue from his mouth are his own, that they express his

ideas, that they have a familiar tone ; and yet he complains of a persistent feeling that it is some one else who is speaking. This remarkable disorder of the perception of speech occurs in a man who has always been shy, uneasy, and troubled in connexion with his own speech. He felt unhappy when he had to speak to his workmen, and became exhausted if he had to continue a conversation. We can readily understand that the depression would in his case, naturally take effect upon speech, since this was his weak point. But that does not explain everything. When he is reading, even when he mentally articulates, and when he talks to himself in low tones, he has no disorder of the kind, and does not experience the sense of depersonalisation. This feeling of aloofness does not affect the articulation of the words, but only his own hearing of what he says. An examination of his hearing did not show anything markedly amiss, nothing more than a definite retardation of auditory reaction. Such prolongations of the reaction time are common in psychasthenics, but they seldom affect audition. We may imagine that the patient had hitherto been accustomed to hear his own voice closer at hand when he was speaking, and that the retardation of the auditory reaction, superadded to the depression affecting the function of speech, has been a factor in inducing this particular form of obsession. But whatever the explanation, the psychological treatment I applied in this case consisted mainly in exercises of speech and exercises of auditory attention.

These observations show that it is sometimes advantageous to attempt the excitation of the subject by the performance of a particular action which the subject knows how to perform (so that he has not to learn it anew), but one which he has ceased to perform, or at any rate to perform correctly. They show that he will gain more advantage from the performance of this particular action than from the performance of any others. We see that, here, excitation has to bear especially upon a particular point, just like education as a form of treatment. In general, however, this is not the case. Depression seems, as a rule, to affect the whole mind ; and the realisation of one particular action is not more important than the realisation of any other. The patients have not themselves discovered what actions interest and stimulate them. " I am a woman who has nothing to do, and is not interested in anything. I have never been in love, and have never been industrious. I have never felt capable of doing anything noteworthy whether for good or for ill, so I have practically given up trying to do anything. If you want to make me do something, choose it yourself for me, since one thing will bore me just as much as another." It would be a mistake, in such cases, to try to find something which will please or interest the patient, for his illness consists precisely in this, that he cannot take an interest in anything. Interest is a form of the activation of tendencies ; it is already the first degree of activation. The tension must be raised to some extent before interest can arise.

We must be guided entirely by convenience when we are choosing the action which is to be a source of excitation. We shall naturally be inclined to choose the action which comes easiest, that which will most readily provide the subject with a success under existing conditions. Sometimes we can insist upon the performance of one of the actions we have just been considering, upon the search for particular sensations, upon the performance of social actions. But in many cases, owing to the practical difficulties involved in actions of this kind, we may encourage the patients to perform other actions, which are more convenient, and which, in my own practice, have often had a stimulating influence.

The simplest of these actions take the form of movements of the limbs which the patient can execute without having to speak, and without having to concern himself as to his associates. Dressing, housework, sewing, walking, bicycling, gardening, carpentry, etc., are occupations of this kind. Emile, a young man of eighteen, erythrophobic, living in a corner of his room quite motionless, his face hidden in his hands (or sometimes absorbed in a book), became able to perform a simple mechanical task such as book-binding. He was quite transformed when he became able to interest himself in the education of a kitten. This had an admirable influence upon him.

More important exercises, and ones likely to have a stronger stimulating influence, are actions in which speech plays a part. It is often useful to compel certain patients to speak clearly upon some subject or other. When they are extremely depressed, there is practically only one subject about which they are able to talk—themselves and their sufferings. Now, strange and even hazardous as it may seem, I think it is often useful to let the patient talk freely of himself, and to lead him on to express his fears and obsessions, though of course we must avoid letting him talk too much about them. What we must insist upon is that the expression of his ideas shall be as clear and definite as possible. As I wrote at the beginning of my book *Les obsessions et la psychasthénie*, these patients, even though they may be inclined to chatter, are apt to express themselves very badly.—Claire, to whom I referred in this connexion, would go on writing as she spoke, and would incessantly repeat " I have already said, as I think I said before ; no that is not it ; " and she was continually in despair because she had said nothing.—Apart from the difficulty they find in expressing their ideas clearly, these patients, especially when they suffer from over-scrupulousness, have to get the better of the discomfort and the shame they feel at having to speak plainly about the strange and often obscene ideas which trouble them.—It was very hard work to make Kl. speak plainly concerning her son's birthmark, and to explain how she was always asking herself whether this birthmark was a real proof that her husband was the child's father and not another man.—Several sittings were needed and a good deal of urging before Da. (f., 22) could be brought to say out loud " I think that God's love has the same effect as man's love. I think that I have become pregnant through God's love. I mingle the human and the divine. I am terrified, when I go to the closet, that I am having a child, and I look round to see what I have passed, for fear that it may be a living being. Is it possible that I am performing the love act with God when I wipe myself ? "—Of course there is a danger that, in certain cases, we may help the patients to fix their obsessions by making them recount these obsessions too often. But this will rarely happen. As a rule, the effect of making the patient express himself clearly is altogether different.

An opposite kind of exercise may advantageously be associated with this one. The patient who relates his sufferings to the doctor, and who learns to describe them completely and intelligibly, must at the same time guard against speaking promiscuously to all and sundry as he has been used to do. He must make an effort to hold his tongue about these matters when he is with the other members of the family, and this will be a great benefit to them as well as to himself. When a person suffering from obsessions has learnt to reserve his confidences for the doctor, and to pretend to be quite well when he is with other persons, he has made an enormous step towards cure. " At last," says Noémi, " I have learned to despise the dull uneasiness which disturbs me, and I pretend that it does not exist. . . . What a lot of things in life there are which we have to treat like that. . . . I do not talk about it now to my husband, and I hardly think of it when I am alone ; . . . but I still feel it, I cannot help feeling it. . . . After all, it does not matter so much if I am not quite well as long as no one else suspects it. I do not want to make myself a nuisance to anybody else." When she begins to talk like this, we know that she is getting near the end of her crisis. An effort of the kind, which is excellent from all points of view, which averts humiliations and gives relief to the patient's family, also induces in the patient a most salutary excitation.

The two kinds of behaviour of which I have just been speaking, will be likely to exercise a tendency which is apt to be in abeyance in such patients—the tendency to confide in a particular person. The patients, in fact, have an urge to confide in some one, and yet they do not really succeed in confiding in any one. They are simultaneously chatterboxes and reserved persons. They speak in season and out of season of certain obsessions, and yet they are extremely reticent concerning their real sentiments and their true preoccupations. In most cases it is a good thing to encourage them to show themselves for what they are. This practice of intimacy is far more difficult to achieve than might be imagined. Time is needed. The patient will have to make a great many efforts before he will succeed, even though he understands the importance of the matter. Many patients are aware how difficult it is for them to speak straightforwardly about themselves, and recognise that it comes as a sort of stimulus to them when they make a successful effort in this direction. " Never before have I said half of what I think. I was quite changed when I was able to speak sincerely about myself."

This particular form of action can be assimilated to a number of other actions which are no less difficult, and the effects of which are extremely interesting. I refer to the becoming aware of sentiments, and to the expressing of sentiments. In general, neuropaths are regarded as sensitive and emotional persons, for they are apt to exhibit for various reasons, and often for no obvious reason at all, emotional derivations of considerable strength. But we must not conclude from this that their sentiments are really, in most cases, accurate and deep. Almost always, imperfectly adapted emotional agitations, continually repeated in inappropriate circumstances, take the place of appropriate sentiments, of sentiments varied as they should be in relation to varying circumstances.[1] The psychasthenic has fewer joys or artistic sentiments, less affection, less hatred, less anger, less fear, even less sadness and less pain, than he would have had if he had been in good health. He is apt to believe that he has checked these sentiments, has prevented their expression, from a sort of shame, and because he is afraid to give utterance to a vigorous sentiment. He fancies that it is by his own free will that he substitutes sportiveness, pretence, or agitation, for true feeling. But this is an illusion. The sentiments comprise particular movements, gestures, and words, which are commonly spoken of as the expression of these sentiments, but are in reality an integral part of the sentiments. They are true actions, and actions performed at a high tension. Now, in these patients, their sentiments are reduced because all their actions are reduced, and especially their higher-grade actions. It may seem very strange that it should be possible to induce persons to feel more acutely than they are in the habit of feeling. Yet the idea is simple enough if we come to regard the sentiment as an action ; if we understand that the expression is an essential part of the sentiment, and that the sentiment is stronger if the expression is more complete and more correct. If we realise that the subject must cease playing the fool when he is expressing a sentiment ; that he must not thwart the expression, but must allow it to develop to the full ; that he must be genuinely angry if he wants to feel angry, or must shed real tears if he feels distressed—no doubt this is a delicate operation which can only be achieved under peculiar circumstances, but more often than might be imagined it gives very remarkable results.

[1] Cf. Les obsessions et la psychasthénie, vol. i, p. 714.

We may also regard as intellectual exercises those in which efforts of attention, representation, and comparison play a part. In educated persons, it is easy enough to organise and guide activities of this kind; and though such actions be less potent than material and social actions, they are none the less extremely efficacious.

Certain actions of this kind are simple, and even extremely depressed subjects can be asked to perform them. I refer to simple efforts of attention bearing upon definite sensations. I have already referred to exercises of attention concerning tactile or muscular sensations, to exercises which are prescribed for patients suffering from depersonalisation, exercises analogous to the aesthesiogenic exercises prescribed for sufferers from hysterical anaesthesia. In this connexion I may mention a number of exercises of attention to parts of the body or to environing objects, exercises akin to those which have already become famous thanks to the method for the reeducation of control advocated by Vittoz of Lausanne. To become fully aware of one's hand, one's fingers, one's feet; to recognise precisely what one feels in one's chest, and to realise by careful attention that there is really nothing but a number of extremely simple sensations where one had imagined there was a terrible pain; to examine attentively the designs on a piece of tapestry and to describe them accurately—such efforts may be most useful, and may dispel a great many algias or doubts. An interesting variety of these exercises takes the form of fixing the attention, not upon sensations, but upon memories, or upon ideas of the future. Some depressed patients, like Eo. (f., 31), feel quite incapable of imagining a situation different from the distressing one in which they now find themselves, and they therefore remain fixed in their obsessions. But human beings need to look forward, need to imagine the future, need to conceive an aim; and such efforts at application are not merely a gymnastic of attention and control, but are also an encouragement. The only criticism I have to pass upon these methods, when advocated with undue enthusiasm, is that they are rather elementary. I think that educated persons can gain more by fixing their attention upon somewhat more exalted mental operations.

Akin to this method is one which I used often to employ in the days when I was trying to make use of hypnotism for the relief of other patients besides hysterics, and in especial for the relief of psychasthenics. What I was particularly struck with at first was that hypnotic practices did not, in these new patients, give the same results as in the others. Except in rare cases, when I had to do with one of those intermediate forms of disorder midway between hysteria and psychasthenia, I could not secure either somnambulism or suggestion in psychasthenics as I had secured them in hysterics. And yet, to my astonishment, I found that these practices, though apparently inefficacious for those particular purposes, had an excellent effect upon the mental condition of the sufferers, raising their spirits so markedly that some of the patients, while noting, as I did, that there was no sign of hypnotic sleep or of suggestion in the true sense of the term, begged me to continue the use of the method which was doing them so much good. It seems probable that these attempts at hypnotism induce, in some of the patients, emotions, and efforts at attention. Patients who allow themselves to be hypnotised think that they are making up their minds to submit to a rather important operation; they make efforts to remain absolutely motionless and to relax their muscles for a certain time; they fix their attention upon particular sensations; and so on. Here we have a certain number of actions analogous to those of which I have just been speaking, actions which have a stimulating effect, although they are quite independent of hypnotism in the strict sense of the term.

A very simple method, one easy to organise, is reading; and we may be certain that the reading of interesting and well-written books can have a powerful therapeutic influence. J. Bourdeau, whom I may take this opportunity of thanking, has drawn my attention to a remarkable passage in John Stuart Mill's autobiography. That philosopher relates that during the winter of 1826–27 he was in a state of intense depression, so that he was utterly weary of life. " I did not think I could possibly bear it beyond a year. When, however, not more than half that duration of time had elapsed, a small ray of light broke in upon my gloom. I was reading, accidentally, Marmontel's *Mémoires*, and came to the passage which related to his father's death, the distressed position of the family, and the sudden inspiration by which he, then a mere boy, felt and made them feel that he would be everything to them—would supply the place of all they had lost. A vivid conception of the scene and its feelings came over me, and I was moved to tears. From this moment my burden grew lighter." [1] Bourdeau has also drawn my attention to a remarkable article by the Rev. Samuel McChord Crothers, entitled *A literary Clinic.*[2] The author imagines a pastor of a church where psychotherapeutic practice is conducted after the manner of the Emmanuel Churches of Boston. But this pastor has a very curious name for his consulting room, calling it " Bibliopathic Institute," and describing it as a place in which patients can receive " book treatment by competent specialists." This doctor of the mind tells us that literature is packed with fine thoughts, expressed in a wondrous variety of forms. Books can provide, not food merely, but medicine as well. In fact, books ought to be classed in accordance with their medical influence upon the mind. A book may be a stimulant or a sedative, a revulsive or a soporific. Some books play the part of a soothing syrup, while others have the effect of a mustard leaf. The author proposes to write literary prescriptions, in which literary passages will function as the ingredients, one being the active principle, another the adjuvant, another the corrective, and another the vehicle, the whole comprising an agreeable potion. The distribution of well-known authors and books among these various groups is wittily explained. Crothers writes jestingly, but there is an underlying element of truth. We can recognise that Jean Jacques Rousseau had an intoxicating influence for several generations, and that certain pessimist poems have a depressing influence on many minds. There can be no doubt that a well-read doctor could turn this moral influence of reading to good account for his patients.

Unfortunately, such therapeutic influences are of a delicate character. They can only be used for a small number of intelligent patients, seeing that the mass cannot be affected in this way. As a rule, we shall have to be content with a more commonplace and simple effect of reading. Sometimes the choice of a book, or merely its acceptance, may be a salutary moral effort. Jd. (f., 19), an intelligent young woman,

---

[1] J. S. Mill, Autobiography, 1873, pp. 140–141.
[2] " Atlantic Monthly," September 1916, p. 292,

but tormented by religious scruples, says that it is difficult for her to read a book (and especially an interesting book) if it is written by an irreligious author, or simply by a Protestant. " I find it distressing," she says, " to take an interest in an author and to know that he holds different views from my own The more I like people, the more strongly do I wish that in all respects they should think exactly as I do." She finds it quite an effort to adopt a complicated attitude so that she can continue to be interested in an author while accepting the fact that he differs from her in certain respects. In most cases, however, the difficulties relate to reading in general, these patients being inclined to let their eyes pass along the lines without understanding or remembering what they are looking at. " There is always a wall between the book and me ; I can never grasp what it is all about." To counteract this disposition, we must ensure that the reading shall be done under test conditions. Some one must be present when the patient is reading, must continually interrupt, ask the patient to recite passages, to explain what has been read, and so on. When I have had to do with intelligent patients I have devised a little exercise which I have called "the paragraphing exercise." It consists in asking the patient to write in the margin of the pages as succinct a phrase as possible, summarising the contents of each paragraph. In other cases, some simple arithmetical exercises may be superadded to the reading ; or the patient may be asked to keep an account of the household expenditure.

Other patients, again, will recognise that they need some difficult intellectual work which will absorb their minds. The reader will remember the case of Bkn. (f., 22), who said that she never felt really well mentally except when she was preparing for an examination. In some cases, too, we saw that the doctor had to encourage the patient to discuss certain moral topics, to reflect upon the problems of life. Apart from these particular cases, various forms of mental work will be found useful in patients whose illness is not very grave, and in those who are on the road to recovery. I have had excellent results, though not of course equally good in all cases, from the recommendation of musical studies, the study of a foreign language, advanced training of various kinds, and even the study of law, literature, philosophy, sociology, and science. It is wrong to suppose that the human mind can conduct itself intelligently without beliefs that are more or less religious, or without systems that are more or less philosophic. A great many persons find it necessary to have a philosophic groundwork before they can appreciate life. The essential thing is that we should not crudely destroy erroneous or unduly simple faiths, but should aid the subject to attain notions in keeping with his or her particular degree of intelligence or cultivation.

8. Performance of Actions.

I need not lay any more stress upon the nature of the actions which may serve as the starting-point of excitation ; for the essential matter is not the content of the action, but the way in which it is performed.   Actions which to all appearance were identical, have shown themselves ineffective in some cases, in others have proved the starting-point of serious depressions, and in yet others have served as stimulants and have raised the psychological tension for long periods. We must try to learn from the foregoing clinical studies what are the psychological characteristics of the actions which have played a favourable part, and we must endeavour to reproduce them.

The doctor finds that he has to pursue two aims which appear somewhat contradictory. First of all, the action must reach the most elevated stage, must attain the highest possible level of psychological tension, and this will necessitate a great deal of work. But, in the second place, the action must be performed without fatigue, without excessive expenditure, for it must not induce exhaustion. In actual fact, however, we are not here faced with a new problem. Every one who undertakes a commercial speculation has to encounter the same problem. The enterprise must be weighty enough to bring in considerable profit, and yet it must not be so speculative that the investment of capital in it will be likely to ruin the main enterprise. In a word, we have to do a good stroke of business. The problems of life are always the same.

If the patient is left to act by himself, he will ruin himself, for he will make foolish speculations. Were psychology a science it would provide the doctor with the means for putting his patient upon the track of a sound speculation without further ado. But psychology is far from being so advanced as this, and cannot do more than furnish some useful hints.

The indications for our guidance will be derived from the general behaviour of our patients, from a study of the way in which they are accustomed to react, from a knowledge of their expression, from little signs which indicate the changes that go on within them.

When the illness is not too far advanced, and when we have to prescribe complicated actions, the doctor will content himself with prescribing the nature of the action, and the time when it is to be performed. He will leave the patient to perform it unaided, being ready to intervene afterwards as a critic, and to advise how the action can be better performed another time. But in a good many cases, when abulia and phobias have supervened, the doctor will achieve nothing unless he gives personal assistance in the performance even of the simplest actions. He will have to compel the patient to act in his presence and in conjunction with himself. A great many of my agoraphobic patients have made their first steps in the street in my own company. Almost always my patients suffering from doubts and obsessions have been in my company when they have taken important resolutions, when they have made efforts of attention and attempts to perform mental work.

An essential point is not to leave the patient to begin the action haphazard at any moment he may fancy, or to continue it indefinitely. It is most important that the action should be begun at a favourable instant, and that care should be taken to avoid circumstances in which the patient is ill-disposed for the action and incapable of performing it. We must, therefore, watch the patient carefully, and note the little depressions which ensue upon fatigue, and the emotions by which the disease is from time to time aggravated. At such times, we must not ask the patient to act. Some patients, as we have just learned, are incapable of acting in the early part of the day, whereas others are indisposed for action in the evening. Some women pass through a period of disturbance just before menstruation, whereas in a great many others this phase of disordered activity comes just after menstruation. Obviously these cycles must be taken into account.

Next, we shall do well to prepare the patient for effort by a preliminary repose, which may have to be prolonged. Lydia cannot gain much by her reflections upon her obsession with her own beauty unless she has been resting for several days, lying down quietly all the time. Such patients must economise their energies, and must not dissipate their forces in subsidiary occupations. " I need to concentrate what little energy I have left upon the performance of one action ; I cannot do several things at a time." We must be careful to avoid letting other preoccupations and other attempts interfere with the action we expect from the patient. The moment must be well chosen, and the patient's mind must be concentrated upon one particular action. These are the essential conditions of the method.

The person who assists in the performance of these actions, and who guides them, has a very complicated part to play. He must aid in the performance of the action without actually doing it himself, although the latter would be very much easier ; and he must do his utmost to conceal his own contribution to the action, for it is essential that the patient should feel that he does the action himself and does it unaided. The guide has chosen the action, has overcome the patient's hesitations, and has taken the responsibility.—" You have insisted upon my making the visit, and if I find that I cannot help passing water in the middle of this lovely carpet, that will be your fault."—" If you compel me to eat in spite of my vows to the contrary, the blame will rest upon you."—The guide settles when the action is to begin, he puts an end to the interminable period of preparations, and as far as possible he takes the patient by surprise and prevents the wasting of energy in prolonged waiting. When we want to make an abulic perform an action, we must not tell him about it long beforehand, for if we do so the patient will be exhausted and agitated before the time comes to act.

The guide will specify the action as precisely as possible, and will analyse it into its elements if it should be necessary to give the patient's mind an immediate and proximate aim.— " When a thing is too far ahead, I cannot picture it in my mind clearly enough to have courage to undertake it."—" I cannot exert myself in the hope of being cured two or three years hence. That is too distant an object, and does not arouse my emotions."—Finally, the guide will favour the complete performance of the action by various gestures and words which will tend to develop the patient's latent tendencies ; by continually repeating the order to perform the action ; by words of encouragement at every sign of success however insignificant, for encouragement will make the patient realise these little successes, and will stimulate him with the hope aroused by glimpses of greater successes in the future. The guide will give various explanations which will reassure the subject about the dangers he apprehends ; and the guide will utter exhortations which will appeal to the patient's sentiments, moral ideas, etc. Some patients are especially moved by signs of intimacy and sympathy. Many authors have noted that we shall not make a success of this therapeutic method unless we ourselves take an interest in our patients, who are persons of a peculiar kind, often with refined and delicate sentiments, persons whose powerlessness for action and expression has made them unhappy and has given them a craving for sympathy. But other patients need strictness and even threats. " Unless I am continually being forced to do things which need a great effort I shall never get better. You must keep a strict hand over me." Thus, in certain cases, we have to use harshness, to put our threats into effect. We may have to isolate the patient in a sanatorium, to suppress the visits of relatives, to feed through a tube, to confine the patient in a padded room. We may have to adopt these harsh methods in order to compel the patient to begin some necessary action. Slight physical sufferings, humiliations, and moral sufferings, are, as we have seen, stimulant phenomena, which in many cases the patients will seek out for themselves. We are certainly entitled to use such methods cautiously in treatment by excitation, just as a pedagogue uses punishment in the course of education.

Must we go even further, must we be bold enough to induce real physical suffering, must we utilise the infliction of genuine pain as a therapeutic method ? Let me point out, first of all, that there is nothing absurd about such a suggestion, for we have seen unmistakable instances of excitation by means of physical pain, and we have noted in depressed patients unmistakable impulses to seek for such pain. In reality, a good many doctors have been accustomed for a long time to make a discreet use of this method without saying too much about it. I remember a case of a patient suffering from abasia who would only hold himself up and walk under stress of threats, but who could walk quite well after I had given him a few smart blows on the legs with a strap. A certain amount of coercion has often been successfully employed in the treatment of nervous and mental disorders.

The problem has been faced far more definitely in connexion with the method of treatment organised at Tours during the war by Vincent, to which has been given the name of " treatment by torpedoing." A good exposition of the method was given by Rimbaud, in " Marseille Médical," on September 15, 1916 ; and an excellent summary will be found in an article published on November 10, 1916, by the " Journal de Médecine et de Chirurgie Pratiques," p. 820. This method of treatment has been especially utilised for patients suffering from what, in my book of 1898, I described as contractures of the trunk—for patients who to-day are sometimes described by the strange names of " camptocormiques " (persons with a bent body) or " plicaturés " (doubled-ups). It is equally applicable in cases of contracture of the limbs, in paralyses, tremors, and mutisms. In a word it is useful in various disorders of movement which are not dependent upon organic lesions, but which appear to be due to fixed ideas in the mind of the subject, and to be connected with the phenomena of psychological depression.

In this method, a continuous electric current is passed through the lumbar region of the patient, being gradually increased from 30 to 50, and even to 100 or 120 milliampères. The pain seems very severe, the subject writhes, protests, sometimes utters loud cries, and in exceptional instances will struggle with the electrician. At the same time he makes defensive movements, and by energetic effort extends his lumbar spine ; or, if the legs are paralysed, he will move these. Then he will remain upright, somewhat astonished, benumbed, and apparently in pain. We must now make him abandon this stiff position, and try to take a few steps. Gradually we shall succeed, though sometimes it may be necessary to make further applications of the electrodes ; and by degrees the subject will start walking. We must make him walk more and more rapidly, but shall only secure this result by issuing a series of increasingly imperative orders. When the patient is undergoing the treatment we must not leave him at rest for a moment. If he stops, the doctors seize his arms, and walk with him, stimulating him in case of need by passing the electric current once more ; then he will walk more quickly, and in the end the doctor will be able to make him run.

Georges Dumas, apropos of neuropathic mutism, also speaks of " impressive and somewhat coercive methods of treatment," of which electrical treatment is the most typical.[1] He, in like manner, remarks that when the patient begins to cry out at the pain, we have only to continue the excitations and we shall make the dumb man speak.

The writers just mentioned give a good explanation of the psychological mechanism of these methods of treatment. They are not, properly speaking, suggestive treatments, although they have sometimes been described under this name. We are not here solely concerned with the automatic and easy functioning of a tendency which has been awakened in an impulsive form, although phenomena of this character play a part in what happens. Nor are they, strictly speaking, methods of education, for we have not here to teach the subject how to perform particular actions, since he knows quite well how to perform them. They are methods of excitation which have a powerful effect, and raise the subject's tension to the level at which effort becomes possible. " The element of pain is indispensable ; it leads the subjects to bring all their will power to work in order to get well, so that they may avoid a further dose of the treatment." The authors even note that in certain cases the subjects utter expressions of joy such as are characteristic of states of excitation. " The face brightens, the patient no longer suffers, he is aware what excellent results have been obtained."

Dumas distinguishes clearly among the influences which are brought into play in these electrical methods of treatment. " First, we make an impression upon the patient by the crackling of the electric sparks, by the noise of the discharges, by the great display of unfamiliar apparatus, and by the physical pain the electric current causes (though this is by no means intolerable)." Secondly, by the electric stimulation, we arouse,

[1] Dumas, Troubles mentaux et troubles nerveux de guerre, 1919, p. 150. With regard to the need for using force in the treatment of certain neuropathic disorders, see Laignel Lavastine and P. Courbon, Prophylaxie et traitement de l'insincérité chez les accidentés de la guerre, " Paris Médical," November 17, 1917.

in the form of a movement or a cry, an automatic reaction in the function which the patient had imagined to be lost. Thirdly, we add energetic and continuous stimulation to the effort we wish the patient to make.[1]

I think there is no reason to spend much time discussing the morality of these methods of treatment, although a good deal of time has been spent in such discussions, even in the Chamber of Deputies. No one denies that the doctor is entitled to apply the actual cautery, or even to perform a surgical operation without giving an anaesthetic, if circumstances make this necessary. Why should we quibble as to his right to give electric shocks, and even painful shocks, if thereby he is enabled to spare the patient a long-lasting and degrading infirmity? Such discussions are childish, like those concerning the " dignity " of suggestion. That is not the question at all. Our business merely is to consider the value of these methods of treatment from the medical point of view, to balance their advantages and their drawbacks.

Treatment by inflicting pain is not dangerous from the physical point of view, but it may certainly and readily become dangerous from the moral point of view. Everyone knows, nowadays, that it is a great mistake to be very ready to inflict serious punishment upon children, for if the punishment fails to secure the effect we desire, we cannot reinflict it, and we cannot increase it. If excitation by pain fails of its effect, it will be difficult to increase the pain without doing positive harm to the subject ; it will be difficult to find some other treatment ʼin which the excitation already applied will be exceeded, and therefore the doctor will soon find himself disarmed. Nor must we forget that pain and fear are only stimulant in their lower grades of intensity and under particular conditions. When these limits are transcended, pain and fear speedily begin to exercise their more usual influence, which is to induce depression and exhaustion. Now, as we shall see more and more, exhaustion is the great danger of treatment by excitation. I regard it as probable that many of the subjects who are treated in this way will subsequently relapse into various forms of depression, and that these, perhaps with other symptoms superadded, will prolong the illness. We have to do, then, with a treatment which is doubtless

[1] Dumas, op. cit., p. 160.

efficacious, but whose application is certainly a ticklish matter. If used, it must always be applied by the doctor in person, and he must keep a sharp watch upon its effects. During the war, when every one was in a hurry and it was necessary to treat a large number of patients speedily, treatment by pain did excellent service, and this " intensive psychotherapy " rendered it possible to send back a lot of good soldiers to active service. When the tempo of life is more tranquil, there will less often be occasion to have recourse to the method. We can avail ourselves of other influences in order to induce the patient to perform actions and to make efforts, which will perhaps be less extensive to begin with, but which will be successful none the less, and the success of which will gradually increase their stimulating influence.

Under these various influences, the patient will begin the desired action, but he is apt to check the action in the initial stages, in the stage of desire, in the stage of a vague idea of future action. Some American writers, advocates of the Mind Cure,[1] seem to think that it may be advantageous to leave the actions incomplete, to check them in an early stage of evolution, in the phase of desire. " What we need is to have wishes, and not to go beyond this. After each repression of a wish, you will become aware of a sensation of plenitude and power. By resisting the force of desire, you will stir up this force, and you will subsequently be able to make use of it in any way you please." I do not think that this remark is in accordance with what I have noticed myself, and have recorded in this work apropos of various cases. My experience is that the patients have improved because they have yielded fully to their desire to thieve, or to indulge in debauchery. As an actual fact, depressed persons are far too prone to repress their wishes ; they always seem to thwart these wishes by inhibitions, and the thwarting gives rise, not to an economy of energy, but to extremely costly derivations. If there is any truth in what Turnbull says, it is in cases in which the repression of the wish has only been part of a higher-grade activity, has been the carrying out of a determination to abstain, to undertake a moral or religious mortification. This higher-grade action is completely carried out, and it is

[1] Cf. W. Turnbull, Course of Personal Magnetism.

precisely because the important action is completely carried out that there is an augmentation of energy and excitation.

If I may summarise here my own observations and my own attempts in the way of treatment, I am inclined to say that, in order to bring about the excitation of the subject, we must first of all ensure that the action shall be really completed in a material fashion, and in such a way that a distinct modification in the objective world or in the situation shall become manifest. That is a difficult thing to secure, for we have to deal with patients who do not finish what they are about, and who usually bring their attempts at action to a close before reaching any obvious conclusion. We have just seen that in the electrical method of treatment, we must not only make the patient straighten himself, but must make him actually walk and actually run. Let us return, in this connexion, to the consideration of some of the cases we recently discussed.—Zoé has not only to make up her mind with regard to the marriage which is proposed for her, but she must really engage in activities which are difficult and important.—The sexual act which has been ineffective must achieve a material result. When a husband is obsessed by the idea of impotence, nothing will produce so great a change in his mind as the onset of pregnancy in his wife.—Shy persons, sufferers from social phobia, must actually remain in company, must say a few words, must take part in a ceremony, go out to dinner, keep their end up in an argument, go on a journey, visit another town for a time, and so on.—Consider the case of Newy. She has not " realised " her marriage, life in common with her husband. What she needs is to perform real and concrete actions in her household. In especial I described the changes which took place in her when she had succeeded in organising a little dinner party for a few friends.—Occupational activities which have been discontinued must be resumed. The chemist whose scruples and phobias were described, must make up some prescriptions.—When we try to make these patients talk, to make them explain what is troubling them, we must not be satisfied with a few vague words ; and we must avoid sparing them trouble by taking up their meaning too readily. We must compel them to express themselves fully and clearly. When we urge them to write a letter, we must see that the letter shall be finished, signed, put into an envelope, addressed, and posted ; for we shall achieve nothing if we let them be content with writing a rough draft. In reading, in study, the patient must do his utmost to achieve tangible results ; he must produce definitely finished work. When we have to do with individuals who are capable of anything of the kind, they must go in for and actually pass an examination.

Success, in fact, is an essential element of treatment by action. I have been amused to read in one of the little American manuals of Mind Cure some remarks anent the moral importance " of actions which earn money." [1] Elsewhere I have told how, when I wanted to make Jean work, I made him write a little review of a book for a magazine, and paid him for it in hard cash—a good deal more than it was worth. The earning of this fee for his work had an amazingly good effect upon him. The chemist who makes up the prescriptions must receive the money for the bottles of medicine. If a servant has lost her place, has become ashamed of herself, incapable of action, so that she is continually repeating to herself " I am an extraordinary creature, a white blackbird," she must find a new situation where she can earn wages, and must be made to realise that she can do her work successfully. In other instances, social success will be indicated by the attitude of the onlookers, by their congratulations, by the answers sent to letters, by all kinds of tangible proofs.

A difficulty arises here. Success is extremely valuable to the patient, but the most trifling failure has a very dangerous effect upon him. Hence the doctor will inevitably be inclined to make the most of the successes and to gloss over the failures. To some extent this is legitimate, and persons who are in need of praise will often be gratified by praise even though they may be aware that there is some exaggeration. (They will not be inclined to admit that there is much exaggeration !) But in other cases we shall have to guard against arousing the patient's susceptibilities, especially when we have to do with one who is over-scrupulous or is a sufferer from doubt. Such persons are fully able to guess that they are being humbugged ; and they may be inclined to exaggerate the extent to which they have been deceived, and may cease to believe in the reality of their actual successes. We must therefore do our utmost to avoid deceiving them ; and, besides, such deceit is useless

---

[1] Atkinson, Thought Force, etc.

more often than not. The doctor must take every precaution to avoid exposing the subject to the risk of obvious failure. He must be on his guard against those weaklings who are avid of fame ; who are continually trying, in season and out of season, to perform actions which they are incapable of finishing, or even of sustaining for any considerable time. We must choose for the patient an act which is within the compass of his powers, and only urge him to the performance of things he is really capable of doing. Furthermore, we must be skilful in the distribution of our praise. In every action performed by a psychasthenic under such conditions, there will be an element of special interest, an element displaying an advance upon the previous behaviour of the patient ; the doctor's business is to make the patient appreciate the real progress.

It is more difficult to ascertain the psychological perfection of the act, and unfortunately we have to decide this by inference from the sentiments expressed by the subject. First of all, therefore, we must ensure that the act shall be conscientiously performed, and that the subject shall be fully aware of what he is doing. This stipulation will exclude from such a method of treatment any kind of automatic action. It is when the end in view is quite different, when the treatment is to be by suggestion, that we have recourse to the encouragement of automatic action. In the cases we are now considering we must be on our guard against semi-automatic actions, which the subjects are only too apt to perform, especially when they repeat the same action an indefinite number of times. In many patients, sewing, embroidery, and even piano-playing, are undesirable practices, at any rate if our aim is to secure excitation by action. When we are treating by suggestion, we allow the subject to distract his attention from the act he is performing ; but when our aim is excitation, we must be constantly urging the subject to give his full attention to what he is doing, and to describe what he feels while he is acting.

We must, then, encourage the patient to act energetically, until, in due course, we witness the disappearance of the sentiments of incompleteness which have hitherto accompanied his actions. New and more desirable sentiments must take the place of these. The patients are perpetually affected with mind-wandering, and it is their way to act without attending to what they are doing.—Agathe (f., 30) is writing a letter to her mother. " I know that I am writing " she says ; " but everything seems so vague to me. I do not know to whom I am writing or what I am writing about ; I do not know if I am writing to order something from a shop, or if I am writing a criticism for a newspaper." What we must ensure is that this patient shall assume the mental attitude of a young woman who is writing to her mother, which is quite a different mental attitude from that of a journalist who is writing a newspaper article. We must ensure that she is well aware of what she is doing.—Lydia knows perfectly well that everything seems vague to her, even though she tries to apperceive clearly ; that she only understands half of what is said to her, and even less of what she reads. She must stop reading, then ; or at least, she must read only a short passage, and must achieve the feeling that she understands what she has read. When she succeeds in this, she is delighted.—In like manner, the feeling of dreaminess or of play-acting must give place to the sentiment of reality. This change is not always so difficult to bring about as might be supposed. The patients know perfectly well how to appreciate the difference between the semblance of a decision and a true decision ; and they are under no delusion as to the fact that in many cases it is idleness which makes them indulge in the sentiment of play-acting.

One of the most interesting among the feelings which arise in the course of action is the feeling of unity, which the patients, when left to themselves, rarely experience, for they always feel a sense of division while they are acting. " It is as if there were within me two persons performing different actions." This division in their mind is often indicated by their behaviour. They will simultaneously laugh and cry, they will smile with part of the face and show an expression of discontent with the other part of the face. This division in the mind is also shown by the strange thoughts to which they give expression during action, to which we have several times referred under the name of repressed wishes, monstrous wishes, sacrilegious wishes. What happens here is an arrest at a particular stage of deliberation, at the stage of opposition and repression. The appearance of this disturbance in con-nexion with an action we ask the subject to perform, shows that the action has not attained an adequate degree of tension, and that we must urge the subject to act more effectively.

Another important characteristic of the completed action, one we must do our utmost to obtain however difficult it may be, is pleasure. There are certain actions which are characteristically pleasurable. For example, the sexual act, when it is not pleasurable, is obviously inadequate ; and we see that pleasure returns to this action when the psychological tension of the patient is reestablished. The development of Pya.'s illness is instructive in this respect. He was a man forty years of age, in whom functional impotence had arisen under the conditions already described, and who had renounced any attempt at coitus for six months. When he tried once more, he first had ejaculations, and subsequently erections, in both cases without any pleasurable sensations attached. Then he had a form of gratification which he called " purely physical, for I had no interest, as of old, in the conquest of the woman." Then desire reappeared, and then the special form of curiosity and interest in gallant behaviour which had formerly filled his life. This ascending evolution of the sexual act in Pya. occupied three months.

It is even more interesting to note gratification as an accompaniment of action in the case of other actions in which, through habit, persons have ordinarily ceased to notice this accompaniment.—Ub. (m., 44), in the course of the education of his urinary function, learned, as we have seen, to pass water at longer intervals, to perform the act more definitely and more correctly ; and the first result of this achievement was that he had no longer any suffering in connexion with the urinary function. He astonished me very much when at length he told me that he had suddenly noticed a great change, that from time to time, now, he experienced a definite pleasure in passing water ; and he realised that in the recent acts of urination, which had seemed perfectly correct, there had still been lacking a very important element, namely, the pleasure which had at length reappeared.—This evolution is extremely characteristic, and I have noted it in connexion with most types of action. When an action is being functionally restored, and when improvement is taking place, we almost always notice at a certain moment that satisfaction reappears in one form or another, a sort of joy which gives interest to the action, and replaces the feelings of uselessness, absurdity, and futility which had formerly troubled the patient in connexion with the action. Many depressed persons who note the disappearance of this interest in what they may be doing, seek to explain the disappearance in a fallacious manner.—A woman of fifty-seven, who has just lost her two daughters, still goes on doing her housework, properly to all appearance, but without any interest. " This loss of interest is quite natural," she says, " for I am in a new house, one which my daughters never knew."—A young girl with marked musical tastes continues to play the piano, but without any pleasure. " I am very careful," she said, " not to grow enthusiastic, not to take any interest in what I am playing, for I should offend God if I were to enjoy a profane pleasure."—We know what is really amiss in these cases, and how the patients are putting the cart before the horse. We shall know that they are cured and that they have been freed from their obsessions when they once more find pleasure in action.

Finally there is a feeling which disappears very readily when activity is repressed ; I mean, the feeling of freedom. A great many patients tell us that for some time they have been acting correctly to all appearance, but that while acting they felt like machines, lacking spontaneity and freedom. We must not always suppose that such patients are suffering from delusions ; we must not imagine them to be paranoiacs with ideas of persecution. Perhaps delusions will appear in the subsequent course of their illness ; but these delusions do not yet exist, and all that we have occasion to note is a certain lowering of the tension of activity. It is this with which we have to contend at the early stage. The foregoing examples will suffice to show that action demands a psychological perfection, as well as the perfection which can be objectively detected. When we try to restore the psychological tension of a patient through action, what we have above all to secure is the perfectionment of these inner feelings.

While undertaking all these labours, we must perpetually watch the expenditure of energy, and must reduce this expenditure as much as possible. One of the great difficulties we have to contend with when we are trying to induce a higher degree of activation of the tendencies, arises out of the phenomena which I have described as phenomena of derivation. As soon as these patients try to act with a higher tension, they exhibit, side by side with and substituting the action we ask from them, a number of motor, emotional and intellectual agitations. When the symptoms are simple, they shake themselves, fidget in their chairs, get up, walk up and down the room, exhibit various tics, or feel an urge to yawn, to urinate, etc.[1] In the graver forms, they shriek, knock about the furniture, try to struggle with their associates.—Ae., when he makes an effort to go near his wife, pinches and strikes her.— Jf. (f., 30), when she tries to attend to what she is doing, begins to tear up all the papers and fabrics within reach. A remarkable detail in this case is that she subsequently attributes these violent actions, for which she is sorry, to evil influences which are exercised upon her, with the result that the derivations in question become the starting-point of a delusion of persecution.—Emotional derivations occur under the form of laughter, tears, anger, dread, anxiety of various kinds, which may pass on into systematised phobias. Intellectual derivations lead to interminable chattering, to the expression of more or less complicated thoughts concerning the character of what the patient is asked to do (which is described as futile and extraordinary), to observations concerning how much better they would like some other occupation (for they always have a predilection for something other than that which they are asked to do) ; or they talk about their powers and their weaknesses, about the wonderful efforts they have made in the past and are going to make in the future, but especially about the insurmountable difficulties of acting here and now.— " It is impossible to set to work until certain preliminaries have been settled. Should I begin work suddenly or gradually ? After deliberation, or passively obeying the first impulse ? With precautions or without ? Ought I not to solve all these problems before beginning to read a few lines ? "—When the illness is already of long standing, and systematised, it is at this stage that there supervene all the mental manias of perpetual seeking and of perfectionment, all the obsessions of over-scrupulousness, crime, and sacrilege.—" It is when I try to do what you ask me to do that the devil invariably comes to take a hand in the game."—" It is when I want to make the

---

[1] Les obsessions et la psychasthénie, vol. i, p. 716.

effort you ask for, that I am tempted to misbehave myself with a little servant who is really repulsive to me, or with a big dog."—All these agitations are obviously disastrous. They interrupt the action which has been begun, and necessitate incessant fresh beginnings. They expend the patient's energy fruitlessly and tire him. They give him pretexts for refusing to continue his efforts and to go on postponing action indefinitely.

Obviously we must do our utmost to strive against these exhausting derivations, simultaneously with our attempts to urge the patient to action. An excitation and education of the power of inhibition must play a part in all treatments of this kind. We must check tics, useless movements, must prevent the patient from continually jumping out of his chair, must from time to time cut short his chatter, his recriminations and declamations, his fits of anger ; must reassure him in his anxiety, and diminish his fears in every possible way ; must check his obsessions by a few well-chosen words summarising and recalling our earlier discussions with him.

Still, I do not think we must attach too much importance to this contest with agitation. The depressed patient whose actions are inadequate, will be agitated as soon as he tries to act with a higher tension. If he keeps perfectly calm, we may be quite sure that he is making no effort, that he is remaining inert, and the significance of this is unfavourable. Emile, a young man whose intense social phobia I have described, tries under my orders to go into a shop and buy some small article. He grows stiff, clenches his fists, makes faces ; he is covered with sweat, his voice is raucous and strange. It would seem as if he could not screw himself up to the required action without getting into a furious rage. But all these agitations are signs of the effort he is making. That effort only appears disproportionate to the action because we ourselves fail to realise how difficult action is for him. We cannot at the outset suppress these agitations entirely unless the patient renounces the desired action, or at any rate renounces the conscious action we want him to perform. We must never forget that the true remedy for such derivations will be successful action. In a series of experiments with Emile, his fury grew less in proportion as he was performing the action more successfully and completely. It was the same thing with anxieties and broodings, which diminished when the act was more complete. Thus, while we must check the agitations as far as may be, so that the subject's efforts shall not be entirely dispersed in fruitless agitations, we have to tolerate them to some extent.

An interesting indication of how difficult work under such conditions is, is the fatigue which results. " It is a strange thing," says Lydia. " Although I can go on talking for an indefinite time to any one and every one upon my fixed idea of beauty, I cannot talk to you, when you make me attend to what I am saying, without quickly becoming exhausted. I get as tired as if I had been talking for a long time in English to foreigners." This fatigue comes on quickly in all such experiments, whatever the nature of the action which we try to make the patient perform more completely. No doubt some of our patients have an obsession and a phobia of fatigue, which may recur at this moment, and which is then a sort of derivation analogous to the foregoing, and a matter to which we must not pay undue attention. But I am convinced that in most of those who are really transforming their mode of action, true exhaustion ensues.

If we are to be able to stop the work before exhaustion grows dangerous, we must become familiar with the signs that herald exhaustion. Sometimes we can be guided by objective modifications, by the little signs of fatigue which have been so admirably described by Galton. Some patients drip with sweat ; in others there are circulatory changes ; the heart beats more rapidly or more slowly, or may even become intermittent ; the face, the forehead, and the ears, grow red or pale. —Lydia complains of a feeling of shocks in the head, which bewilder her.—Af. suffers from a beating in the temples, of which he is very much afraid.—A good many patients, like Irène, have genuine fainting fits.

We must be careful to familiarise ourselves with the psychological modifications which indicate relaxation of tension by exhaustion, and which are peculiar to the subject with whom we are dealing. In some we may note an increased difficulty of attention. " My thoughts grow shorter ; I can no longer connect my ideas ; everything in my mind grows confused once more. I again feel as if I had a gimlet boring into my head." The symptom of a " butterfly-like flitting of ideas " to which I have more than once referred, is a typical sign of this real fatigue. In other patients we may notice an increase of all the automatisms, the more frequent appearance of the tics, of the mental manias peculiar to the subject. In many, the feeling of vacancy in the head, a strange sense of sadness, the various sentiments of incompleteness and unreality, are the most characteristic signs. When they appear, we must break off the sitting, even if the results have been incomplete. Moreover, we must be careful to ensure that the subject does not continue his efforts for an indefinite time. These symptoms of fatigue do not disappear in a moment. In some patients they will last for days after the sitting.—Lise always finds that she needs a great expenditure of energy in order to make any progress, and that after this she feels ill for several days. I noticed a good while ago in connexion with the treatment of Lise that a more active life, which relieved her of her obsessions, was distressing to the patient because of the fatigue it induced. "This cure is horribly fatiguing. Nothing could be more distressing than to have to keep one's thoughts perpetually on the stretch." [1] With her, it was, I may say, as it is with ourselves when we are preparing for a difficult examination ; and we all know how distressing it is to have to keep ourselves for a long time at an unaccustomed level of tension. During these periods she does not digest her food so well as usual, and she grows thin. She can only get a rest by relapsing into her obsessions.—We see the same thing in Le. (m., 41), timid and agoraphobic, who makes speedy and remarkable progress, but whose efforts I am obliged to check from time to time because he becomes affected with enteritis, and rapidly loses flesh.—The same thing happens in the case of Emile, whose efforts have also to be checked for a considerable time.—The onset of fatigue, when well marked, restricts the utilisation of treatment by excitation. When fatigue comes on too rapidly and lasts too long, it may make the treatment impossible, and may compel us to return, for a time at least, to treatment by rest and by the economising of energy. But, in most cases, the onset of fatigue is merely a sign that we must take certain precautions. We can reduce the fatigue if we can reduce the fruitless agitations. We can also reduce it by varying the exercises and avoiding too regular an effort. We must be

[1] Les obsessions et la psychasthénie, vol. i, p. 533.

on our guard against the enthusiasm of certain subjects who, in the hope of curing themselves more quickly, will exhaust themselves by unduly prolonged effort, and whose last state will then be worse than the first. We must only allow them to work for short periods at a time ; and, if we are ourselves guiding their efforts, we must be careful not to let the sittings last too long.

One observation of especial value must now be made. It has a bearing alike on the precautions needed to prevent exhaustion and on the measures which must be taken to secure a complete action. First of all, we must be careful to allow for the slowness with which high-tension actions are performed by depressed patients. Slowness of action and slowness of progress are fundamental characteristics in all neuropaths, and the doctor must never forget this when he is trying to secure such actions and such progress. The patients work slowly ; understand slowly ; adapt themselves slowly. I shall only select a few examples out of an interminable series.—Aj. can look after her little household just as well as anybody else, but she takes five hours to do what any one else would do in half an hour.—Paul (m., 30) is able to take a journey, but he must be prepared slowly for the idea of the journey. For a month before he starts he must go to have a look at the station every day ; must get used to the aspect of the train, which he examines without getting into it. Give him time enough and he will bring himself to start.—It was through an accident that Zoé was rendered incapable of coming to a decision in connexion with her betrothal. Ordinarily she can decide well enough, if she is given plenty of time.—Irène must be acquainted with any one for years before she can experience a feeling of affection.—Anna needs hours before she can understand a letter she has received.—Some of these patients require months or years before they can grow accustomed to a situation, before they can adapt themselves, before they can perform useful actions and definitely acquire the tendency to perform these actions.—Wkx. needed two years to make himself at home in his new flat ; and Ka. needed fourteen years to get used to his wife. It is true that at long last Wkx. found his new flat charming ; and that Ka. cannot now bear to be out of range of the rustle of his wife's skirt.—Nf. (m., 29) can turn his hand to anything, provided that he is given a sufficiency of time to adapt himself to his occupation ; what he regards as a sufficiency being, in many cases, very long indeed.— Uk., who has just bought a business, begins by being over-whelmed and extremely agitated. He is full of feelings of incapacity. He suffers from obsessive over-scrupulousness, dread of ruin, and even has thoughts of suicide. " I know that I shall be able to work this business very well. It is what I have always wanted. But I need time to get fond of the place, time to set to work. What has disturbed my mind is the suddenness with which I have had to begin."—Bfa. (m., 27) says : " I must get used to persons and things by degrees. No one suspects how long a time I need for this. That is the source of all my troubles and of all the misunderstandings that arise."

These last patients are perfectly right. Other persons do not allow for the deep-seated reasons for their slowness. Other persons try to hustle them, and this makes them incapable of action, so that they can achieve nothing. The patients always complain when they are hustled, when any one is waiting for them to do something. " It is impossible to get on, for some one is always trying to hurry me."—" I do not think it suits me at all to consider things so quickly or to go so quickly." —" One has no time to instal oneself."—" People hustle me, so that I have no time to see what I ought to do."—Zoé expresses the matter very well : " Simply to urge me to do anything quickly, makes me nervous, and incapable of coming to a decision of any kind. I cannot bear that any one should be waiting for me to do something, for if I try to go more quickly I always make a mess of it."—It is the same with all such patients. When circumstances are pressing, action is replaced by hesitations, resistances, and a sense of bewilderment.

And yet we are apt to be puzzled when we recall some of the peculiarities in the behaviour of such persons. Sometimes we see them act rapidly, even more rapidly than ordinary people. Irène, who usually hesitates and tergiversates for weeks before she can make up her mind to leave the house for a few months, suddenly determines upon a long journey when she has received a letter (one of no great importance), and she cannot find time to warn any one that she is going away. —Oda. (f., 40), over-scrupulous and affected with doubts, " will from time to time engage in some tremendous undertaking," says her husband ; this meaning that she hurls herself unreflectingly into enterprises that are complicated and too difficult for her.—I have just had occasion to point out that if we want to get anything out of these patients we shall do well not to warn them, but to take them by surprise. Does not this conflict with the foregoing remark ? Anna herself notices the contradiction. " It is amazing, I need a tremendous time to do anything, and yet I can be induced to act better, if I am suddenly urged to do it without being given a chance to think things over." But this contradiction is more apparent than real, for we have to do with very different kinds of actions, in the two cases. The actions that are performed rapidly are more or less automatic, and lack the characteristics of the complete action. They are often very dangerous for the patient. Irène's journey, which closely resembled a hysterical fugue, was the starting-point of disorders and obsessions ; and the same thing happened in the case of Oda.'s impulsive actions. In other cases, such actions were trifles and did not do the patients any good. The actions which were slowly undertaken, on the contrary, were complete actions exhibiting all the characteristics of the highest degree of activation of tendencies. None but such actions can be the starting-point of useful excitations, but they are far more difficult to achieve, and they can only be realised after prolonged labour. They are important actions, and they are disordered and become impossible if the subject is hustled, and cannot be given a sufficiency of time.

If this be so, we can understand why these patients so rarely succeed in performing a correct and complete action unaided, even though they still possess the power to do this action. The rapid change in circumstances, and, above all, the rhythm of social life which is imposed by the far greater speediness of other persons, seldom leaves them a sufficiency of time. At the outset of their malady, they are always behind time. They are never ready as soon as other persons, and for this reason they are continually being chided for their supposed idleness. After awhile, when the illness has become more serious, they completely lack adaptation to the happenings of life. By the time that they have got ready to begin an action, the wheel has turned, new circumstances have arisen, and other persons are asking of them a different kind of action.

Other persons actually thwart them and make fun of them when they talk of beginning the first action. " People come to visit me. They stay for an hour and find me sulky. They go away just about the time when I am beginning to realise that they are there, and to like them."

This slowness of action, in conjunction with the change that occurs in the circumstances while the psychasthenic is preparing to act, complicates action in yet another way which is even more serious. It imposes upon the subject, who desires in spite of all difficulties to achieve the complete realisation of the action, an enormous amount of additional work. Since the delayed action is no longer stimulated by the extant circumstances, if the preparation for the action is to be continued the idea of it must be persistently retained in the mind for a very long time. The subject must himself keep the tendency in a state of moderate activation for a considerable period. It is precisely this which constitutes a peculiar form of action, the action of waiting, which is always superadded to all the other actions of these patients. Now, waiting is always a difficult matter, and for them it is extremely difficult and costly.—" Waiting is what tires me most. I do wish that everything could be finished promptly. I should so much like to arrive all in a moment at perfect joy, with the feeling that I had got through once for all."—" I should like to do everything at once, and that everything should be finished instantly. But this is precisely what I am unable to do."—The difficulty of waiting, thus superadded to all their complete actions, makes it more and more difficult for them to effect the tedious preparation of actions, though such tedious preparation is unavoidable in their case. Some of them, as we have seen, precipitate themselves into an automatic and incomplete action which is harmful to them, and they allow the act to come to a conclusion despite insufficiency of tension. But most of them give up the struggle. More and more they renounce the performance of complete actions, and are apt in the end to renounce action of any kind. When a tendency awakens, and even reaches the first stages of desire, they do not try to go any further ; they allow a relaxation of tension to occur, and permit the tendency to return into the latent condition, making no attempt to push further by means of an effort which they know will be fruitless.

This relaxation of tension after the tendency has been awakened, this abandonment of the action before it has been begun, are very important phenomena. In days to come, when there is a real science of psychiatry, they will play an essential part in the diagnosis of the intensity of the illness. At the present time, these phenomena demand from the doctor a particular form of behaviour if, in such conditions, he wishes to secure a complete action. He must do his utmost to ward off the influence of unfavourable circumstances which may check the slow excitation of the tendency, which may demand a supplementary effort of waiting from the subject, or may lead to the abandonment of the action. First of all he must do his best to maintain around the subject an unchanging situation, so that the circumstances may continue for a long time to demand the same action. Subsequently, by his attitude and his words, he must persist in arousing in the subject's mind the same tendency, must prevent the dispersal of effort, must maintain concentration upon the same point, must prevent forgetfulness of the stimulant idea and abandonment of the action. His work, as I have said, consists in maintaining the idea of the action before the patient's mind as long as may be necessary to bring about the complete evolution of the tendency. He will render the action possible notwithstanding the slowness of the activation. The doctor will enable the subject to perform complete actions by placing him in an artificial situation in which he will find himself equal to the occasion, whereas he has lost the power of acting in the circumstances of normal life, whose tempo is too rapid for him.

In order to give a clearer explanation of the work the doctor has to do, I will give some simple examples. Let us consider the patients whose minds are " attached " upon an intellectual difficulty.—Lise has for years been confronted by the problem of expiation for the soul of her uncle, or by that of her responsibility in another world for the souls of her children. —Lydia for twelve years has been " attached " upon the problem of the loss of her beauty.—Both the patients imagine that they are continually thinking of these questions, that they are perpetually striving to solve these problems without ever reaching a solution. This view of the matter is not quite correct. They merely begin the work. They make a few efforts to get their cart out of the rut, but are continually turning aside to other things, so that each effort is transformed into sterile agitations. The circumstances of external life, which from moment to moment are presenting new problems, and the difficulty of keeping the same thought before the mind in the absence of an external stimulus, make these women speedily withdraw their attention from what they regard as their primary aim, so that they abandon the effort without having achieved a solution. Then, since the same difficulty in the intelligent interpretation of life persists, their efforts begin again a few moments later, to fail as before, and so on da capo.

The doctor isolates them from other persons and other circumstances. He persistently shuts off from them the thought of other problems, and compels these patients to look squarely at the difficulty which is obstructing their mind. The first result of this is to induce all kinds of contortions, to lead to disorderly chattering concerning all possible topics.—Lydia, who imagines she is actually studying the problem of her beauty, brings a dozen pages which she has just written, which she wants to read aloud and comment upon. It is not difficult to discover that in these dozen pages there are not a dozen lines which really bear upon the question.—We shall do well to allow the agitation to find vent for a time, since we cannot completely suppress it. Then, when we see that the subject is beginning to abandon his problem, we must bring him back to it once more. There will be little efforts, and consequent mental agitation.—" It is very difficult. I think I understand the words, but the ideas do not seem to enter my mind."—" I think that I understand, and that I believe for a moment, and then everything slips from me."—" My ideas are like the objects which I look at when I try to fix my eyes upon anything ; they dance off into the water or into the void."—" You must repeat the same phrases to me again and again, must give me the same explanations over and over again."—In these conditions, the patient does not work in the same way as when he is left to himself. He attends longer ; and, above all, he attends to the same point much longer than before. By degrees, he simplifies his problems. The dozen pages shrink to half a page. Gradually he advances in his work, and does not continually begin at the same point once more. Similar considerations apply to any action which we want the patient to do. We keep the tendency awake for a long time, since a mind of this sort needs a long time, and such patients are not capable, unaided, of keeping up their attention for as long as is necessary.

There does not seem to be any great drawback to spacing out the sittings. Lydia says : " I need to be alone, and to turn over slowly in my mind what you have said to me." The work which has been begun appears to go on at a slow pace almost unconsciously. The acts of human beings, as I have often pointed out, are like physiological advances, physiological evolutions. They take place slowly, just as new organs are formed slowly. When, after a few days interval, we try once more to fix the patient's attention upon the same point, we are surprised to find that the work has become much easier, and that the patient has made a great deal of progress.

Unfortunately these indications are extremely nebulous, for such psychological operations remain ill-defined, and a large amount of individual groping is still needed. All I have tried to do is to show in what way I have attempted to carry out treatment by the excitation of complete action. Such methods of treatment have been vaguely indicated in a good many works on psychotherapeutics, and I think their value is borne out by the observation of certain spontaneous cures that have followed particularly fortunate actions.

9. THERAPEUTIC RESULTS.

It is interesting to study the results of these methods of treatment, in order to draw certain conclusions as to the psychological nature of such phenomena, and as to the future which may lie before such methods of excitation. The results are more difficult to appreciate than might be imagined. The mental modifications are ill-defined, are far from easy to observe, and vary under so many influences that it is hard to ascertain which of them are determined by our intervention. I shall, therefore, give only a general impression, classifying my cases in three groups : first of all, those in which the therapeutic effect seemed insignificant ; secondly, those in which the effect was considerable but transient ; thirdly, those in which the beneficial effect lasted for at least a year.

Treatment which takes the form of inciting to activity is obviously not applicable to every case. It is necessarily unsuitable to patients who seem too much enfeebled physically and morally to bear a new and considerable expenditure of energy without danger. Unfortunately, such patients form the majority, and this greatly restricts the application of the method. Even when the patients can make attempts at action without serious danger, we shall rarely and with difficulty succeed in having these attempts made under satisfactory conditions.

A treatment which almost always demands considerable personal effort on the part of the patient will be far from agreeable to the majority of such patients, since nearly all of them desire a treatment in which they can remain passive. All sorts of vague ideas concerning psychotherapeutics have been diffused through the public mind, and these patients are apt to demand treatment by hypnotism and suggestion, which, they think, will transform them in a moment, without their having to make any effort themselves. But a curious thing is that hysterics, who are hypnotisable and suggestible, are often afraid of suggestion and refuse it. Depressed patients of any kind, doubters, obsessed persons, melancholics, for whom hypnotism and suggestion are of little use, are almost always persistent in demanding it, this being a consequence of their abulia and of their desire for the minimum of effort. A young man of twenty-seven, intelligent, timid and phobic, tormented by obsessions of bodily shame, prayed me to hypnotise him, and, when he had been put to sleep, to read out loud to him a statement which he had prepared, and which ran as follows : " When you speak to any one you must never feel bashful. Be satisfied that you are always a better man than your interlocutor. When you find yourself in the company of a young woman, you cannot fail to be at your ease, agreeable, well-mannered. Your gestures will be suitable and thoroughly natural ; your conversation will be bright and witty ; you will never make any forced witticisms ; and, though you will obviously be a well-mannered man, you will carefully avoid making any parade of the fact." His idea was that it would suffice to repeat this suggestion to him when he was in the hypnotic sleep, and he would thenceforward be freed from all his shyness and awkwardness. Could there be a more naive expression of the desire to be transformed by a wave of the enchanter's wand without having to make the least effort on one's own part ?

When, instead of making to them the sort of suggestions they expect, we ask them to collaborate in their own treatment, they take fright directly they hear a word about a change of behaviour. They are convinced that they would grow much worse at once if they were to change their manner of life, absurd though this generally is. They declare, in fact, that they really want to retain their illness, that they dread losing their scruples, that they are afraid their hearts would dry up if they were to occupy themselves with any other things than their obsessions or their regrets. They invent all kinds of pretexts to conceal their fear of having to make an effort. Although we do our utmost to avoid frightening them, and although we try to hide from them the efforts they will have to make, we do not always succeed in getting them into a favourable frame of mind. If we fail to obtain any appreciable effect it is because we have not really been able to make a fair trial of the method.

That is why we must not be surprised if we have a good many failures. Many patients who declare that they have made the efforts we ask for, have secured no definite result, and have rapidly grown discouraged.—Lch. (m., 36), affected with doubts and phobias, but otherwise still fairly well, abandoned his occupation without any adequate reason, and since he has been idle has been much more ill than before. Twice I tried to make him resume work, but, when he did take up his work again for brief periods, he never carried anything through and always gave up the attempt far too soon.—The same thing happened in the case of Cq. (m., 22), a morbidly shy young man, given to all kinds of obsessive reveries, who relinquished his activities one after another because he conceived some scruple in connexion with them. The other members of his family are unintelligent persons and are likewise timid. They indulge him in all his whims. Backed up by them, he makes this an excuse for the speedy abandonment of all his efforts, and never achieves anything.— If we undertake this method of treatment we must always bear in mind such a possibility.

Good will on the part of the patient and his associates

does not always suffice, and we encounter cases in which the exercises cannot be continued because they have a bad effect. In many instances, the fatigue which ensues upon the work of excitation is extreme.—Sd. (m., 53) is familiar with the method, and has instinctively had recourse to it on his own account. In a first and very serious crisis of depression, he spontaneously adopted a more stimulating life, and informed me : " I cured myself by going on the loose, and by doing a lot of work." In his second crisis, which supervened twenty years later, he tried the same plan, but without success, for it led to a considerable loss of flesh and made him more depressed than ever.—In the patients about whom I have just been writing, the fatigue which came on when a stimulant treatment was adopted, was attended by digestive disorders, enteritis, and great loss of flesh, so that it was necessary to stop the treatment, or at any rate to suspend the exercises for a time. In two cases I found it necessary to rescind the advice I had given young husbands to practise sexual intercourse, for in their cases attempts at sexual indulgence induced prolonged agitation and delusional crises.

In other patients we note the onset of symptoms closely akin to the nervous paroxysms and attacks of migraine observed as a sequel of aesthesiogenic treatment, attacks which were regarded as indications of relaxation of tension and of discharge. By exhortations and discussions it was possible to make Clarisse grasp the futility of her fears regarding microbes and hooligans ; she could be induced to get through her toilet more quickly, she could be made to feel a greater sense of security and even to admit the reality of her environment. But, after having led a higher-grade existence for twenty-four hours, she would have a great agitational crisis, suffering from extreme anxiety, attended by convulsive movements and delusional dread. Nothing could check the development of these symptoms, and they led to a relapse into the condition of phobia and doubt. Here we have the phenomenon of relaxation of tension which we have just been studying. We must always bear in mind the likelihood of this relaxation of tension when we are prescribing treatment by excitation ; and we must be careful to avoid too rapid and too extensive a relaxation of tension, as a result of which the patient may become worse than before. Clarisse declares, probably with good reason, that several times she has had very severe and almost irreparable lowering of tension which has come on a few hours after making great efforts under medical orders. For instance, she was urged to enter a large drawing-room full of people, although the thought of doing so filled her with doubts and terrors. Still, she succeeded in doing what she was asked to do, and even felt over-excited, and more lucid in consequence, for several hours. But then there supervened a long delusional crisis ; and thereafter for several years, she was affected with psychasthenic delusions, and her general condition was far more serious than it had been before this effort.

This observation brings us to consider one of the most remarkable of the symptoms which may supervene as a sequel of excitation by completed action. I refer to the onset of epileptic fits during efforts to raise the tension. This is certainly rare, but when it does occur it is so interesting from the physiological and psychological point of view that it deserves special attention. In connexion with treatment by rest and by the simplication of life, I would draw attention to the remarkable case of Paul. This young man, thirty-four years of age, has been a typical psychasthenic since youth. He is abulic, affected with doubts, tormented by a dread of women, dread of journeys, and even dread of any change of domicile ; he is obsessed by questionings concerning human destiny, the value of life, etc. ; his own existence is gloomy, retired, and almost inert. If we try to shake him out of this inertia, to make him take an interest in something, to act with fuller consciousness and more energy, he will tell us that he thoroughly understands our advice, that long since he has himself divined the importance of such treatment, and has spontaneously tried to apply it. He knows quite well what happens when he is keenly interested in anything, when he takes pleasure in an action or a sensation, when he " lets himself go " and gives himself up to admiration of a sight or a picture. When he does any of these things, he first of all becomes affected with an agitation which is mainly mental, finding himself " obliged to imagine symmetrical thoughts ; " he relapses into broodings concerning the future life, concerning the question whether a man is entitled to enjoy pleasure, and the like. If he does not pay too much attention to these agitations, and succeeds in transcending them, he feels an intense joy, " a sort of delightful ecstasy." Up to now, in Paul's case, we are dealing with familiar facts, with phenomena which are characteristic of the excitation of psychasthenics.

But, unfortunately, Paul does not stop long at this stage. Speedily a transformation takes place. He begins to suffer from slight pains in the head. He finds that objects assume a strange aspect, an aspect that is at once gloomy and terrible. All the details of what he is looking at become significant, they have an intimate relationship with himself, they are the revealing signs of a dreadful catastrophe which threatens him. Simultaneously, he is astonished to notice that these objects and this situation have already been perceived by him before, in the same manner, and in all their details. This fact, or rather, this fancy, makes them more terrible even than before. He thus suffers at one and the same time from the feelings of pseudo-recognition and of mournfulness. Sometimes, though rarely, Paul can still break away at this stage. If he remains perfectly tranquil, without looking at anything, and as far as possible without thinking of anything, the trouble will gradually disperse. In most cases, however, he has no further knowledge of what happens after this stage has been reached, for he falls down in an epileptic fit.—The case of Td. (f., 24) is analogous. If needs must, she can make a vigorous physical or moral effort. For instance, she will run to catch a train ; she will get the better of her shyness when she has to make an important visit ; she will talk energetically in defence of a friend who has been unjustly accused. Her efforts are successful. The action is fully accomplished and satisfies her completely. When it is over she will be gratified, and will be in a thoroughly characteristic condition of high tension; but inevitably, twenty-four or thirty-six hours later, this excitation is followed by a severe hystero-epileptic paroxysm. The nature of the paroxysm may perhaps be called hysterical, but at its inception it is typically epileptic.

These patients, and especially Paul, know well enough what they have to do in order to escape having such fits. " This is a much surer method than taking bromide." Paul knows that he must avoid pleasures, expectation, enthusiasms of all kinds. He must never let himself admire anything, love anything, do anything, completely.   His dread of journeys, changes, new circumstances, is the outcome of his depression, and of the terror he feels of what may be the result of excitation. He himself remarks that without very much danger he can enjoy a speedy and elementary pleasure like the pleasures of the table, or the pleasures of coitus, provided that he does not prepare for them, and does not give himself up to them too much.   Here we note a remarkable detail, which confirms the observation already made regarding the difference between automatic actions performed at a low tension and complete actions performed at a high tension.   Certainly Paul's observations on his own case would seem to be justified by results, for whereas formerly, under the conditions described, he had a great many epileptic seizures, since then, by adopting the precautions he has found necessary, he has succeeded in avoiding even a single attack during several years.   Quite recently, he was imprudent enough to allow himself to be persuaded to go and see an aeroplane rise into the air.   He was close to it, and was greatly impressed by this new and remarkable sight.   The result was that, despite his efforts to shake off the crisis when he began to suffer from the feeling of pseudo-recognition, he had a fit after this long interval. Are we to encourage him to brave the danger ?   Are we to encourage him to try and find an escape from his persistent depression with obsessions and phobias, when the escape can only be made at the risk of such grave symptoms ?   Must we not rather advise these patients to walk warily ?

We draw the conclusion that, not only in patients who are greatly enfeebled, but also in patients who are timid, who lack the requisite good will either through disposition or as the outcome of their illness, in patients who too quickly become agitated or exhausted to a dangerous extent, treatment by excitation is inapplicable, or cannot be expected to give useful results.

Fortunately, however, I have in my case-books notes of cases in which the treatment has been more valuable.   Among the patients previously mentioned, there are some who have been able to carry out the treatment successfully.   They have been able, at times, to perform, in a more or less satisfactory way, the actions demanded of them, and I have often had

occasion, in these patients, to note the occurrence of remarkable mental modifications as a result.   I shall first lay stress
upon the psychological phenomena which have immediately
followed the experiment, during the next few hours or days
after the performance of the action.   These immediate sequels
are perhaps the least important from the therapeutic standpoint, but they are extremely interesting from the psychological outlook, for they are analogous to the remarkable
phenomena we have already noted in connexion with the
aesthesiogenic treatment of hysterical patients.   In my first
work upon patients suffering from obsessions,[1] I devoted a
chapter to the study of stimulant emotions, in order to
demonstrate the reality of the oscillations of psychological
tension in these patients.   Incidentally, I draw attention to
the therapeutic effects of certain moral excitations.   " On the
first occasion on which Claire comes to see me after her return,
if I threaten her and make a violent scene, so that I succeed
in making her cry, the effects are remarkable, for her obsessions
vanish for a whole week."   I made similar observations in
the case of Lise.   " It was sometimes necessary to threaten
to put her under restraint, for that was the only thing which
would raise her mental tension.   She herself said, apropos
of the good effects of this threat :   " Certainly nothing but fear
can really move me."   After reading, conversing, making an
effort, this patient no longer felt herself to be so much divided.
She said :   " I am no longer split up into little pieces."   The
restored unity of mind would last for several days.   Facts
of such a character must now be reviewed with greater accuracy
as regards the patients who have been subjected to the before-
mentioned experiments.

Let us consider the series of various actions which we have
tried to make the patients perform completely.—In Sb., after
excitation by exercises of breathing and swallowing, we see
that she is tranquillised, breathes freely, and looks with astonishment at her pillows, asking herself how she could possibly
have fancied that she had swallowed them.—We see a similar
transformation plainly enough after sexual acts in the patients
who describe their very remarkable impressions.   The enthusiasm and pride of Ae. when he has succeeded in touching
his wife with somewhat less disgust, are quite amusing.—

[1] Les obsessions et la psychasthénie, vol. i, p. 538.

The education of Pya., which I have already described, was not merely successful, in the course of three months, in restoring his psychological sexual functions to their primitive condition, and in reorganising his life of amorous adventure ; but, after each success, after each advance, there was to be observed for a day or two a complete transformation of his mind, the disappearance of his obsessive ideas and in especial of his thoughts of suicide, the development of activity and memory and feelings of joy.—As far as this matter is concerned, I have notes of the confidences made to me by eleven women in whom the effects of sexual excitation were absolutely definite, effects both upon the physiological and upon the psychological functions.—Bkn. (f., 24) relates how much energy she had to expend in order to " manage things a little better," how she had to experience contortions, fits of weeping, and to endure a great deal of pain in the head ; but after a success she was thoroughly cheered up, and was even freed from her enteritis for several days.—Uf. (f. 45) was astonished to find that her ideas of persecution vanished in similar circumstances.—The excitation of urinary phobics has similar results. When Vor. and Ub. were able to urinate " correctly and pleasurably," the improvement not only affected the urinary function, but extended to the whole mind.

I shall not lay any stress upon the phenomena of the same kind which can be frequently observed during the treatment of phobias of contact or of occupational phobias. I shall merely refer to the enthusiasm of patients who are able to gain a certain amount of money by their work, and who are transformed for several days by a success. But it is necessary to dwell for a time upon the results of efforts to perform social actions, for these results are often important.—I pointed out before how Jean was metamorphosed for a fortnight after attending a dinner party when I had insisted upon his going. I have observed the same sort of thing in many other cases. —Vd. (m., 30) observed that, whenever he had been able to make the necessary initial effort, he felt quite well throughout the evening party, and that he remained free from his customary troubles, from his tremors and hesitations. All the patients to whom I have referred in the foregoing paragraphs as subjects whom I had urged to undertake social efforts, derived satisfactory results from these efforts, at least for a time. The transformation of Emile after he had made one of the efforts which were so distressing to him, and had gone out, and after he had made one of those incursions into a shop which cost him so much labour, was really interesting. The young man became quite different ; the illness from which he had suffered for years seemed to have disappeared. He was no longer so much embarrassed or so stiff ; his movements had become more supple ; he held himself up better, no longer hid his face in his hands, and would from time to time look people in the face ; he ate with more appetite, ventured to call the other members of his family by their pet names, and could talk intelligently without uttering improprieties and in a voice which was no longer raucous. Usually, when he wanted to speak to his parents in the evening before going to bed, he would forget himself so far as to go into their room half undressed. Unfortunately, most of his troubles returned next day, and he had to make the same effort once more, and to advance slowly and gradually.

I gave an even longer account of the remarkable case of Zoé, whose indecisions had to be cured, and who had to be induced to make up her mind with regard to a proposal of marriage. As soon as she had made up her mind, she showed herself both energetic and clever in resuming the engagement, in spite of the difficulties of the case, and although, before, she had been hesitant and discouraging. The change in the patient's physiognomy was remarkable. For months prior to this time, her face had been stiff and cold, with a disagreeable expression ; now, it was almost unrecognisable, so pleasant did she look whenever she had made a fresh step towards the solution of the problem.—Newy, whom I tried to induce to become accustomed to her husband and to her household, always improved suddenly after any successful action. " I was much more tranquil after making that effort," she said. " All the afternoon, I felt that I was really at home in the flat ; or rather, that I was really at home in the kitchen and in the dining-room, but not yet in the bedroom. . . . There are moments when I can really believe myself to be married. . . . Do you think that I am going to become just like other people ? " One evening, after having successfully organised a little dinner party for a few friends, she felt thoroughly at home in her flat, even in the bedroom. She succeeded in loving her husband ; and she succeeded in doing what she had thought would be impossible, in sleeping for a whole night by his side. I have seen the same sort of thing in several other cases of the kind.

Efforts at attention bearing upon tactile and kinaesthetic sensations, gave rise, in a specially obvious manner, to modifications of the sense of depersonalisation in Wc. (m., 18), who, after a sitting, found that he felt thoroughly master of himself for a day or two. Work at reading, writing, or the piano, has not seemed in my cases to bring about any more than trifling modifications of tension, for I have seldom noticed, where these minor occupations were concerned, the production of characteristic feelings of wellbeing. Such activities only exercise an influence when frequently repeated.

On the other hand, I have been struck by the extremely stimulant effect of confession, and of confidingness, which are, indeed, generally considered to be forms of action able to affect the emotions strongly. The case of Kl., which I recorded as typical, comes into this category. In at least a dozen other patients, I could note a manifest excitation, sometimes lasting for several days, when I had been able to induce them to confide in me, and to express themselves freely. The inverse kind of action, which consists in imposing upon them a certain amount of discretion in the utterance of their stereotyped complaints and of their obsessive queries, has often had a similar influence.

The complete expression of the emotions, which is rarely achieved in these patients (who are reserved alike by system and because they are impotent), often has a remarkable effect when it does occur. Many of the patients become unrecognisable if we can only make them cry. After a fit of weeping, which is sometimes very difficult to induce, their obsessive ideas of persecution, the airs they put on, their stiffness, their incessant doubts, and their resistances, will disappear as if by magic. They assume a different expression of countenance, speak in a different way, utter different kinds of thoughts, and express a frank delight at having rediscovered themselves. This excitation often lasts several days. Then it vanishes, and the patient resumes his previous condition. Thereupon we have to set to work once more ; to make the patient feel emotion, and give expression to this emotion.

As I said before, I have often tried to make the patient understand his own obsessions, being convinced that an obsessive idea is, in many instances, an idea which has been incompletely elaborated, and one in which obscurity and mystery play a considerable part.—I have already pointed out how greatly Lise was relieved when she became able to understand the nature of her reveries concerning expiation for her uncle's soul, and her responsibility for her children in the world to come.—I could add a score of cases in which efforts of attention bearing upon the patient's obsession had a similar effect. Some of these patients give interesting expression to the sentiments they experience when, for a moment, they have come to understand a little better.—" It is strange," says Jd. (f., 20), " I have only spoken of my scruples of mortification, and not of my other scruples, and yet this has sufficed to dispel all my disquietude. Although I was continually troubled by scruples, even in my dreams, I no longer suffer from them, and my dreams are pleasant ones. . . . I feel a sense of expansion in my life, and have an urge to activity such as I have not known for a long time. . . . It is a pity that it does not last."—" After this work," says Yd. (m., 30), " I have a remarkable feeling that the day has become brighter, and I feel as if I were seeing things more distinctly. I see them as clearly existing outside myself, and I am interested in them, whereas ordinarily I see myself in outward things, and I see them badly."—In similar circumstances, many other patients have recovered the sentiment of reality. " How good it is to be able to think just like every one else, and to recover reality. It sends a glow all through me."

The slowness with which this work sometimes takes place shows us that we have to do with a deep-seated transformation. The case of Lydia, upon which I have already laid considerable stress, is very characteristic from this point of view. If her obsession with her own beauty were a purely intellectual phenomenon, the discussion of this obsession, and even its dispersal, would have purely intellectual results, and would simply give her other ideas. How can it be, then, that, after a certain number of sittings, during which she has been studying this idea, her whole behaviour should undergo modification ? She finds a new interest in her toilet. She is willing to show herself to others and to go out, but of course we may regard these changes as a consequence of the change in her idea concerning her looks. In addition, however, her movements have become quicker and more precise. She is interested in household occupations. She once more tends her flowers. She takes an interest in the other members of her family, who, before that, to use her own words, " had no longer existed for her." She is now able to read, and to understand what she reads ; to eat her food with enjoyment ; and even to sleep. She has a keen sense of wellbeing. " Now that I no longer feel the gimlet boring into my head, I have a strange sense of happiness. It seems to me as if I were beginning to live, and yet I know perfectly well that I am forty years of age. Have I really been alive for the last twelve years ? How is it that the sun seems quite new to me ? The sun really existed just the same during all those years." Whereas other patients, Lise, for example, were able to advance very quickly in this process of excitation through an understanding of their obsession, but speedily relapsed into their depression. through a revival of the old obsession or through the adoption of an equivalent, Lydia takes a long time before the excitation appears, but can then pass a much longer period without relapse. In her case, the excitation is slower and more lasting.

Other kinds of intellectual work, provided only that the actions are completed, have a like stimulant effect. This was evident in a number of cases. Madame Z., after studying attentively for an evening, exclaimed : " I have the impression of being alive ; I enjoy a sense of wellbeing ; this has made marks, has created waves, in the thick mass of my brain."

The foregoing brief summary shows that a real though often transient excitation is common in depressed patients after the complete performance of certain actions experimentally imposed. We see that such excitation is frequent enough if we take the trouble to detect it and to induce it. It exists even in some of the cases in which at first sight we have been inclined to regard the effects as negative. Treatment by excitation, we think, is unsuitable for Paul, seeing that in him a rise of tension rapidly leads to exhaustion, and brings on an epileptic fit. This is true ; but it is no less true, from the psychological outlook, that the complete performance of an action gives him intense delight, and enables him for the time to shake off his depression. Thus the phenomenon we are considering is an important one ; and it is one of general occurrence, since we observe it in so many cases under varying circumstances.

In trying to understand the phenomenon, I am especially struck by a comparison which forces itself on my attention. All the facts described in this chapter were seen under a different form in connexion with complete somnambulism and with the aesthesiogenic treatment of hysterical patients. It is a remarkable fact that successive therapeutic sittings in psychasthenics, who show no signs of the phenomena of suggestion or of hypnotism, give rise to oscillations perfectly identical with those which we have just been noting in the case of hypnotisable hysterics. In a great number of these patients we can observe that therapeutic sittings lasting for about one hour each, seem to fall naturally into two parts of unequal duration, the duration of the respective parts varying from patient to patient, and the parts being characterised by a different disposition of the subject. In the first part, the subject, on arrival, is in a bad humour, out of tune with himself and with the doctor. He is tormented by various troubles, by a sentiment of incompleteness and by a feeling of discouragement. He fancies that the doctor does not understand him properly, or does not tell him the truth. He wants to begin his interminable explanations over again, and he will not believe what the doctor says to him. Often this state of mind makes him morose and irritable ; sometimes, even, aggressive and rude.

It is apt to be difficult, when this mood prevails, to act efficiently upon the patient, and to induce him to make any effort at attention. We have to let him talk freely for a time, while listening sympathetically. He will go on complaining interminably about his doubts concerning " the principle of identity," concerning " dreams of a more complete life," etc. ; but, soon, he grows excited, is transformed by the very fact of talking, by the fact that what he says is being listened to ; he will lend himself better to efforts of attention and discussion ; he will more readily perform some of the exercises we have been considering. As soon as the patient has succeeded in understanding something, in believing something, in experiencing a definite sentiment, he will be completely transformed, and the second part of the sitting will be utterly different from the first. The patient will declare that he is " delighted to be understood " ; he will be contented with himself, and, by a satisfactory reaction, he will be well content with his doctor.—Simone (f., 26), tormented by scruples, ideas of damnation, and ideas of persecution, when she first comes to see me always has an icy expression of countenance ; she knits her brows ; she speaks in an irritable and rather rude way, and utters long tirades upon the clever folk who dupe trusting persons, and upon the universal wickedness of mankind. But in the course of about half an hour she invariably changes so as to become hardly recognisable, assuming a gentle and childlike attitude, and thanking me with tears in her eyes.— I could add a dozen similar cases to this one. Many of these patients, at the outset of a sitting, suffer from a fatigue which is closely analogous to that of hypnotised hysterics. In some of them the fatigue is manifest even at the close of the sitting if this has been too long. We see that they do not understand so well what we are saying, that their faces becomes drawn, and that sometimes they shed tears. In many of them the fatigue will last for several days, and be extremely distressing. Then there ensues a well-marked period of euphoria, which, as before, may be spoken of as a period of influence. Now, the patients, more or less completely freed from their obsessions, have recovered their powers of will and attention ; they are again capable of acting, of adapting themselves to social conditions, and even of doing useful work. They feel happy and they express their happiness with the same enthusiasm in the same picturesque language as the other patients. " I live more vigorously ; I find time for all I want to do and can do it in an orderly way ; to the amazement of all my associates I have become accurate, I have recovered my individuality ; it seems to me as if my life had entered a new springtime." These patients, likewise, have the remarkable feeling that they are seeing things more brightly, that the daylight is more brilliant, that they are beginning a new life.

Unless we have to do with subjects whose illness is already drawing to a close, this happy period does not last indefinitely. After a time which varies, but which is ordinarily very short, they complain that a fog has enveloped them once more, that they no longer have any energy for action ; and their customary follies are resumed.   This relapse is usually explained as being the outcome of the patient's weakness, of the readiness with which fatigues and emotions once more lower the patient's tension.   It is said to be due to the ordinary course of life, which speedily brings up new problems and provides new occasions for exhaustion.   That is why, at the next sitting, they appear once more in the state of depression and discontent. That is why this cycle of oscillations continues.

In reality, except for the essential modifications connected with the restriction of consciousness in the hysteric, and except for the anaesthesias, the paralyses, and the amnesias, connected with the alert period of influence, we note once more the difficulty the subject finds in preparing for special conditions, the varied agitations at the outset, the rise of psychological tension which renders possible actions performed at a higher tension, and which enables the patients to attain a higher grade of activation, the sentiments of ecstasy which often find the same sort of expression, and the slow or sudden descent after a longer or shorter time, so that the patient returns to a condition of more or less intense depression.

The most striking difference between the two groups of phenomena is that in the hysteric such oscillations of tension induce modifications of memory, and give rise to a duplication of the personality, whereas these other patients usually present nothing more than simple modifications of disposition and character.   We must not exaggerate the difference.   We have seen that the characteristic amnesias of complete somnambulism can be more or less attenuated ; on the other hand, it is not rare to note that persons suffering from simple depression may have had a period of excitation with diffuse amnesias and the early stage of a duplication of the personality.   This phenomenon is clearly seen in Lise, who, when she comes back to visit me, has often forgotten the previous visit and the intervening days ; has forgotten, that is to say, the period during which she was in a state of excitation.   But towards the end of the sitting, when her tension has been reestablished, these memories return.   The accentuation of this characteristic is due to the disposition hysterics have to suffer from a restriction of consciousness, whereas this disposition is much less marked in psychasthenics.

There appears to be another difference as regards the

procedures employed to bring about such changes of state, but I do not think the difference is one of much importance. Aesthesiogenism is only a form which these methods of excitation assume when we are dealing with patients who suffer frequently from disturbance of sensation and of movement, and whose attention can readily be concentrated upon elementary sensations and movements. The same method can be utilised for psychasthenics, as we have seen in certain cases of depersonalisation. Even in hysterics, excitation of sensibility is not essential in order to bring about the second state. In the description I published some time ago of Marceline, a very interesting case, I remarked that emotion sometimes had an excellent effect upon her. " Four or five times in succession my notes contain the description of violent scenes which others and I myself had perforce with the poor girl. She had become absolutely intolerable, and we were obliged to tell her so rather roughly. . . . Why was it that, when this happened, her spirits were raised, whereas other emotions only depressed her ? She recovered her powers of sensation and her memory, she ceased vomiting, she ate well, she did her work perfectly, and she seemed to be cured for a fortnight at least." [1] The same thing was noticable in the case of Irène, in whom, moreover, complete somnambulism was usually induced by directing her attention to memories rather than to sensations. In her, likewise, reproaches or threats uttered to make her abandon her resistance or to compel her to act, had a stimulating effect, and gave rise to complete somnambulism.[2] In these various cases the method of excitation was the same in both groups of patients.

All these phenomena, which are still very little understood, are of the same kind, despite certain differences in form. They enable us to glimpse a very important notion, namely that in the course of mental depressions, whatever their kind or their origin, we sometimes have a means of artificially modifying the psychological tension and of bringing the subject into a condition of greater activity ; in a word, we have the power of inducing excitation. Although, in most cases, this

---

[1] Une Félida artificielle, " Revue Philosophique," 1909, vol. i, p. 329 ; L'état mental des hystériques, second edition, 1911, p. 610.

[2] L'amnésie et la dissociation des souvenirs par l'émotion, " Journal de Psychologie Normale et Pathologique," September 1904 ; L'état mental des hystériques, second edition, 1911, p. 542.

transformation is not extensive, and although the change is only transient, it is still important to know that we can bring it about, and the fact is encouraging.

These temporary modifications are extremely interesting to the psychologist and to the theoretician, who is glad to be able in this way to link up phenomena which ostensibly are very different, such as duplicate personality, the therapeutic effects of metallotherapy or aesthesiogenism, the psychasthenic's urge to seek stimulation, excitations by action, epileptic discharges, etc. But these reflections do not solve our therapeutic problem; we still have to ask whether treatment of this kind, perseveringly continued for a considerable period, can bring about in our patients changes sufficiently durable to be of real value.

We have to admit that in these methods of treatment (as, indeed, in all others) we experience many disappointments. The most distressing are the ones that occur in the treatment of certain patients, young people as a rule, who seem at the outset, and sometimes for long periods, to present a very remarkable condition of psychological depression, assuming either a hysterical or a psychasthenic form ; but who, more or less rapidly, despite all we can do in the way of treatment, grow worse, until they become affected, either with special forms of delusion, or else with a peculiar condition of dementia which is tantamount to delusional insanity or asthenic dementia.

But, even in patients belonging to this category, treatment by excitation will sometimes give encouraging results. I have more than once remarked how Simone, an abulic, tormented by recriminations and by obsessions of persecution, would be transformed if she was able to experience a complete emotion which reduced her to tears ; she then became active and amiable for forty-eight hours at least.—The same thing happened in the case of Xd. (m., 24), whose illness was of a similar kind.—A remarkable case was that of Yh. (m. 50) who has always been a social abulic, tormented by the longing to find friends, but incapable of getting to know any one or of making himself known to any one ; incapable of adopting a natural attitude in society, where he masked his extreme timidity by paradoxes, disdainful assertions, and rudeness. After the most trifling emotion he became affected by serious depression, and then he was inclined to regard all his discomforts as the outcome of his enemies' machinations. His wife, and subsequently his daughter, devoted themselves for years to the difficult task of trying to restore his spirits at these times, to make him discuss his delusional affirmations for hours, to compel him to understand his ideas of persecution. For a time they succeeded in freeing him from the onset of these delusions, in restoring his confidence and serenity for several days or weeks. For twenty years, in their care for him, they played the part of the doctor who stimulates the patient's attention and restores his mental level by inciting him to complete action.

In the foregoing studies I have also alluded to the remarkable cases of Adèle and Agathe, twin sisters, who, at the age of sixteen, both fell ill in the same way, and whose symptoms for fifteen years have displayed a remarkable parallelism. At the outset of their trouble, both these young women, under suitable guidance, could be freed from their inertia and their recriminations, and could be induced to achieve the complete performance of an action, even a complicated action. After the performance of this action, a sense of satisfaction and a condition of excitation supervened, lasting for several days.— Qg. (f., 20) exhibited sentiments of incompleteness, doubts, a sense of play-acting and unreality ; she was constantly asking herself whether she was telling the truth or lying, and whether objects were real or unreal. In her, and also in the similar case of Zb. (f., 23), by stimulating attention, doubts could be dispelled, and the patient could be induced to make precise observations on things and people, and to affirm them with confidence.—In all these cases, excitation by action had an obvious and a successful influence.

But what is especially characteristic of such patients is that the progress achieved is not lasting, and cannot be intensified by repeating our efforts.—In Simone's case, after a few months, it became more and more difficult to induce emotion, and the emotion was incomplete.—Yh.'s wife and daughter were able to restore his spirits again and again for twenty years, but the task became increasingly difficult. " I know quite well what I have to do to help father," said the daughter ; " but it is hard to spend so many hours in order to secure a single hour of tranquillity. I get so tired of it at last that I lack courage to begin again." More and more the patient tended to succumb to delusional insanity, whose onset had been postponed until he was fifty years of age. Asthenic delusional insanity and asthenic dementia are not necessarily precocious, as many people imagine ; they sometimes come on comparatively late in life, but present the same characteristics as the precocious types.—In Adèle and Agathe, after five or six years, excitation by action became more difficult, and had a less marked effect. When Agathe was twenty, an hour's work would induce her to write a short letter to her mother. By the time she was twenty-five, the same amount of work was requisite to induce her to take a sweet out of a box. Now, when she is thirty-two, with my utmost efforts I can hardly make her lower her arm when it is stretched out in one of those catatonic attitudes which are the expression of her profound inertia.—In Qg. and Zb. the decadence was more rapid. Within a few months, efforts at attention became increasingly difficult, and could no longer take effect except for very simple things, and for a few moments. Ere long it became impossible to get any effect whatever.

This progressive diminution of the action, even when it is ordered and stimulated by an assistant, seems to me of great importance. Some day it will be regarded as an essential element of the diagnosis of progressive depressions, tending towards asthenic dementia. When we make such experiments upon a patient who is seriously affected, we can note a peculiar form of behaviour which I regard as characteristic. I wish to stress the point, for the appearance of this form of behaviour is a definite contraindication to continuing the treatment of excitation by action.

To demonstrate this form of behaviour, let us compare two of the patients we have already studied, Zoé and Agathe, at a moment when circumstances are arousing in them a tendency to some special action.—Zoé has just received a letter from some one who is busiest in the matter of her engagement to Monsieur X. Since, in actual fact, she is in love with Monsieur X., and wants to marry him, she is inclined to answer by writing an amiable letter.—Agathe is in a sanatorium where she is ill at ease, and from which she wants to get away. She is told that her mother is coming for her and that she must dress, so that she can be ready to leave the sanatorium and to return home. Naturally, she is delighted to hear this, and understands the proposal perfectly well and accepts it.—In these two patients, at the outset, things seem to happen in exactly the same way. The tendency awakens, it enters the first phase of activation which I have called the phase of erection, and even passes on into the second phase, that of desire. Movements related to the development of the tendency begin. The patient gets up, walks up and down the room. Zoé touches her pen. Agathe her hat, and each of them seems about to begin the proposed actions. But now there ensue various kinds of agitation, for already the energy of the tendency which cannot be properly activated is undergoing various kinds of derivation. The patients move about restlessly, breathe irregularly, complain of feeling stifled and anxious ; they talk of all kinds of ideas awakened by the action under consideration, and, generally, of ideas opposed to this action. Zoé tells us that she has an impulse to kill Monsieur X. Agathe assures us that she loathes her home, and has never had any wish to go back there.

Here resemblance between the two cases comes to an end, and marked differences are speedily displayed. Zoé may remain for a long time, hours or even days, in the same condition. She perseveringly endeavours to increase the tension of the tendency which has been awakened, or, rather, this tendency is in itself endowed with sufficient energy to remain awakened for a long time, and even to undergo a further activation, so that it passes into the third phase, that of effort. The excitation, in fact, has been enriched by other tendencies : the tendency to be amiable towards an important person ; the longing to get married ; the wish to have a house of her own, independent of her parental home ; even the sexual tendencies are now awakened side by side with the principal tendency, and supplement that tendency by the energy peculiar to themselves. It is true that, notwithstanding these reinforcements, the tension is barely adequate ; but the derivations continue to manifest themselves in increasing numbers, and in more complicated forms. The patient has symmetrical ideas, contradictory ideas, manias of interrogation, manias of making vows and resolutions, and all these symptoms are inextricably interlaced. If I may use such an expression, the energy of the tendency lacks tension, but does not lack quantity. That is why the inferior activations can be continued so long ; that is why all these agitations can be sustained.   The assistant who is trying to bring the action on to a higher level turns to account this quantity of available energy and this persistency of effort.   He can canalise the forces, can check the excessive derivations, can awaken the higher forms of the tendency ; and, sooner or later, he succeeds in bringing about a complete activation.   In a word, by means of the various methods previously described, he is able to get Zoé to write her letter, and even to achieve that this action shall be made consciously, decisively, and cheerfully.

It is quite different with poor Agathe.   We might have imagined that her wish to leave the sanatorium and to return home had been intense, for in perpetual recrimina- tions she had talked of nothing else for months past.   We are not surprised that this tendency does not secure prompt realisation, for we know that in these patients complete activa- tion is a difficult matter.   But we look for a prolonged struggle, enduring agitations, intense efforts to satisfy this urgent wish. In reality the tendency does not transcend the stage of an apathetic desire, and it simply leads to a few trivial derivations ; laughter, anxiety, recrimination against her family—that is all.   The tendency to quit the sanatorium does not reach the stage of effort, it does not call other tendencies to its aid, it does not induce complicated agitations.   On the contrary, it seems to be rapidly exhausted, and after a few moments the patient passes into a condition of complete relaxation of ten- sion.   She resumes her ordinary posture, and continues her endless repetitions, as if there were no longer any question of going away with her mother.   We have to stimulate the ten- dency anew, by explaining the situation once more, by remind- ing Agathe how much she has been wanting to see her mother and to leave the sanatorium with her mother.   Under this influence the tendency reawakens, but more feebly than before. She does not get up, hardly touches her hat, is very little excited, and relapses into the same oblivion.   If we try again, we shall have even less success, and we shall no longer be able to shake the patient out of her indifference.   This rapid relaxation of tension after the tendency has been awakened, this loss of interest in the action after the first phases of activation, this impossibility of reawakening the tendency which is so speedily exhausted, seem to me characteristic traits of asthenic dementia. It is not merely that tension is insufficient, as in simple depression ; what is wanting here is a sufficiency of available energy, for there is not enough to give the tendency a higher tension. Without going far into the discusssion of these problems, which belong rather to a study of delusional insanity and asthenic dementia, I may be content to point out that the illness has assumed a peculiar form, and that in this form excitation by action will soon become impossible. It follows that the methods and experiments we have been describing can, in such cases, only play a part of minor importance in the treatment. Their main value must be to help us to an accurate diagnosis.

Side by side with these cases, the study of which is as interesting as it is discouraging, we are glad to be able to note a good many others in which the patients have behaved quite differently. Let us consider once more the cases of various patients in whom we had noted temporary excitation after treatment, and let us ascertain what was the subsequent course of their illness under the influence of the same treatment, frequently repeated.

The first case, that of Kl., which we have regarded as typical, is a definite example of the transformations that occur in a patient subjected for a considerable time to this treatment by excitation. I pointed out that wc had to do here with a patient who had been subjected to the same treatment fifteen years earlier. The result of the treatment in her case was a disposition to be stimulated after a successful effort of attention, expression, or reasoning, together with a disposition to preserve this excitation. This is what we note when we see her transformed after going to confession. Thereafter, she will retain her mental balance for a considerable time, and, in some instances, for years. Obviously this was not the case fifteen years earlier, when she was first treated in the same way, for at that time the desired effects were difficult to obtain, but they were obtained far more easily in subsequent crises.

The same transformation has been observed in quite another set of instances.—The complete cure of Pya. by genital excitation required ten months before he was fully restored to his previous condition, but it soon became plain that the sexual endeavours of the patient were being transformed through repetition. Not only, as I said before, were they perfected in the sense of an elevation towards higher-grade sexual phenomena ; but also they became less and less difficult, and induced mental ameliorations which were more extensive and lasted longer.—Similar advances are easily noted in other cases of the same kind, when we compare the confidences made by the patient at successive epochs. Ub., suffering from a urinary obsession, who had spent eighteen months in a sanatorium without any improvement, found after three months' treatment by excitation that he " could urinate properly and pleasurably " ; simultaneously, he had completely emerged from his condition of depression. The powerful emotions induced by the war did not cause relapse in this patient.

The social actions which have been made the object of interesting endeavours in a considerable number of cases, did not always remain as difficult and distressing as they were at the outset.—In Emile's case, his expeditions from the house and his incursions into the shops were not always so dramatic and did not always demand the immense amount of work which I described in my earlier account of his case. This young man, who grew stiff and dripped with sweat on the occasion of his first expeditions, was able five or six months later to make similar expeditions without suffering any inconvenience. He made such satisfactory progress that the following year he was well enough to go in for his university examinations, and to pass them with brilliant success. Since that time he has been able to continue his advanced studies.—Efforts of attention bearing upon the sensations were successful in four months in bringing about a modification of the sentiment of depersonalisation in Wc. Subsequently this young man was able to perform his military service satisfactorily. He had no relapse during the three ensuing years.

Seven months were required to free Zoé from her condition of doubt regarding her engagement. Still, during the last two of these months, she could hardly be regarded as ill, and she was able to perform delicate and difficult social actions. She remained quite well for three years. Then, indeed, she relapsed into a state of depression, and was troubled with obsessive questionings, these symptoms being induced by the emotion from which she suffered on account of her mother's rather sudden death. She was cured more rapidly than the first time by a similar treatment.—Newy had her powers of action fully restored in a year. Since then she has retained a moderate amount of will power and energy, which suffice for the affairs of her little household.

Jd.'s crises of over-scrupulousness were cured in a few months.—In Lydia's case, her interminable discussions concerning her fixed idea of beauty became gradually easier and more lucid. The patient, who had not left her room for twelve years, now began to go out regularly, and to see a few people, this improvement manifesting itself after seven months' treatment. For the next three years, she remained perfectly well, and during this period she recovered an amount of energy which enabled her to do good service to her family in distressing circumstances.

It would be needless to enumerate many more cases of the kind. I find in my case-books the report of forty-five instances in which the general course of events was of the same kind, being the precise opposite of what we have noted in the downward progress of patients suffering from asthenic dementia. Excitation by action was at first difficult to achieve, and gave rise to nothing more than temporary improvement, analogous to " lucid intervals." By degrees, however, thanks to repetition, and thanks to the cumulative effect of advantages which were ever more easily obtained, the effect was prolonged, the complete transformation of the patient occupying a time varying from one month to twelve. The symptoms of depression were dispelled, and psychological activity regained a tension that bordered on the normal.

In other cases, of which I have fifteen among my notes, the course of events was somewhat different. Patients like Lise, Lox., and Daniel, never attained a complete cure in this way. Not one of these cases satisfies the condition which I have laid down as indispensable if we are to regard a method of treatment as truly efficacious ; not one of them remained well enough for a whole year to have no need to consult a doctor. After a few sittings of this kind, they would be a great deal better, and the improvement would last for several weeks or even several months, but, as if by an inevitable fate, the depression would then recur, and further guidance and renewed efforts would be needed. Still, I must not say that stimulant treatment had no effective action in these cases. The patients had to be given a fresh impetus from time to time, but, in actual fact, by this impetus, their tension could be restored, and could be kept at a sufficiently high level by occasional sittings. In ordinary social life they carry on normal activities, and most of their associates would be very much astonished to learn that they require this peculiar form of medical treatment every fortnight or so. They would be unable to lead such a life if they were allowed to remain persistently at the low level in which they were before the excitations. If the treatment is not curative, it is at least palliative, and succeeds in masking an infirmity.

When we consider these facts, we have to ask ourselves if we are entitled to attribute a large share in such permanent or transient improvement to the treatment by excitation. I cannot, at this stage, undertake a general discussion of the worth of psychological methods of treatment, for that matter must be reserved to the Conclusion. Suffice it to recall a few facts, a knowledge of which will be useful when the time comes for that discussion. Many of these patients had suffered from disturbances long before the treatment began.—Lydia had suffered from obsessions for twelve years, and had given up going out and seeing any one for ten years.—Mnd. (f., 40), tormented by scruples and by imaginary impulses to perform shameful actions, had lived in complete retirement for seven years.—A good many of the other patients had been ill for at least two years.—A change of disposition was clearly marked in Lydia after seven months' treatment ; in Mnd., after three months' treatment.—The way in which the cure speedily ensued upon the treatment cannot but be significant. In the patients who had had numerous crises, we could note that the antecedent crises had been very long, whereas new attacks of depression treated in the same way were of much shorter duration. Finally we had occasion to note that these patients had tried other methods of treatment.—Lydia had tried a rest cure, and had stayed in bed for two years.—Newy had on two occasions been isolated in a sanatorium.—The coincidence of improvement in the mental condition with the change in the method of treatment and with the adoption of treatment by excitation, should be noted. In view of the fact that such coincidences have been frequent, I feel that I have been justified in devoting so much space to a historical and psychological study of a method of treatment which is still little known, and which it is not easy to describe in precise terms.

Such a method of treatment is surprising at first sight, for it appears to be absolutely opposed to certain methods of treatment which seemed reasonable and useful, to the methods that we studied in a previous chapter under the name of treatment by rest and by the economising of energy. When we have to do with an individual suffering from exhaustion, it seems strange that we should be able to cure this invalid by making him work, and that we should save him from bankruptcy by advising him to undertake fresh expenditure. Still, the results are not inexplicable, for we have seen that action is not simply a matter of expending force, inasmuch as in many cases action may renew the energies. A good investment, a fortunate speculation, may prove to be a very remunerative expenditure. In actual fact, such methods of treatment are only contradictory in appearance, and may both of them be equally reasonable and useful.

It would be a very good thing if we could be certain which of these two methods of treatment is most expedient in any given case. Here we encounter a very difficult problem, and it is one whose importance does not seem evident to the majority of psychotherapeutists. If I mistake not, whether the doctor orders complete rest or prescribes distraction by occupation will usually depend upon his doctrinal preferences, and his decision will not be based upon a carefully considered psychological diagnosis. We find that some doctors advise in all cases : " Stop working, abandon your business, lie down on a sofa, take refuge in a sanatorium." Others advise in every case : " Shake off this numbing inertia, go out for a walk, work hard, amuse yourself, sursum corda ! " Some day, we may hope, these prescriptions will not be made in so haphazard a fashion, but will be dependent upon a serious psychological analysis. Unfortunately we are still far from the attainment of such an ideal, and for a long time to come we shall continue to grope in the dark, and to guide our steps by vague indications. We shall certainly do well to take into account the apparent energy of the patient. When the sufferer has symptoms of organic weakness, when he has lost flesh, when he has digestive and circulatory disorders, when he obviously suffers from muscular asthenias, we shall unquestionably be wise to recommend treatment by rest for a time. On the other hand, treatment by excitation will be indicated in a patient who appears vigorous and agitated. We must also take into account the degree of depression. Simple sadness, accompanied by a loss of the higher grades of activation, with suppression of the triumph and of joy after the performance of the action, must not be treated in the same way as true melancholic depression, with a lowering of activation below the stage of desire. Treatment by excitation is much easier in cases of the former type than in cases of the latter type. We must recognise that rest is especially indicated when the disturbances occasioned by psychological depression are more generalised, that is to say, when the symptoms of depression (such as inadequacies of activation, sentiments of incompleteness, derivations taking the form of agitations and phobias, and mental manias) occur not only in connexion with certain specific actions, but in the case of a great number of actions, which are the expression of different tendencies. An interesting indication may be furnished by the development of agitation, which may appear in all grades of depression, and which in each one of them assumes a characteristic form. The occurrence of these agitations often shows us that a considerable quantity of energy has been retained, although the tension has been lowered.

It is a regrettable fact that such indications are far from easy to discover, and often lead us astray. In most cases we shall have to experiment with different forms of treatment ; we shall have to grope our way. In general, I am inclined to begin the treatment of depression by the application of the methods of economy and rest ; and we must never completely abandon these methods, for it is rest which economises the force that excitation can make use of. Only by degrees can we add to treatment by repose, various attempts at excitation by action. The excitations will be continued, increased, or diminished, according as they are easily applied, according to their results, and according to the manner in which the phenomena of relaxation of tension and discharge present themselves.

Some patients have already instinctively tried to apply treatment by excitation, having had impulses to perform this or that action. The doctor must begin by studying and regulating these impulses, which almost invariably contain, or have contained, an element of useful excitation, but which undergo transformation by abuse, so that they become dangerous. Of course we must check any kind of action which is dangerous to the patient from the social or hygienic point of view ; and we must also counteract the impulses which I may term " erroneous," the impulses in which the patient seeks an excitation which these particular impulses cannot supply.

On the other hand we shall find it well to encourage, to some extent at least, certain impulses which represent a search for love, domination, success, etc.—impulses which in point of principle are not absurd. The patient is no longer securing good results from such impulses ; first of all because he acts unskilfully and does not succeed in achieving his desire ; and secondly because he repeats the action too frequently, so that the tendency becomes exhausted and is no longer vigorous enough to bring about complete activation. The role of the doctor must be to regulate these impulses rather than to suppress them. As we have seen, the chief danger of impulses is their narrowness, their exclusiveness. Instead of trying to bring about excitation through the repeated performance of the same action, we must try to induce excitation by various actions attaching to different tendencies, for in this way we shall achieve a larger number of successes at less cost. In this connexion I may refer to a letter written by an interesting patient whose case we have already studied and whose amorous impulses were described above. Under guidance, she improved a great deal, and was able to gain a better understanding of the advantages which could be derived from the search for love. To begin with she had constantly been in pursuit of the dream of an ideal of complete and absolute love incarnated in a single personality. She made considerable progress when she became enabled to understand that it is possible to distribute the affections among several persons in such a way as not to exact everything from one person. " I have found it necessary to cut up my heart into little bits ; nobody wanted all of it, for it is so exacting and so large. My husband is glad to accept the offering of my domestic virtues ;

my parents like my good temper ; my children have a taste for my purse ; and my friends are fond of the pleasures I can give them, which do not empty their purses. Every one I come into contact with wants a little bit of me from time to time ; no one wants all of me. At long last I have learned how to love people without trying to absorb them." Guidance of this kind will succeed more often than might be imagined in transforming morbid impulses into instruments of cure.

In many cases we have to do with depressed patients who have no impulses, and then the doctor's part (if we may summarise all we have been just studying) must often take the form of an attempt to create impulses. He must point out to the patients what actions they are capable of performing, and what actions can be beneficial to them. He must teach them to perform these actions correctly and completely, and in the way which will make the actions most stimulating. A man can enrich himself in another way than by economising on his expenditure ; he can also enrich himself, perhaps even more rapidly, by learning how to increase his income. Notwithstanding the obscurity of these phenomena, and notwithstanding the inadequacy of my explanations of them, we shall often succeed in bringing about notable and permanent cure or improvement by interesting the patient, after this manner, in his own cure

CHAPTER FIFTEEN

PSYCHOPHYSIOLOGICAL METHODS OF TREATMENT

PSYCHOLOGICAL methods of treatment have often been regarded as opposed to other methods of treatment which appeal to the resources of physics and chemistry, and are founded upon a knowledge of physiological laws. In the days when a great enthusiasm for suggestion prevailed, in that delightful epoch when it was enough to say to our patients " sleep and get well," well-informed doctors could not disguise their sorrow at seeing that all their arduous study of physiology and clinical medicine had been fruitless, and to many of them it seemed that psychotherapeutics was a useful house of refuge for doctors who had had no real medical education. Paul Dubois, in his book on the psychoneuroses, which from so many points of view is of great interest, has said a good deal which might seem to confirm this opinion. Not only has he advised a moral system of therapeutics, but also he has condemned the majority of the examinations, the operations, and the remedies which form part of physiological therapeutics. " We must do away with all this " he writes. " We must advance against the illness without weapons and without drugs. Then the patient will be convinced that there is no real danger, and that is a matter of enormous importance.[1] . . . The doctor's only weapon must be his encouraging words.[2] . . . His only weapon must be his concise, imperturbable, benevolent argumentation."[3] No doubt these authors had in mind the exaggerations of contemporary surgery, for the surgeons of their day " were cutting, cauterising, and scarifying numberless hypochondriacal neuropaths." Or they had in mind the pharmaceutists, "who were poisoning these patients by the administration of innumerable

---

[1] Dubois, Les psychonévroses et leur traitement moral, 1904, p. 487.
[2] Op. cit., p. 302.   [3] Op. cit., p. 544.

1030

drugs." None the less, the advocates of dialectic were demanding a very unfortunate restriction of the resources of therapeutics in such cases of neuroses, and their conception of psychotherapeutics was mischievous and unscientific.

Psychological disorders are disorders of behaviour, and behaviour is simply a totality of the outward reactions of the living being. How can we possibly suppose that these outward reactions, which take place through the limbs, the mouth, and the tongue, can be completely independent of the inward reactions which take place in the interior of the same body, and the study of which comprises physiology ? Is not the satisfactory adaptation of the outward reactions just as much a part of life as the satisfactory adaptation of the inward reactions ? A man whose behaviour is disordered is a man who is not living either correctly or completely. At bottom, however contradictory appearances may be, we must never cease to consider the insane person as a sick person. I cannot but be astonished when I see a lunatic, who has suffered from delusional insanity since the age of twenty, nevertheless attain advanced old age, and exhibit even in old age an aspect of sound physical health. Here we are faced with an extremely complicated problem, complicated by our ignorance concerning the true longevity of man, concerning the causes which restrict the normal duration of life, concerning the appreciation of vital activity ; and obviously we must be deceiving ourselves when we wonder at the apparent good health of these insane persons.

All that we can say is that in many cases of this kind disturbances of health are not manifested by gross lesions of the familiar organic apparatus ; that there are no obvious disturbances of the heart or the lungs, and even that there are no obvious lesions of the brain. Behaviour, and the psychological phenomena which depend upon behaviour, are not an isolated manifestation of the activity of the heart, lungs, or brain ; they are the expression of the entire organism, of its growth, of its evolution and its involution. The organs and the functions which play their part in the production of these phenomena are little known to us, and their disturbances are hardly suspected ; but they exist, and will have to be studied more carefully. Psychology is not independent of physiology, but it needs a more delicate and more profound physiology than that of digestion and respiration. The study of nervous and mental diseases, far from being able to dispense with physiological and medical knowledge, will to an increasing extent demand a very abstruse physiology and medicine. The treatment of these patients, far from being undertaken after no more than a summary medical study, will be the work of a highly instructed clinician, and will necessitate the use of all possible methods of examination, and of extremely delicate procedures.

Should methods of treatment of this kind be still classed as part of psychotherapeutics ? I think so, for several reasons. First of all, the application of such methods of treatment will demand psychological knowledge, and procedures based upon psychological laws. In the case of ordinary illnesses which do not disorder behaviour, it is enough to give the patient a little advice and a prescription ; to say to him, " you must undergo such and such an operation, must adopt such and such a regimen, must take this or that medicine." Is it enough to give prescriptions of this kind when we have to do with a neuropath ? Is it enough to tell a sufferer from hysterical anorexia to eat more ; or to tell a psychasthenic with bulimia to eat less ? It is not enough, when we are dealing with such patients, to give advice or to correct an error. We have to make our advice understood by patients whose intelligence, powers of credence, and will power are disordered ; to get them to accept our advice and to carry it out. This is a very different thing, and our treatment will, to a preponderant extent, remain a psychological problem.

But there is something more to be said. The diagnosis of these disturbances of the organism, the choice of methods of treatment, and the appreciation of the effects of treatment, can only be made with the assistance of psychological studies, and thanks to psychological methods. If we are to appreciate the significance of these disturbances in the evolution of the organism, we must recognise the characteristics and the degrees of depression, must study the excitation induced by certain methods of treatment, must distinguish depression from agitation (always a difficult matter), and so on. Moreau de Tours, when he had studied the effects of hashish, proposed to employ this drug in the treatment of melancholics. If his advice to use such a method of treatment had been adopted, quite a number of psychological studies would have resulted, and the knowledge gained thereby would have formed a permanent part of psychotherapeutics.

Far from wishing that the psychotherapeutist should approach the patient "without weapons and without drugs," I should like him to furbish up all the weapons he can get hold of, for he can never overestimate the formidable powers of his enemy, and can never be too well equipped. In the treatment of the psychoneuroses, he must avail himself of all the knowledge which the medicine and physiology of his day can supply. This knowledge, which, unfortunately, is gravely restricted, can be classed under two heads : first of all, observations concerning the bodily diseases which often accompany disturbances of behaviour, this study enabling us to investigate the more or less intricate methods which aim at favourably influencing the neuroses by the simultaneous treatment of the physiological disturbances of the organism ; in the second place, certain observations concerning the effects of particular chemical substances and particular physical phenomena which seem to modify the psychological tension and the behaviour, these studies giving us indications as to a direct medication of psychological disturbances.

I. PHYSIOLOGICAL DISORDERS RELATED TO THE NEUROSES.

General Diseases. It seems probable that all diseases, of whatever kind, must have an influence upon the psychological tension, seeing that this tension must depend upon the satisfactory functioning of the entire organism. The ancients summarised this belief in their celebrated aphorism "mens sana in corpore sano." Very frequently, doctors have applied the axiom to the study of the neuropsychoses by diligently searching in the patient's organism in order to discover some kind of morbid lesions with which the obvious disorders of behaviour might be connected. "If we want to cure the neuroses," wrote Lewellys Barker, " we must especially take into account local processes, diseases of the ears, the eyes, errors of refraction, disorders of the sinuses, genito-urinary diseases, tuberculosis, arteriosclerosis, syphilis, alcoholism, larval forms of

Graves' disease, etc."[1]—" We must," said Henri Damage, " pay great attention to tuberculosis, gynecological affections, infectious diseases, inflammatory disorders, suppurations of every kind, organic inadequacies, chronic bronchitis, Bright's disease, etc."[2] I need hardly say that the importance which tubercular and syphilitic diseases have assumed in pathology has directed a great deal of attention to these processes, and it is difficult to realise how many neuropathic disorders have been connected by one doctor or another with tuberculosis, and still more with syphilis. As for syphilis, people have obstinately endeavoured to discover evidence of its existence, often despite the absence of all the characteristic symptoms.

Seductive though these physiological explanations appear to be, it is easy to show that even to-day they are inadequate, and that no scientific treatment of the neuroses can possibly be founded upon them. The fundamental adage " mens sana in corpore sano " which underlies such studies, is itself very difficult to apply when we are concerned with disorders of behaviour and of thought. How many patients in the last stages of consumption seem to be perfectly healthy as far as their mental functions are concerned, whereas a great many dements appear to enjoy perfect physical health !

One remarkable point in connexion with this matter concerns the influence which age exercises upon these maladies which take the form of psychological depression. I have already shown by statistics which agree perfectly with those of Pitres and Régis that psychasthenic disorders occur mainly during youth.[3] Their maximum frequency and severity is found between the ages of twenty and thirty-five years. The frequency, and perhaps also the gravity, of the illness begins to diminish from the age of forty ; and if we do not confound these depressive types of disorder with mental affections of a different kind, we shall note that they become rare in old age. Deschamps is even led to conclude " that the nervous system of asthenics improves with age, so that many of these patients recover health towards the age of sixty."[4] Many of the serious

[1] Barker, On the psychic Treatment of some of the functional Neuroses, 1906, p. 4.
[2] Damage, Les affections mentales curables et leur traitement, " Journal de Neurologie," April 20, 1911, p. 141.
[3] Les obessesions et la psychasthénie, 1903, vol. i, p. 614.
[4] Deschamps, Les maladies de l'énergie, 1908, p. 265.

cases I have had under observation for years ran a course which fully justified Deschamps' remark. Jean, Nadia, Lise, and Lox., who have been my patients for twenty years, are certainly less ill than when I first made their acquaintance, and their present troubles are hardly comparable with those from which they suffered when they were young. Lise, who is now fifty years of age, elderly, suffering from serious biliary lithiasis, and having undergone a gallstone operation, is, mentally speaking, much better than she was in the days when physically she was quite strong. A very remarkable case is that of Xe., who from the age of eighteen up to the age of sixty was obsessed with excessive scruples to the verge of delusional insanity, was a persistent doubter, and, above all, an agoraphobic absolutely unable to leave the house. At the age of sixty he underwent a complete change of character ; thenceforward he was free from doubts and phobias ; he was able to travel alone, and boldly to make long journeys ; he enjoyed a green old age, and was thoroughly happy until his death took place at the age of eighty-two.

In former days I explained these facts in a way which I still regard as partially sound. I said that in old age life requires fewer new adaptations, is simpler, less costly. In old age, it is therefore easier to meet the now diminished expenditure even though the patient's resources are still slender. The obvious improvement resulting from the menopause in such women as Lise and Lox. would seem to justify this interpretation, for the expenditure necessitated by the sexual functions, and even by the amorous tendencies, has been enormously reduced. Perhaps we may also admit that in these patients there has occurred an evolution which has favoured the production of psychological energies. As I have repeatedly insisted, such persons are sluggish, their physical and mental evolution is very slow, and they do not attain their complete development until extremely late. I could adduce evidence to show that in several of them mental puberty, sexual interest and curiosity, did not occur until the age of thirty ; that social activity and a desire for independence, which arises in normal young people at the age of seventeen or twenty, did not arise in them until the age of forty. It may well be that there are a great many other energies as yet hardly suspected whose activity is a factor of psychological tension, and that in these patients such activities have likewise developed late. Whatever we may think of the hypotheses in question, it is certainly a remarkable fact that these individuals come to display a far more complete psychological activity at the very time when the onset of old age impairs their physical health and entails various infirmities.

I have frequently had occasion to point out another fact which has always seemed to me very remarkable. I refer to the obviously beneficial influence of pregnancy in neuropaths. I have recorded thirty cases in which severe psychasthenia was mitigated by the onset of pregnancy, and was completely relieved by the time the fourth month of pregnancy had arrived. It is true that two-thirds of these patients relapsed into a similar condition of depression shortly after delivery. I have recently had under my care a dozen or more cases exhibiting the same sequence. Among these patients, two women who for years had suffered from tics, manias, and obsessions, were completely freed from such symptoms during the later months of pregnancy, only to relapse after childbirth. —Héloïse was never normal except during pregnancy and during menstruation.—X. (f., 27), abulic and tortured by all kinds of phobias since the age of thirteen, is herself greatly surprised to find that she can behave just like other people, and that she is no longer afraid of anything when she is pregnant. Shortly after delivery she begins to ask herself whether she really loves her baby; she is afraid she will injure the infant, and all her troubles begin over again. In two cases the influence of lactation was favourable, this continuing for six months the good influence of pregnancy. I have only observed three cases of a contrary kind, in which the evolution of pregnancy induced no amelioration in the psychasthenic condition. I could not find any other differential characteristic by which these three women could be distinguished from the far commoner cases in which the effect of pregnancy was beneficial. Without laying much stress here upon the possible explanations of this influence of pregnancy, I shall be content to point out that many of the pregnancies in these cases were attended by distressing symptoms, that they induced weakness and general disorder of the physical health, and that nevertheless there was a great improvement as regards the neuropathic condition.

The problem becomes still more complicated when we pass from normal or physiological conditions like old age and pregnancy, to obviously pathological conditions, which are nevertheless accompanied by a similar improvement in the mental condition. Simple febrile disorders, transient illnesses, will induce obvious improvement.—Pepita, when attacked by influenza became perfectly reasonable and happy for ten days ; during the intercurrent illness she menstruated, and though it is usual with her to have her mind especially disturbed in the days following menstruation, on this particular occasion she was free from that trouble.—The same thing happened in three other cases ; the patients were free from a sense of shame, from tics, and from hysterical symptoms, when they were suffering from fever.—If we find that Wd. (f., 16) does not pass water in her bed, or does not suffer from sleepwalking during the night, it is because she has an attack of fever.—Bul., a woman of fifty-six, with the strange and persistent obsession that she is in a black tomb surrounded by dead persons, has an attack of bronchopneumonia, and her temperature ranges between 100° and 103.° " It is extraordinary," she says ; " your face is no longer smeared with black ; you no longer look as if you were dead ; and I myself am no longer in a black tomb." A fortnight later, when she welcomed me with lamentations because she was once more living in a black cave, and because all the people around her were dead, her temperature had fallen almost to normal. In other patients who, after an attack of pneumonia or an attack of typhoid, remained very weak for a considerable time, the obsessions and phobias, and even epileptic fits, did not immediately recur. During convalescence, the mental condition seemed quite satisfactory, and the will was energetic. The mental disorders did not reappear until the physical force had been fully reestablished.

The case of Mba., suffering from quinsy, a case we have already studied, was extremely characteristic. It is possible that febrile disorders give rise to stimulant toxins which raise the psychological tension. But this explanation cannot apply to periods of convalescence, when there is no fever, and when the only morbid change is a condition of extreme weakness. We have better grounds for connecting these phenomena with those which have given birth to the theory of the discharge. I refer to observations akin to those which are made upon melancholics in asylums, who are sometimes found to be worse after a good night, and who seem to be clearer in mind after insomnia and fatigue ; also upon neuropaths who are improved by grave convulsive crises, after long walks, and after prolonged and exhausting labour. In all these cases, the weakness or the exhaustion restores the balance between the quantity of energy and the psychological tension, and thus diminishes the neuropathic symptoms.

There is no doubt that many authors have been inclined to exaggerate the part played by the tubercular infections in the neuroses. Beyond question there are numerous cases in which the patient has more or less severe symptoms of tuberculosis in addition to neuropathic disorders ; but this conjuncture is far from being the rule, and in certain remarkable cases reported by myself the development of pulmonary tuberculosis seems to have the same sort of effect as the exhausting illnesses of which I have just been speaking, for it induces a favourable transformation of the mental condition. —Claire, whose case was reported at great length in my book *Les obsessions et la psychasthénie*, was troubled by obsessions of sacrilege, and by all kinds of disturbances, from the time she was sixteen until she was thirty-two, but as soon as her pulmonary tuberculosis became severe, and from then until her death (for more than two years that is to say) her mind was perfectly clear.—Vea. (m., 35) had been tormented from the age of ten by superstitious obsessions, anxious self-enquiries as to whether he was " a religious man or a criminal," and by vague thoughts of domination which resembled the delusion of persecution. When tuberculosis supervened, and he was bedridden, his mental calm was restored for three years.

Still more often, doctors have exaggerated the pathogenic importance of syphilis in connexion with the neuroses. If we put aside the special affections in which well-marked specific lesions play an incontestable part, we cannot find that there is any regular relationship between the true neuropsychoses and syphilis. No doubt it is correct to say that congenital syphilis, by its effect in producing organic degenerations, exercises a predisposing influence ; and no doubt it is true that the onset of syphilis may give rise to intense emotion, and in certain instances to exhaustion ; but these influences are not specific.

Such reflections concerning various general disorders show us that it is far from easy to apply to the neuroses the old adage " mens sana in corpore sano." We are not entitled to find a facile explanation of all mental disorders in everyday organic affections. Much further study will be requisite before we can be certain as to the precise disturbances in the working of the organism which may play a predominant part here.

Gastro-intestinal Disturbances. There are, however, certain groups of disorders, or, if the phrasing be preferred, certain groups of physical symptoms, which accompany the neuroses with a far greater regularity ; which seem to have more importance in the actual evolution of the neuroses ; and the treatment of which, therefore, must greatly concern the psychotherapeutist. Among these I may especially refer to gastro-intestinal disorders.

Unquestionably, a great many patients who suffer from various forms of mental depression, have already suffered from, or still suffer from, disorders of the alimentary system. A certain number of neuropaths are badly nourished, take their food badly. These patients used in former days to be almost invariably spoken of as sufferers from hysterical anorexia. To-day this ill-defined group has been subdivided, and, side by side with genuine hysterical disturbances, we distinguish various obsessions, impulses, and delusions relating to the process of taking food. Speaking generally, we must be on our guard at the very outset against the restriction of diet practised by neuropaths under some pretext of regimen, or upon some idealist excuse. The patients will soon go too far in this direction, and will restrict their diet to an increasingly serious extent. Even more frequently, in neuropathic patients, we see a tendency to overeating ; far more often we have to do with neuropaths who eat too much than with neuropaths who eat too little. Apart from the sufferers from high-grade bulimia, who are driven by an obviously morbid impulse to eat all day long and to consume enormous quantities of food, we see a great many patients who make a practice at their meals of eating far more than the average quantity of food, and certainly far more than the quantity they ate before they were ill. This behaviour is connected with their persistent feeling of depression, and with the instinct people have to connect this weakness with want of food and to treat it by taking a great deal of food. The patients who eat too much are, in fact, inert patients, who suffer from sentiments of incompleteness; whereas the anorexics are usually restless patients in whom agitation masks depression, and who, precisely because of their agitation, suffer very little from sentiments of incompleteness. We often see subjects exhibiting successively these two contrasted syndromes, according to the stage their illness has reached. For instance, Ug. (f., 20) conducted herself at first as an anorexic, moving about a great deal, riding on horseback, spending whole nights at dances, and absolutely refusing to eat. Then after eighteen months, rather suddenly, she changed her ways, declaring that she was tired, and that she would do no more work. She refused to leave her bed, but went on eating all day, and insisted on having supplies of cold meat and bottles of wine on her bedside table. Such an evolution is quite common; I have seen it in about a dozen cases, and it generally signifies that the illness is growing worse. The overfeeding usually practised by these patients has a very bad effect. Far from reducing the depression, it increases the depression owing to the fatigue imposed upon the digestive organs, and owing to the resulting complications.

A great many neuropaths, especially at the outset of their illness (it may be as a sequel of overfeeding, or it may be independently of any disorder in the process of food-taking), suffer from disturbances of gastro-intestinal digestion. "Every neuropath" writes Gilles de la Tourette,[1] "suffers more or less from intestinal troubles." Looking through the notes of the various cases to which I have so frequently referred, I find that there were about sixty patients who were continually complaining of serious digestive troubles, simultaneously with their psychical disorders. They had gastralgia, heartburn, acid regurgitation, vomiting, and salivation. This salivation would sometimes be extraordinarily profuse, as in the case of Te. (f., 30) who filled whole basins with her saliva.

[1] Les états neurasthéniques, 1900,

Sometimes they suffered from anorexia, dislike for food, slow digestion with flatulence, gastric distension, stagnation of the food, and various other symptoms of disordered stomach. In technical terminology, these symptoms are classed as hyperacidity, hyperchlorhydria, gastric hypersthenia ; or else as gastric insufficiency, gastric hyposthenia, gastric fermentations, gastric intestinal ptoses ; but the various symptoms merge into one another, and alternate one with another. In many cases they lead in due course to grave diseases of the stomach. I find it very difficult to believe what some declare,[1] that gastric ulcer is always the primary cause of these troubles ; but there is no doubt that in many cases it is their sequel.

The disturbances of gastric digestion, the intestinal atony, the ptosis of the transverse colon, and the flexures or kinkings connected with the ptosis, often lead to chronic constipation. In a hundred or more cases, there were the disturbances of intestinal digestion which have been made familiar to us by the studies of Maurice de Langenhagen[2] under the name of " muco-membranous enteritis." The chronic constipation which is so common in neuropaths, especially in those who suffer from gastric hyperacidity, gives rise to abdominal spasm and to meteorism. The stools, which are infrequent, hard, laminated, and scybalous, are accompanied by the voiding of mucus, false membranes, and often blood. Sometimes the mucous discharge is attended by severe pain. In many cases, bleeding piles complete the picture. These disturbances of the stomach and intestine are very serious in neuropaths. They cause a great deal of pain ; they induce spasms of all kinds in the thorax and the abdomen, troubles which are not always satisfactorily diagonised, and which have a great deal to do with the causation of the algias and the phobias. Many of the patients who believe that they are suffering from heart disease are merely affected with gastric hypersthenia.

I shall be content with describing one interesting case, that of Pepita, whose remarkable mental condition has already been considered. She exhibited all these gastro-intestinal disturbances in a most typical way. She is now fifty years of age, and declares that her gastric and intestinal troubles

[1] Pauchet, Traitement de l'ulcère chronique de l'estomac, " Presse Médicale," October 9, 1916.   [2] " Presse Médicale," 1898, p. 7.

began when she was nineteen, when she had a severe attack of choleraic diarrhoea as a sequel of indigestion. In reality, however, her troubles began much earlier, for she had anorexia when she was twelve years old, and refused all food at the boarding school she was attending. Since then, she has continually been complaining of troubles in the stomach and the abdomen, where all sorts of extraordinary sensations are localised. From time to time she has painful crises, feeling in the thorax and the abdomen shocks which drag her to one side or the other " as if with cords." " These movements throw me off my balance and make me feel as if I were going to fall. Hold me up, I feel I am going to fall." Such shocks, such spasms of the trunk or limbs as sequels of hyperchlorhydria, are common. A woman of forty, Sea., has been fixed in her chair for two years " because heartburn induces shocks in the stomach which would throw me to the ground if I were to try to stand." Rf. (f., 56), after a prolonged attack of gastric hypersthenia, suffers from a sense of pulsations throughout the body and from spasms which, she says, pass down into the vagina and the anus, so that she no longer dares to move for fear of falling. Similar phenomena, descibed in similar terms, were met with in seven cases.

Returning to the case of Pepita, we find that soon after she has been affected by these violent spasms, she has a strong desire to go to stool, and that she then passes a large, loose, and evil-smelling motion. She has been subject to such diarrhoea ever since youth, and has rarely had a normal motion during the last thirty years. Her digestion will not tolerate a great many kinds of food. Milk, cream, eggs, beef tea, certain vegetables such as carrots, even when taken in very small quantities, and hidden amid other kinds of food, always induce violent symptoms within two or three days. After she has had terrible pains in the abdomen, there comes a violent serous or even haemorrhagic diarrhoea, with suppression of urine, extreme chilliness, and symptoms of the imminence of collapse. These phenomena may reasonably be compared to those of the anaphylaxis described by Richet. —Such mucous and evil-smelling diarrhoeas occur in a great many neuropathic patients. In Aln. they first appeared when she began to menstruate at the age of thirteen, and continued till her death at the age of thirty-two.—The same thing happened in the case of Ac., who, after the suppression of menstruation at the age of eighteen, suffered from intractable offensive diarrhoea until her death took place at the age of thirty.—A good many patients, like Ar. and Te., pass a large quantity of sandy material in the stools, suffering to a marked extent from the oxalic diathesis which has been so well described by Loeper.

Intoxication of alimentary origin is manifested in Pepita by an abnormal condition of the skin, by an extreme degree of the phenomena of dermographism. On one occasion, after one of the violent anaphylactic reactions I have just been describing, she suffered from an extraordinary outbreak of erythema which covered almost the whole of the body. The eruption appeared upon the face, the external genitals, the outer surfaces of the arms and the hands, the front of the thighs and the legs, taking the form of large symmetrical plaques, which, after a few days became covered with thick crusts, these subsequently falling off without leaving any trace. The eruption was preceded, accompanied, and followed by pains in the skin and in the muscles, pains which the patient persistently compared with that of bites, of rubbing with stinging nettles, or of rubbing with sandpaper. We can find descriptions of similar eruptions in the books of dermatologists, and especially in the treatise of Monsieur Brocq, where it is described as erythema ferox.—Such dermographic troubles as erythemata, lichens, eczemas, and urticarias, are fairly common in neuropaths, and I find notes of about twenty such cases in my books. Can we connect with these skin troubles the remarkable phenomenon of the blackening of the tongue which occurs in Irène during very severe depressions ?

Notwithstanding all these symptoms, notwithstanding the obstinate diarrhoea and the difficulties connected with nutrition, Pepita is obese. Although of small stature, she weighs over thirteen stone. I found it very difficult to thin her down, for there was no loss of weight in spite of extreme restriction of diet. I had to keep her under strict observation for two years and to diet her almost continuously in order to reduce her weight by as much as two stone. The same characteristic was to be found in Noémi and Ar., and in a dozen other patients, all of whom became extremely stout in the early stage of severe attacks of depression. Finally, I must point out that, in a great many cases, such patients have characteristic disorders of the liver, which accompany the psychosis. In especial, biliary lithiasis is common in psychasthenics.

These gastro-intestinal diseases which accompany the symptoms of mental depression, develop under the same conditions as the mental disorders after fatigue and emotion. It is hardly necessary to remind the reader that neuropathic anorexia and bulimia almost always appear as the sequel of emotional upsets.

In Noémi, crises of gastric hypersthenia appear during the night following emotional disturbances, just as her obsessions appear at this time. In Ph. (f., 20), they supervened after disappointments in love. In Oe. (m., 45), they appeared during the days which followed a medical consultation and the decision that an operation would be necessary. In Sea., they appeared after she had received news of her son's death. In a great many patients, attacks of enteritis recur whenever there is an emotional disturbance, and often the same period of incubation is observed in the case of the enteritis as in the case of the mental symptoms. For instance, Ng. (m., 30) sustained a serious injury of the left hand when he was out shooting, and had to have the thumb amputated. A month later there began a severe muco-membranous enteritis which lasted for years. The cure of these visceral symptoms (except in certain cases to the consideration of which we shall return) is apt to accompany the complete cure of the neuroses. Many of our patients have been freed from enteritis when they have been freed from their obsessions. During the periods of temporary cure, which I have spoken of as periods of excitation, Lise, Pepita, and a great many other patients, were able to digest perfectly ; and the circumstances which led to the cure of the digestive troubles were the same as those which led to the cure of the mental troubles. Many doctors are familiar with such cases as that of my patient, a woman, who had suffered from enteritis for years, and who was completely cured after her house had been burnt down. The reader will remember how in Héloïse the enteritis disappeared after she had read a love letter.

Cases of this kind, instances of which could easily be

multiplied, have inspired a theory which might be called the *gastro-intestinal theory of the neuroses*. Even without considering the extreme types of "delusional wasting" and of sitiophobia, we must admit that insufficient nutrition will certainly have an effect upon the development of an illness whose main characteristics are weakness and lowered tension. Recently, A. F. Plicque referred a number of neurasthenic disorders to inadequacy of nutrition.[1] On the other hand, many authors, such as Pascault, of Cannes, Guelpa, and Vigouroux, have studied the bad effects of the overeating which is also common in neuropathic patients, being inclined to regard neurasthenia as due to excessive nutriment, and especially to excess of animal food. J. Laumonier, in an interesting study of the treatment of laziness in children,[2] states that idlers are persons who are poisoned by excess of food, and by overstimulating food, which causes undue functional activity and exhaustion. It is usually agreed that intoxications of external origin may give rise to mental disorders. For a long time, too, proof has been forthcoming that intoxications of internal origin play an important part in the causation of certain psychoses. Lasègue,[3] in former days, and Chaslin [4] more recently, have shown that states of mental confusion and of dreamy delirium must be regarded as due to the phenomena of the kind. Many authors, following the line of enquiry suggested a good many years ago by Bouchard in his animadversions upon Charcot, tried to extend this notion, and were inclined to consider most neuroses as due to autointoxications resulting from intestinal disturbances. Interesting though such theories are, I regard them as premature. Too much stress has been laid upon autointoxication as a cause of the psychoses. Sometimes autointoxication actually does exist in these cases, and is manifested by the ordinary clinical signs such as disturbances of the liver, skin affections, neuritis, mental confusion, etc. Undoubtedly such a clinical picture is to be seen in a fair number of neuropaths, and this shows that in these patients intoxication readily

[1] Maladies par insuffisance d'alimentation, " Journal de Médecine et de Chirurgie," November 10, 1917.
[2] Traitement de la paresse, " Bulletin général de Thérapeutique," February 23, 1913.
[3] Lasègue, Catalepsies partielles et passagères, " Archives Générales de la Médecine," 1865 ; Etudes médicales, vol. i, p. 899.
[4] La confusion mentale primitive, 1895.

occurs and that it is apt to complicate and aggravate the neuroses, but we certainly cannot say that it is a constant complication, and that every neuropathic condition is identical with a state of intoxication. From the mental point of view, we must not confuse the depressions of neuropaths with the confusional states of those suffering from intoxication; the two mental conditions are entirely different. We can sometimes distinguish them in the same subject. I have described elsewhere the symptoms of stercoraemia (faecal intoxication) in Nadia, a young woman who suffered from the typical mental condition of psychasthenics. The symptoms of faecal intoxication continued for three months, inducing neuritic symptoms and mental confusion, with a tendency to reverie. The noteworthy point is that these symptoms were superadded to the ordinary condition of the patient, who, after the superadded mental confusion had been dispelled, returned to her customary obsessions. From the physical standpoint, we must recognise that there are a great many persons whose behaviour is that of neuropaths, but who are entirely free from the symptoms and the general aspect of those suffering from intoxication.

It cannot be said that all neuropaths suffer from disorders of digestion, or from enteroptosis; there are numerous exceptions. When such symptoms are present in neuropaths, there is not always a coincidence between the two kinds of disorder. I have previously referred to the remarkable form assumed by the illness of Mf. (f., 50). For years she suffered from severe nervous enteritis without, during this period, exhibiting any very definite mental symptoms. Then she became affected with grave mental depression and with hypochondriacal obsessions which especially concerned intestinal digestion; but the strange, I might almost say ludicrous, fact was that at the time when her delusions were bearing upon her intestine, this organ was functioning satisfactorily, and the neuritis had absolutely disappeared.

I think it will be of interest to recall in this connexion a remarkable clinical observation, namely that these troubles of the stomach, the intestines, and the skin, these autointoxications which so frequently accompany the slighter forms of neuroses, are much rarer in the severe forms of psychoses. Whereas gastric hypersthenia, abdominal ptosis, mucous enteritis, and skin affections, are common in town practice and in hydropathic practice, they are rare in lunatic asylums. This is a matter which I have frequently discussed with Monsieur Arnaud, in his establishment at Vanves. There, dietetic precautions, alkaline treatment, and intestinal lavage, are quite exceptional, whereas they are a regular part of the regime in sanatoria for neuropaths. Nay more, the very patients who, in the early stages of their illness, when they were suffering only from obsessions or phobias, were affected with digestive disorders, ceased to present these troubles when they were admitted to a lunatic asylum in a condition of well-marked melancholia or delusional insanity. Sophie, a psychasthenic from the age of sixteen onwards, suffering from obsessive over-scrupulousness, obsessions of independence, and an inclination to fugues, was constantly complaining of her stomach and bowel ; for ten years she had had to diet herself for enteritis. When she was twenty-seven years old, she became affected with grave depression and with well-marked asthenic delusions ; but now there was no disorder of the stomach or bowel. When, in her delirium, she would try to eat her own faeces, these were of a perfectly normal consistency, whereas ten years earlier the stools had been always loose and full of mucus. The same remarks apply to Emile, who, during the two years in which he suffered from asthenic delusions, was free from enteritis, and who, when his insanity had passed off, began to suffer from enteritis once more.

I have noticed the same phenomenon in patients passing from psychasthenic depression to asthenic dementia. There was no longer any question of disorders of digestion in Adèle and Agathe as soon as they became affected with dementia, whereas such disorders had been persistent in them previously. When they were living at home or in hydropathic establishments, and were still suffering from neuropathic troubles such as abulia, doubts, and obsessions, these twin sisters were both affected with a remarkable disorder of the secretions which gave their room a strange and unpleasant smell like that of a wild beast's den ; in the morning, although their bedroom was kept scrupulously clean, this smell was extremely disagreeable. When they had both become dements and had been removed to an asylum, the smell was no longer noticeable. The same fact can be recorded as regards Sita (f., 28), and as regards Noémi. The last-named, at the beginning of her crises of depression and obsession with the thought of death, diffused a strange odour of burning indiarubber, this being partly derived from the skin and partly from the stools. When the depression was further advanced and had become serious, no smell of this kind could be detected. I could quote a number of additional observations to show that digestive and secretory disturbances which have existed over and above the true neuropathic symptoms, or which have accompanied the first stages of psychological depression, have often to a large extent disappeared when more serious psychological perturbations have manifested themselves.

Although in the light of our present knowledge it is difficult to give a complete explanation of this phenomenon, it need not surprise us very much, for we have studied kindred phenomena, especially in connexion with hysterical crises, and with attacks of migraine. Certain reactions occur in the early stages of the depression, when attempts are still made at the restoration of tension, when rapid changes of tension are occurring in one direction or the other, when there are discharges and relaxations of tension; but nothing of the kind is noticed when the tension is definitively lowered. Whatever the explanation may be, the recognition of these strange phenomena must make us cautious, and must disincline us to regard digestive disturbances and autointoxications as persistent and essential factors of neurosis. No doubt if we contend apriori that all the functions of the organs depend upon chemical changes (and such a theory is probable enough), if we consider that every change for the worse in this functioning is connected with an intoxication of nerve cells and muscle cells, then we are entitled to regard the neuroses as intoxications. But these are general and theoretical propositions, and they have no practical importance. In actual fact, intoxication does occur in the course of the neuroses, and it even occurs easily; but neurosis in its totality does not run the course of the intoxications with which we are familiar, and unfortunately the treatment of neuroses is far more complex than the treatment of intoxications.

Circulatory and Glandular Disturbances. The circulatory functions may be studied in the same manner, and this study will some day give even more interesting results. I am not thinking of grave cardiac lesions, for these, curiously enough, are rarely accompanied by neuropathic disorders. I am thinking of functional affections of the heart, of changes in the frequency and the force of its pulsations, and especially of modifications in the peripheral circulation, depending upon contraction or relaxation of the smaller bloodvessels. Changes in the frequency of the pulse are very common in neuropaths, and ought to be more carefully studied. I have noted a permanent reduction of the pulse frequency in five cases. In Noémi the pulse ranges between 50 and 65 ; and, in this patient, every fifth or tenth beat, or thereabouts, there is an intermittence, the heart beat failing to occur, or being so slight that it cannot make itself felt at the periphery. Increased frequency is even commoner. I exclude, here, genuine cases of Graves' disease, which have been put in a class apart (perhaps erroneously) ; but I will refer to twenty-two cases which can be grouped under the name of spurious Graves' disease, without goitre and without exophthalmos. In these cases of mine, just as in those which have been so carefully studied by Alquier, the pulse ranged from 90 to 120 ; and the patients were subject to flushes of heat, to sweats, and to attacks of diarrhoea. Pepita comes in this category, for the pulse ranges constantly between 90 and 100 ; and Céline and Jsa. belong to the same group. The increased frequency of the pulse is especially marked when the patients are standing, this being what Pron had also observed in sufferers from gastric and intestinal dyspepsia.

The blood-pressure in neuropaths, as measured by Pachon's oscillometer, is extremely variable ; and in a great many patients it is abnormal, and inclined to oscillate. Some patients show excessive pressure ranging from 18 to 23, as in Pepita's case. But more often, I think, especially in young psychasthenics, the pressure is too low. In Irène, Vv., and Ej., it is difficult to detect the very slight movements of the needle ranging between 10 and 8. These patients, who are always chilly and whose hands and feet have a bluish tint, are prone to syncopal attacks. I cannot venture to assert that different neuropathic manifestations are associated with the

respective types. Identical abulic and other symptoms
occur in Pepita, in whom the blood-pressure is 23, and in
Irène, in whom it is difficult to record a blood-pressure of 8.
Perhaps there is some evidence that low pressure is commoner
in asthenic dements.

In a small number of well-defined instances, and especially
one remarkable case, I have recorded modifications of the
internal temperature, and state them here with all reserve.
Céline, a young woman thirty-four years of age, who has been
under my care for ten years, is suffering from asthenic
depression, with abulia, inertia, doubts, scruples, sexual
manias, and obsessions with love ; her mental condition is
simple and typical. When I examined her for the first time
(she was then twenty-three years of age) I noticed, not only
that her pulse ranged from 100 to 110, but that her temperature was constantly about two degrees above the normal.
Although her pulse suggested good health, and although there
were no appreciable stethoscopic signs of disease, I was led by
this to arouse the disquietude of her family by speaking rather
incautiously of my suspicion of tuberculosis. I have now to
admit, without attempting to explain the fact, that as far as
bodily health is concerned Céline's condition is exactly what
it was eleven years ago. She has made a certain amount of
progress as regards her mental condition, and physically she
seems perfectly well. She is well nourished, and is of a fair
average weight, or is perhaps a little heavy for her height.
She never coughs, and there have never been any suspicious
physical signs on auscultation. She does very little, but her
actions are reduced by her mental condition and not by her
physical health. At the outset the treatment was one of
almost complete rest, but for several years she has been going
about in a nearly normal fashion. Nevertheless, throughout
these years the temperature, taken in the vagina or rectum
when she was lying down, has ranged between 99·6° and
101·4°. The highest temperatures are recorded just before
menstruation, and for several days while menstruation is in
progress it rarely falls below 100° ; but as soon as menstruation is over it will sink to somewhere near 99·6° A very
short walk will send it up to 101·6°, but it falls rapidly after
a few minutes' rest. This abnormal temperature does not
seem to inconvenience the patient in any way ; whereas she

complains of fever if she has a slight attack of influenza, in consequence of which her temperature rises a very little above what seems to be normal to her. In a word, for eleven years this young woman, whose physical health seems in every respect satisfactory, has persistently had a pulse of 100 and a temperature about two degrees above the normal. Are we to suppose that these symptoms are due to a latent glandular tuberculosis ? Are we to class them with the temperature disturbances of spurious Graves' disease ? Earlier writers on hysteria used to speak of " hysterical fever " ; was this designation so absurd as we have been inclined to imagine ?

Disorders of the peripheral circulation taking the form of passive dilatation of the bloodvessels or of vasomotor spasm, are far more important, and are much commoner. A great many of these patients are continually becoming affected with redness or pallor of the skin of various regions, and when this occurs we can detect in the affected parts notable changes of peripheral temperature. Irène, whose case I have studied very closely in this respect, almost always has a rather low internal temperature, the thermometer registering from 97·2° to 98·0° in the vagina or the rectum ; and her hands and the other uncovered parts of the skin are always rather chilly to the touch. When she is indisposed at the outset of her serious attacks of depression, her internal temperature falls yet lower, so that upon one such occasion I found it as low as 95·8° ; and at these times she has great red patches on the face and the hands, which grow hot, this distressing her very much. During the period of depression she complains simultaneously of these hot patches and of other cold patches which appear on the knees, the buttocks, the chest, and the neck. Some of the cold patches are apt at times to become painful. She has a feeling as if great drops of water, sometimes very hot and sometimes icy cold, were falling upon her arms, and the patches where this sensation is felt become red, or pale. Occasionally, these same regions will appear bluish on the following day, and will exhibit actual ecchymoses. The appearance of such ecchymotic patches heralds a bad period, and Irène's relatives look forward (in a sense !) to her having a crisis of depression when she has a bluish patch on the left cheek.

Some time ago I published the remarkable case of a young

man who complained of a persistent sensation of cold on the outer side of one of the legs, and I showed that there was a remarkable relationship between this localised sensation of cold and the memory of an impression he had received when sleeping upon the frozen ground one night. This case is by no means exceptional. I showed twenty years ago that in a great many cases of extensive paralysis, even when the paralysis is incomplete, we can detect a remarkable difference of temperature between the two limbs, and we find that the paralysed side is definitely colder than the other.—We see this in Lydia, who, in almost all her attacks of depression, suffers from weakness of the right side. The chilliness is not due to the absence of movement, for she continues to move the right arm although it is weaker than the other. Besides, such local chilliness can be noticed in cases in which there is no paresis.—Kf. (f., 46) and Ej. (f., 41) have for several years been liable to crises of chilliness on the right side without any disturbance of movement.—Gt. (m., 30) often suffers from cold patches between the shoulders. When his nose grows white and when he has a red and burning patch on the nape of the neck, he rapidly passes into a condition of serious depression. It is then that he tells us that the sun is no longer the same, that everything has become grey, that everything is incomprehensible, as if he were in a dream. Pepita, in like manner, has icy patches on the front of the legs ; she has patches which at first are red and hot, and then pale and very cold, on the arms, the ears, and the cheeks. She notices, like Irène, that these patches, especially when on the arms, are apt to become blue on the following day, and that for a long time in these areas a marked bruise is left, although she has not had any blow. Since my attention was first drawn to these phenomena I have been able to record among neuropaths a dozen instances of the kind, for disturbances of the peripheral circulation are fairly common in such patients.

These disturbances of circulation may attack the deep-seated organs. Madame Z. and three other patients complain of very distressing crises of chilliness, and say that they cannot keep their eyes warm even by covering them up with cotton-wool. Two of the patients likewise exhibit phenomena of asthenopia, and I have several times had occasion to refer to the strange disorders of vision from which Madame Z.

suffers. But such symptoms are not general, for in the three other patients the chilliness in the eyes is not accompanied by any disturbance of visual perception. On the other hand, another patient, Emma, who suffers severely from asthenopia, is not affected by the chilly sensation in the eyes. Pepita suffers from terrible crises of cold or heat in the anus or in the vagina. She has also suffered from very severe crises of uterine congestion, although there was no infection properly so called. The attacks of congestion of the uterus were attended with very remarkable symptoms, analogous to those from which she now suffers in connexion with the stomach. The slightest movement of the body gave her the impression that some great displacement was going on in the pelvis, this being accompanied by a sense of vertigo and of projection of the body to one side or the other. Irène suffers from congestion or livid pallor of the pharynx and even of the vocal cords, this last having been verified by laryngoscopic examination. These disturbances brought on sudden attacks of aphonia, which disappeared just as suddenly when the circulation was reestablished. Similar disturbances of the circulation could be detected in all the organs accessible to observation.

In women, menstruation is interconnected with the regulation of the peripheral circulation and with the functioning of the incretory glands. It is important to note the disturbances of menstruation which almost invariably present themselves in the course of the neuroses. Very seldom does a woman suffering from serious depressive neurosis continue to menstruate in a perfectly normal fashion. Sometimes, menstruation will simply be painful, and will be attended by all kinds of spasms of the abdominal organs. Dysmenorrhoea, inducing fainting fits, vertigos, and other kinds of paroxysm, is often the first manifestation of the onset of a neurosis. At the same time, the periodicity of menstruation becomes irregular, menstruation occurring too frequently or too seldom. In the latter event, when menstruation recurs after an unduly long interval, there is apt to be a flooding. Irène had no definite catamenial periodicity, the flow sometimes recurring after six weeks and sometimes after three months, its reappearance being heralded for ten days or so by abdominal spasm, and then by marked abdominal ptosis, and at the same time by extremely painful swelling of the breasts, and by congestion of the throat and the lungs, often very severe. From the beginning of each menstruation the flow was excessive, and speedily became haemorrhagic. For ten days, the flooding continued, the patient passing great clots. The same sort of menstruation, irregular, delayed, preceded by congestions in the thorax, and extremely profuse, is common in these cases. It occurred with almost precisely the same characters in Pepita, in whom this severe menorrhagia was said to have preceded the onset of obesity. Six other patients presented similar symptoms.

In other patients, or sometimes in the same patients at other times, we observe phenomena of the opposite kind. Céline menstruates once a fortnight, the flow being very scanty, and lasting only one or two days. Not infrequently, this diminished flow will cease altogether for a considerable period. In Sophie we have a remarkable instance of the alternation of the two types of disturbance. Ordinarily, during the periods when she is simply abulic, scrupulous, and obsessed, she suffers from painful and haemorrhagic menstruation ; but when she passes into the phase of agitation with asthenic delirium, she stops menstruating altogether, and on one occasion the amenorrhoea lasted two years.

All these disturbances of circulation may be summarised in the phrase which was already used by Alquier. We note in such patients a complex of vasomotor troubles with cardio-vascular instability. It is sometimes possible to render these disturbances evident by certain methods of verification. The study of the vasomotor reaction after pressure upon the skin or upon the finger-nail, the study of the diffuse flushing which follows vigorous pressure upon a small area of the skin, and the detection of dermographism, serve to confirm the importance of this disturbance of the vasomotor equilibrium.

Finally, there is a little difficulty in detecting a relationship between these circulatory disturbances and the modifications of the mental condition. The crises of tachycardia from which Jg. (m., 30) suffered, were induced by the destruction of his factory during the war. We know, moreover, that the emotions attendant on the war led to a considerable increase in the number of cases of Graves' disease and spurious Graves' disease. Most of the other vasomotor troubles were originated or aggravated by emotions. In certain cases, as in that of Irène, there could be observed an extensive change in, the circulation during complete somnambulism and during periods of excitation. In most of the cases, menstruation was modified by one of these phenomena, which acted also upon the mental state ; and we have again and again had occasion to describe changes in the neurosis which were associated with menstrual periodicity.

These remarks naturally lead us to stress the importance of circulatory disturbances in the neuroses. Without transcending the limits of legitimate hypothesis, we are inclined to regard circulatory disturbances as causal factors in the case of a good many other neuropathic disorders. When patients like Uk. (m., 40), and like Adèle and Agathe, are continually complaining of " spots before the eyes," and saying " I always have the feeling that rain is falling before my eyes, or that hail is falling, or I see a jet of water falling continually, and this makes me feel so miserable," must we not suppose that there is a congestive disturbance of the membranes of the eye? When the patients complain, as they often do, that the nose and the throat are always dry, or when, on the other hand, they suffer from rhinorrhoea or from hay fever (which play a great part in Lox.'s crises), are we not entitled to suppose that there are disorders of the circulation in the nasal cavities and in the pharynx ? Finally, in many of these patients we note attacks of oedema, usually brief, but sometimes prolonged. Too much scepticism has been displayed as regards neuropathic oedema, for although it is difficult to explain, its occurrence cannot be denied. Qi. (f., 40), to take one instance among many, suffers from marked local oedema as the outcome of the slightest pressure on the skin, or without any obvious reason whatever. She cannot carry a light basket on her arm, or hold a flower in her hand, without having a great hard weal on the arm, or having her fingers swollen for several hours. Besides, every one knows that many of these patients exhibit the phenomena of dermographism, and the symptoms we are now considering belong to the same category. It is most probable that such oedema is the outcome of the same sort of peripheral circulatory disturbances as the other symptoms we have just been discussing.

If we push the hypothesis a little further, we shall not hesitate to suppose that attacks of migraine, a disease which plays a strange part in such disorders, are due to arterial spasm of the cerebral circulation. Such a theory is a very probable one. To all the familiar arguments in its favour, we may add another, namely that, in many of these cases, the attacks of migraine are intermingled with phenomena in which the influence of circulatory disturbances is manifest. At certain times, Lox. is subject to attacks which begin with rhinorrhoea, with watering of the eyes and congestion of the face—with obvious circulatory disturbances. Then, when the congestion of the nasal cavities passes off, and the nasal mucous membrane dries up, she becomes affected with asthma and circulatory disturbances of the bronchial tubes ; and frequently the asthma alternates with migraine.

Cannot we go further ? Certain crises of anxiety are accompanied by lividity of the face, by a feeling of shocks in the head, vertigo, terror, and a sense of faintness. " It seems to me that my vitality passes away, I lose the sentiment of my own personality, the effect is deadly, I feel as if I were about to die." Are we not concerned here with spasm of the cerebral vessels and perhaps with spasm of the vessels of the medulla oblongata ? Such patients as Lydia cut short the anxiety by drinking champagne, which has a congestive influence. I have several times noted a remarkable fact in Irène and Lydia, namely that we can check severe crises of anxiety by making the patient inhale nitrate of amyl, which gives rise to extreme vascular dilatation in many of the organs. May we not suppose that in the digestive disorders previously described, phenomena of the same kind play their part. We can see the intense congestion of the pharynx. Is it not probable that there is the same congestion in the oesophagus, the stomach, and the intestine, when disorder of these organs is prominent ? Various authors have agreed that muco-membranous enteritis is due to disturbances of circulation. When Ac. (f., 25) suffers from severe serous diarrhoea because some one has come suddenly into her room, may we not say that under stress of the emotion the mucous membrane of her bowel has blushed ? The explanation of the neuroses by circulatory disturbances may be applied just as widely as the explanation by autointoxication.

It is natural therefore, that these observations should have given rise to a second group of physiological theories of the neuroses. Savill, in especial, in his book *Clinical Lectures on Neurasthenia* (1906), pointed out that marked modifications of function can appear, without any modification of the structure of the organ, when the flow of blood through the vessels of the organ is insufficient ; and he remarked that the quantity of the flow is regulated by the vasomotor nerves. In nervous attacks, he said, it is probable that there is anaemia of the brain simultaneously with congestion of the splanchnic area. Most of the neuroses, he contended, depend upon circulatory disturbances of this kind, and can therefore be reasonably termed vasomotor neuroses or angioneuroses.

The various observations relating to dysmenorrhoea, menorrhagia, or amenorrhoea, preceded or followed by general disturbances, lead us to-day to think, not only of a disorder of the peripheral circulation, but also of disturbances of the internal secretion of certain glands. It is possible that variations in the incretion of the ovaries, variations which are connected with menstrual periodicity, may have an independent effect in the periodic disorders we have been considering. Disturbances of menstruation, paraesthesias, and flushes of heat, such as are noted in these patients, are probably due to disturbances of the ovarian incretion. The continual sense of fatigue which so many of the patients describe, their weakness, and the instability of the arterial blood-pressure, lead us to suspect disturbances of the adrenal incretion.

The most complete demonstration of such phenomena has been made in the case of disturbances of the thyroid incretion, these being the best known phenomena of the kind. Patients who digest badly, who suffer from constipation, muco-membranous enteritis, obesity, great liability to autointoxication, recurrent attacks of sore throat, enfeebled circulation, chilliness, transient attacks of localised oedema, painful menstruation, delayed menstruation, menorrhagia, etc., seem to present the picture of hypothyroidism which has been so carefully studied by Léopold Lévy and de Rothschild. We could even detect, in these patients, other symptoms of hypothroidism : such as migraine, the importance of which has already been signalised ; dryness and fragility of the hair ; and even, in some, the eyebrow sign. Other patients, who suffer from local congestions, diarrhoea, loss of flesh, persistent frequency of the pulse, rise of temperature, sweats, and inadequacy of menstruation, remind us of sufferers from Graves' disease and hyperthyroidism. Finally, a good many patients, whose symptoms exhibit remarkable alternations, are obviously suffering from what may be called a loss of thyroid equilibrium.

The remarkable modifications that take place in the neuroses during pregnancy can be interpreted in like manner. To explain these modifications, people have sometimes spoken of changes in the position and equilibrium of the abdominal viscera. Gastroptosis, and enteroptosis of the transverse colon, have been supposed to be temporarily cured by the enlargement of the uterus which plays the part of an internal pad. This remark may apply to certain cases, but I have to point out that none of the patients in whom I myself noticed pregnancy to have such an influence of the neurosis, had suffered from visceroptosis before pregnancy. We know, moreover, that during pregnancy there occur important changes in the internal secretions, and especially in the incretion of the thyroid ; such changes are manifested by numerous signs, and it is probable that this temporary increase in thyroid activity modifies the course of the disease for a time.

In some patients we can be fairly confident that there is a primary change in the endocrine glands. Lema (f., 37), an abulic with a phobia of fatigue, etc., and the typical aspect of hypothyroidism, appears to have been normal up to the age of sixteen. Then she had a bad attack of mumps, and after this illness she was affected by severe inflammation of the throat and neck. Immediately afterwards, menstruation became haemorrhagic, and the neurosis ensued. Is it not possible that the attack of mumps was the starting-point of ovarian disturbances, and of disorder of the thyroid incretion ? A great many patients have suffered for years from chronic pharyngitis with loss of the sense of smell ; the inflammation has passed down into the trachea and there have been frequent attacks of laryngitis. It is perfectly plain in Irène's case that chronic pharyngitis has induced definite changes of the mucous membranes and has caused atrophy of the tonsils. Is it not likely that these changes have also affected the pharynx and the thyroid, and that in youth they gave rise to lesions which were the cause of the obvious condition of hypothyroidism ?

Inasmuch as the neuroses appear to be disturbances in the development of the individual, it is natural to connect them with changes in these organs whose function it is to regulate the development of the organism. Léopold Lévy and de Rothschild, who have made a special study of the thyroid, regard neuro-arthritism as dependent upon a disorder of the thyroid balance. They consider that the inheritance of the arthritic diathesis is an inheritance of thyroid peculiarities. " The thyroid can be compared to a source of energy capable of setting the nervous system to work, but incompetent to endow this motor with its peculiar qualities." Inasmuch as neurosis is not a defect in the motor itself, but a reduction of the tension of the activity of the motor, a sort of hypo-function, it would seem, in the view of these authors, to consist mainly in an inadequacy of the thyroid.

I regard such circulatory and glandular theories of the neuroses as very important, and it is possible that the physiological explanation of the neuroses will gradually have to turn in this direction. Unfortunately, at the present time, these theories are still too general and too vague for any practical conclusions to be drawn from them. To speak simply of congestion or anaemia of the brain, or even of certain parts of the brain, does not help in any way to explain abulias, obsessions or delusions, and gives us hardly any indications as to treatment. On the other hand, before pushing such conceptions of the neuroses any further, we should have to ascertain more precisely what is the correspondence between these physiological troubles and the changes in behaviour.

Can we assert that all the individuals who suffer from circulatory disorders, or that all those that are affected with disturbances of the thyroid incretion, are neuropaths ? I cannot say that I myself have sufficient materials for a conclusion. I can merely recall the case of a woman of thirty, who, from childhood onwards, had presented typical symptoms of myxoedema, and who had been transformed by thyroid treatment. She needed continual dosing with thyroid extract, and when this substance was withheld for a time she exhibited symptoms of hypothyroidism ; nevertheless at such times she had no neuropathic symptoms. We must devote a good deal more work to the study of the changes in the incretions of the ductless glands before we shall arrive at clear notions concerning the influence they can exercise as accessory pathogenic factors of neuroses.

All that we can say at present is that the neuroses and the psychoses represent a reduction in the activity of the evolution of the living being ; that this reduction simultaneously affects the nervous and muscular functions, and thus influences the behaviour and the digestive, circulatory, and trophic functions which regulate the activity of the viscera. All these functions are disturbed in the same way, the disturbance taking the form of disappearance of the higher portion of the function and exhaustion of the lower portion. We see arrest, agitation, and derivation of function, and cannot always be clear as to the meaning of the details. In some cases modifications of behaviour, and in other cases visceral disturbances, seem to predominate ; but we cannot invariably ascertain the relationships between these two kinds of disturbance. Both categories alike depend upon a deep-seated disorder of vital evolution, a disorder of which we know very little.

One of the before-mentioned cases enables us to summarise, as it were, this discussion. Ie., up to the age of twenty-five, was in good physical health, and her mental state was normal. After some family quarrels and a decline in the family fortunes, she left home, went to live with a lover, became pregnant, and gave birth to a child clandestinely. Then, after various distressing adventures, she took up with a new lover, who himself was an invalid, abulic, unstable, suffering from obsessions. She gradually became changed in two ways. She grew unhappy, sluggish, incapable of action, uneasy and jealous ; she talked too much about herself, was always looking out for compliments, became authoritarian and violent, and was continually making scenes ; she complained that she was not loved enough, and was not flattered enough. " What I need is that some one should be perpetually helping me and affectionately tending me ; but here I have to wear the breeches, and that irritates me." We are familiar with this evolution, which led her to obsessions of self-depreciation and jealousy. At the same time, she suffered from increasingly frequent attacks of migraine ; she was constantly complaining of her stomach, of heartburn, acid eructation, and the like, symptoms which were only relieved by taking large quantities of food ; she suffered from obstinate constipation which brought on piles, and from time to time she had motions which were highly charged with mucus and the passing of which was extremely painful ; she grew very fat, so that although she was quite short she weighed more than thirteen stone ; menstruation was irregular, delayed, and profuse ; she complained of a perpetual feeling of cold, and was affected with the circulatory troubles which have already been described. Are we to suppose that her unhappiness, her sense of boredom, gave rise to the digestive troubles and affected her circulation and her thyroid incretion in this serious and persistent way ? Are we to suppose that when she was about twenty-seven years old she accidentally began to suffer from a disease of the thyroid which modified her circulation and her nutrition ? To me it seems a better way of explaining what happened to say that this young woman, whose vital activity was already of low grade, when she found herself in a false, difficult, and exhausting situation had not sufficient energy to adapt herself to it properly, and that therefore her whole vital evolution was disturbed. The exhaustion acted at one and the same time upon the visceral and glandular functions and upon the mental life. Although my explanation is vaguer than the physiological explanation, at any rate it does not attempt to mask our ignorance, and it leaves the field open for various attempts at treatment.

2. INDIRECT METHODS OF TREATING NEUROSES.

Many doctors insist, not only on the need for a complete examination of the neuropath, but also on the need for a complete treatment of all the organic affections from which he may suffer, being convinced that the proper treatment of these latter will lead to the disappearance of the neuroses.

The advice is sound. There is no doubt that we shall do well, whenever we can, to cure all the morbid affections, trifling or serious, from which our patients suffer in addition to their mental depression. We have just as much reason for curing an attack of blenorrhagia in a neurotic as we have for getting a decayed tooth stopped. In this way we shall restore the patient's general health, and that will be a good thing to do, even if the patient remains insane. Furthermore, it is a logical supposition that better general health, the reestablishment of bodily energy, will assist the patient to restore psychological tension. Unfortunately, however, in these questions, simple logic does not take us all the way. Our conclusions as to the value of a method of treatment must be based upon the statistics of cases, and it is often very difficult to draw up accurate statistics.

No doubt, like the writers I have mentioned, I have had a few successful cases. In some instances, a dozen perhaps, the treatment of diseases of the nose or throat, the treatment of metritis, or of persistent blenorrhagia, seemed to be one of the causes of improvement in patients suffering from hypochondria, algias, crises of psycholepsy. I have thought it best, in these cases, to have the local treatment carried out by the doctor, and not to allow the patient to go on treating himself, as he has been accustomed to do. When the patient has no longer to carry out these troublesome measures, when he has faith in a speedy cure, and when the local conditions improve, rest is facilitated, continued expenditure is lessened, and a rise in mental tension is possible.

Where syphilis is concerned, diagnosis is a delicate matter. Some very serious mental disorders, such as syphilitic dementia and the varieties of general paralysis of the insane, are directly due to syphilis. In such cases, the direct treatment of the syphilis is obviously essential. Happily we are often able to record improvement under antisyphilitic treatment in cases of mental disorder connected with specific arteritis, and in mental disturbances such as are sometimes connected with paralytic troubles. I have to admit that I have not myself been successful in the treatment of general paralysis, whatever the method employed. I regard the hopes expressed by certain authors as unduly sanguine. But there is no doubt that we must continue attempts in this direction, and that the treatment of the causative syphilitic affection is of primary importance. But apart from these strictly specific affections, there are various ways in which syphilis is linked with different neuropsychoses. In such cases, too, antisyphilitic treatment has sometimes had good results. In six of my own cases, psychasthenic patients suffering from obsessions were benefited in this way. It is true that three of these patients were suffering from obsessions bearing upon general paralysis and locomotor ataxia, and that treatment by salvarsan had a reassuring effect upon their minds, exerting a great moral influence as well as a physical one. Still, it is likely that in these three cases, and in the three others, the restoration of general health had a good deal to do with the mental improvement.

However this may be, we must not be too ready to generalise from a few successful cases. As a rule, the treatment, nay, the complete cure, of intercurrent or superadded disorders, seems to have a minimal influence upon the neuroses. The treatment of affections of the throat, the skin, the genital organs, the teeth, even when it cures local lesions, does not transform the mental state to any notable degree. Plenty of instances might be given in support of this assertion. As regards syphilis, the following case is of interest.   Ha. (m., 35), abulic, timid, phobic since youth, contracted syphilis at the age of twenty-six and had a certain number of secondary symptoms. An intensive antisyphilitic treatment caused rapid improvement as far as the bodily disorder was concerned. But neither the onset of the syphilis, nor its treatment, nor its cure, had any effect upon the mental condition.—A great many other patients suffering from severe mental depression mentioned that they had had syphilis and were therefore subjected to antisyphilitic treatment. I could not satisfy myself that the depression was modified in any way by the treatment. It ran its ordinary course.—In four very definite cases, the patients, who had formerly suffered from syphilis, were simultaneously affected with psychasthenic disorders and with well-marked syphilitic symptoms. Gf. (f., 36), in especial, suffered simultaneously from a crisis of psychasthenic depression with a phobia of contact, and from incomplete hemiplegia due to syphilitic arteritis. In all four cases antisyphilitic treatment was perfectly successful as far as the relief of the syphilitic symptoms was concerned, but it had no effect upon the neuropathic disorder.—In another case, that of Pk. (m., 28), a constitutional neuropath, malaria existed as a complication. He suffered from hysterical crises with somnambulism and fugues, and at the same time from intermittent fever with anaemia and symptoms of hepatic disorder. The treatment of the malaria relieved him of his bodily symptoms, whilst the nervous symptoms persisted. Subsequently the nervous troubles were greatly relieved by hypnotism and suggestion, which had a much better effect than quinine.

Many of these patients themselves recognised that the various methods of treatment which improved their general health did not relieve their mental disorders; and they even declared that their obsessions and phobias were more troublesome when their general health was better. " You can hardly imagine," says Rk. (m., 40), " how terrible my dread of matches becomes when I am well; I suffer less when I am weakly and out of sorts." Douches and cold baths, while strengthening to many patients, may render their obsessions more distressing, and such patients will soon come to dread fortifying treatment. These observations make me less inclined than the writers I have mentioned to trust in the efficacy of treatment of the general health. Certainly we must always attend carefully to the general health, but we must not be under any illusions as to the efficacy of such an obvious method of treatment.

I am inclined to attach more importance to treatment of digestive, circulatory, and glandular disorders, for these are far more closely connected with the neuroses. They are, I think, symptoms, expressions, of the vital depression in the same way that the disorders of behaviour are symptoms of the vital depression. The treatment of such disorders, therefore, will certainly reduce the complications of the neuroses, and will sometimes alleviate the neurotic disorder itself.

The first thing we have to do when our patient suffers from indigestion and from obsessive ideas concerning diet, is to regulate the diet. It is almost always a mistake to leave the decision as to diet entirely in the hands of the patient, when the latter's tastes, appetite, and ideas concerning health are completely disordered. I shall not here reconsider the various psychological methods of treatment, such as suggestion, the dissociation of fixed ideas, rest, isolation, and excitation. One or other of these will modify the patient's ideas, increase his energies, raise his tension, and facilitate the act of food-taking. Enough, now, to speak of food-taking itself, and all the means whereby it can be facilitated when it is still difficult. I have dwelt at considerable length upon the varying degrees of complication and difficulty of actions, and upon the need for simplifying actions, when they have to be performed by persons whose tension is lowered. The act of food-taking is one of those to which an especially large number of complications have been superadded by civilisation ; one of those actions which were very simple primitively, but have now become extremely difficult and artificial. Eating has become a social function, attended by excessively complicated rites ; but this higher-grade behaviour is not an essential part of food-taking, and is not indispensable to the absorption of nutriment. We must know how to dissociate from the act of food-taking the elements that have been superadded, and that are not really essential. No doubt, if our aim is to raise the tension of a timid psychasthenic and to apply the method of excitation by social activity, we shall prescribe for him the practice of social feeding with all the refinements of polite behaviour ; but we must remember that when we do this we are demanding from our patient an act of high tension, and must only prescribe the practice in full awareness of what we are doing. Where we are concerned primarily with the feeding of one in whom for various reasons the act of food-taking has become difficult, we can discard these refinements, which are a needless exaggeration of the difficulty of the action In one of my cases, a young woman of twenty-five was taking less and less food, and was finding more and more difficulty about the matter. She declared that eating made her nose red and generated gas in her intestine. Since the other members of her family insisted upon her taking her meals in company, her mind became completely disordered. She said she would rather throw herself out of the window than be exposed to the danger of breaking wind in company. She therefore starved herself. The relatives often do a great deal of harm to young women suffering from anorexia owing to their absolute disregard of these psychological ideas anent food-taking.

Instead of trying to cure, as is too often done, by refinements of cookery and table furniture, we must enormously simplify these patients' meals. As soon as the illness becomes rather serious, we must, to begin with, suppress all social complications, and especially, must forbid the presence of other members of the family. We must make these invalids take their meals alone, of course under the supervision of a nurse, who should always be the same nurse, and who must not eat her meals with the patient. Most of these patients masticate badly, swallowing their food too soon, or keeping it for an indefinite time in the mouth. Many of them suck in air, and swallow it with every mouthful of drink; others swallow incompletely, keeping the food for a long time in an oesophageal pouch. We have to effect a thorough reeducation of mastication and deglutition. Almost always, the feeding of these persons, whose food-taking function is affected by their abulia, is an extremely slow process. They must be given a sufficiency of time, even while they are guided, stimulated, and assisted with discretion and skill. Some nurses become remarkably competent in making such patients take their food. In many cases simple measures of this sort enable us to make anorexics take sufficient food, and will even enable us to avoid the use of forced feeding in patients suffering from sitiophobia. Still, we must be ready to have recourse to forced feeding when the nutrition is manifestly too slow and is inadequate. In many cases, moreover, it will suffice to pass the oesophageal tube a few times, and then we shall be able to return to the before-mentioned methods. Whatever method we employ, we shall often find that two months' good feeding will do more than any other therapeutic method to reestablish the psychological tension in these patients.

It was the observation of this fact which inspired the idea of treating neuropaths by hyperalimentation. Weir Mitchell, and more recently Seguin, of New York, added this method of treatment to treatment by rest.[1] In the sanatoria where this method is practised, the patient has to undergo not only a " rest cure," but also a " fat cure." We cannot but be surprised when we read the diet table of the patients in some of these celebrated establishments. For my part, I regard the fat cure as an exaggerated method. We must not pay too much attention to the loss of flesh in some of these patients

[1] Lectures on some Points in the Treatment and Management of the Neuroses, 1890.

unless we have to do with deliberate refusal of food ; we need not interfere if a reasonable quantity of food is being taken. The loss of flesh, when persistent, is dependent upon intoxication, upon depression of nutrition ; it can easily be overcome by the ordinary ways of treating depression, and need not be treated by hyperalimentation. The attempt to fatten the patient rapidly at all hazards, at a time when he is digesting badly and assimilating with difficulty, is to my mind futile, and in many of these cases is positively dangerous.

Often enough, hyperalimentation, or food-taking under bad conditions, is the cause of autointoxication. A few years ago, various writers, and in especial Pascault, of Cannes, and Guelpa, carried on a vigorous campaign against hyperalimentation, contending that it gave rise to arthritism. Vigouroux, in his book on the dieting of neurasthenics, maintains the same thesis. He writes : " The best way of treating these patients is by a restricted diet." [1] Laumonier, in his essay *Traitement de la paresse* (1913) regarding idleness as a minor degree of chronic depression, considers that it is essential to prescribe in these cases a diet which is less abundant and better chosen. We must suppress soup, meat, alcohol, tea, and condiments ; the meals can be numerous, but must be very small, consisting mainly of farinaceous food, eggs, cheese, milk food, dry biscuits. " This diet will not give rise to glandular hypersecretion or to hyperacidity ; it will not exhaust the digestive organs, and will only demand from them the minimum of work ; it is not toxic, being almost purin-free. Nevertheless it contains sufficient roughage to prevent constipation."

Many of my own cases confirm these observations. A great many psychasthenics, hypochondriacs, phobics, algics, and even epileptics, manifestly improve when their diet is considerably restricted. To take only one example among hundreds, this is particularly conspicuous in Lema. A woman of forty, suffering from frequent attacks of migraine, always complaining, immobilised for twenty years by the phobia of fatigue, she was continually suffering from disturbances of the stomach and intestine due to over-feeding. A marked reduction of the quantity of food for several months gave her more energy, and, strange to say, led to an increase in weight. All

[1] Vigouroux, Neurasthénie, etc., régime alimentaire, 1893, p. 44.

the more, then, this reduction of diet is essential when there are physical and mental signs of grave autointoxication. A restricted diet, and sometimes a very liquid diet for a time, are indispensable elements of treatment by disintoxication. This treatment was strictly applied for more than a year to some of my patients, as to Pepita and to Ie. (f., 35). I have already pointed out how difficult it is in such cases to reduce the fat. These women could stay for weeks and even for months on a starvation diet without any appreciable loss of weight. Much pains and a great deal of perseverance were requisite to achieve disintoxication and to induce loss of weight. But even in cases of this kind, the treatment required is as a rule more complicated. A mere reduction of diet can be but one élement of it, though perhaps the most important element.

Should we, in these patients, pay special attention to the nature of the food, and prescribe some particular diet ? Generally speaking, in my opinion, the nature of the food is in such cases less important than the quantity. It is the quantity, above all, which must be watched and reduced. Still, we may point out that, except in special cases, when the patient's age, the condition of his energies, or the nature of his disease, definitely demands this or that diet, we shall find it advantageous to prescribe a modified vegetarian diet. Lagrange was one of the first to recommend a vegetarian diet in the treatment of fatigue. The cutting off of alcohol, the reduction of the amount of meat and other albuminous food, and sometimes the prohibition of common salt or of bread, seem to have a good effect. Milk foods, farinaceous foods, vegetable foods, and fruits, are certainly good for most of these patients, for they tend to reduce intoxication. In some cases I have been able to note a great improvement in the bodily and the mental condition after several months of a strictly vegetarian diet. The most remarkable instance of this was that of Fe. (f., 32), a neuropath suffering from over-scrupulousness and hypochondria, who had been feeding to a gross and ridiculous excess for several years. She had a preference for the most indigestible forms of food, and was rather inclined to exceed in the matter of alcohol. Her mental state was far from undergoing improvement upon this liberal regimen. She suffered from crises of psycholepsy, with anxiety, and a sentiment of depersonalisation ; also from hysterical paroxysms, obsessions of jealousy and of persecution. In addition she had various kinds of gastro-intestinal disorders. Her skin was cold, dry, and pulverulent, and in the end became covered with urticaria. This eruption of urticaria, which lasted for more than a year, was very remarkable. The slightest friction of any part of the skin, or simply exposure of the skin to the air, would lead within a few seconds to the appearance of enormous urticarial weals, the eruption being accompanied by intense itching. It was the distress caused by the skin eruption which finally induced the patient to accept a strict regulation of the diet. A vegetarian regimen and a great restriction in the quantity of food, led to the disappearance of the urticaria after a month, and in three months helped to transform the physical and mental state.

In certain cases, which it is not easy to explain, but which remind us of the phenomena of anaphylaxis described by Charles Richet, there is a marked idiosyncrasy as regards particular foods. Many patients, like Irène, bear milk very badly, even in small quantities. Very soon after they have taken any milk they suffer from severe serous diarrhoea. I have already mentioned how Pepita became affected with marked intoxication when she took milk, eggs, or meat soups, in any form. There are, then, cases in which these articles, once their ill effect has been definitely recognised, must be carefully excluded from the patient's diet. Very remarkable in this respect was the case of Ef. (f., 10), who for several years had been suffering from epileptic seizures and hysterical paroxysms. She was agitated, unstable, and intolerable. After having fruitlessly tried various regimens, a perusal of Loeper's article upon intoxication in children led me to withdraw milk and eggs altogether from this child's diet. The change thus brought about was amazing, and during the ensuing years not only was there a marked improvement in character, but the child remained entirely free from convulsive seizures.

In few cases, however, is it necessary to be so strict. Most of the patients can take milk food with advantage ; and eggs and meat in moderate quantities at one meal every day are well tolerated. Detailed indications concerning the way to diet these patients, both as regards the restriction of food and as regards the composition of actual meals will be found in the writings of de Fleury and Deschamps, and in the bills of fare published by Leon Derecq and G. Gallois in the " Journal de Diététique."

Guidance in the arrangement of these regimens is furnished by the analysis of the faeces, which has to-day become an important and instructive matter. Such analyses ought always to be made in cases of muco-membranous enteritis, and in cases of persistent autointoxication. Not only do they disclose the abnormal elements of the intestinal excretions ; but they also inform us as to the final state of digestion of the principal articles of food, of connective tissue, muscular fibres, cellulose, starch, fat, acids, soaps. According to the indications thus furnished, we can easily regulate the patient's diet by withdrawing for the time being articles which are imperfectly digested and by substituting others. These precautions enable us to check the crises of enteritis and help us to await the day when the reestablishment of energy and the reestablishment of normal circulation will have cured the tendency to enteritis.

Of course all these disorders of the stomach and the intestine may require at the same time drug treatment. This is not always very effective when we have to do with neuropaths, and it must invariably be subordinated to the general treatment of the neuroses and to dietetic treatment ; but it has its uses. Certain gastric stimulants, certain adjuvants to the gastric secretion, bitters, phosphoric acid, ipecac, pepsin, papain, etc., will do at least temporary service. A reduction of the amount of fluid taken at meals, lying down after meals, an abdominal belt, Glénard's belt, etc., may do a great deal of good to patients suffering from visceroptosis. A good deal of epigastric pain, marked nervous reactions, will be suppressed by this simple method of treatment. I also lay stress upon giving large doses of bismuth, and upon giving alkalies, which are especially useful in neuropaths, for they have a calmative influence upon the pains and upon the reflexes due to the gastric hypersthenia, the importance of which in these patients we have already recognised. Not only gastric acidity, but also pains in the chest and the back, tics, hiccough, vertigo, and even crises of sleep, can be suppressed by simple dosage with bicarbonate of soda or carbonate of calcium. Here, too, we must guard against the exaggeration characteristic of neuropaths, who readily acquire a craze for any medicine which relieves their troubles. I have often noted the onset of a true alkalinomania, which is itself dangerous. To-day there is a tendency towards surgical intervention in many cases of chronic disorder of the stomach, and in the various forms of visceroptosis.[1] We must not be too ready to take this course when we are concerned with neuropaths, in whom it is often difficult to appreciate the true gravity of the symptoms. I think, however, that in certain cases we must not hesitate to adopt surgical measures. Rereading the notes of one of my early cases, that of Marceline, I regret that I did not have her operated upon early for a chronic ulcer of the stomach.[2]

Certain medicinal measures do good service in cases of nervous enteritis. Useful are : laxatives, intestinal lavage (though this method must not be abused), and, more especially, lavage with oil, which gives a great deal of relief ; calmatives, opium, and, above all, belladonna, in spasmodic affections ; stimulants of the biliary secretions, various biliary extracts, amylo-diastase, etc. Of great importance is purgative medication, in patients suffering from severe intoxication. Although I do not go so far as Guelpa, who purges his patients freely for several days in succession, while at the same time giving them a very full diet, I have often prescribed repeated purgation in patients suffering from mental confusion and from various forms of intoxication, and also in obese patients. I think the results have always been favourable. In at least a dozen of my patients suffering from mental confusion, purgation has given unmistakable relief ; and the same method has also been useful in cases of obesity and of intoxication. Many of these patients, like Pepita, never feel so well as when they have been sharply purged. This is an important indication which must not be overlooked in the treatment of neuropaths.

The treatment of circulatory disturbances may seem to be even more important. Unfortunately, we still know too little about this matter, and I can merely summarise the results of certain attempts which seem to me to have been of interest.

[1] Cf. V. Pauchet, Gastroptose, traitement, " Presse Médicale," April 11, 1918.
[2] Une Félida artificielle, L'état mental des hystériques, second edition, 1911, p. 567.

Cardiac stimulants and cardiac tonics, when the circulation is sluggish, are of more help than is usually imagined. Small doses of strophanthus or digitalis often have an excellent effect. On the other hand, I have frequently had occasion to prescribe drugs which regulate cardiac pulsation and the arterial circulation ; and I am glad to be able to confirm the statement of various authors that the effects of quinine are sometimes remarkably good. The case of Jg. is typical. A young man of thirty, abulic and timid, he had for two years after the bombardment of his factory been affected by a persistent emotional condition, with hypochondriacal obsessions, continual tremor, extreme tachycardia (the pulse-rate ranged from 110 to 130), digestive disturbance, and marked enteritis, aggravated by the practice of aerophagia. In a word, this patient presented, in addition to the psychasthenic mental condition, the physical condition of a person suffering from spurious Graves' disease, without goitre and without exophthalmus. Treatment by rest and excitation played their part here, but the quinine was the most important factor in bringing about his rapid restoration to health. It is very remarkable how long such patients can continue to take this drug. Jg. began by taking large doses ranging from 25 to 30 grains daily for a month ; 15 grains a day were taken for a whole year ; and it was only during the last months of the treatment that the dose was reduced to 10 grains daily and then to 7 grains daily. After the quinine had been given for a few days, the pulse-frequency rapidly diminished, and after the first month the pulse-rate was normal, but the tachycardia speedily reappeared if dosage with quinine was intermitted. The mental state was transformed just like the physical condition. It was amazing to see how the patient could play his part in family councils concerning his affairs, and how he was able to preside over the work of rebuilding his factory. Only a little while before, he had been unable to see any one coming into his room without having severe and dangerous attacks of palpitation.—Quinine also had a most useful effect in two other patients of the same kind, though here the influence of the remedy was perhaps less striking. In certain other patients with similar symptoms calcium salts and especially chloride of calcium gave very satisfactory results in my experience. Calcium chloride is a most valuable drug in neuropathic disorders, for it regularises the circulation and reduces agitation. Medicines which relieve passive congestion, such medicines as hamamelis virginica and hydrastis canadensis, are no less useful. In four of my patients they had a well-marked effect. Recently, injections of emetin have been recommended. I think they have had a remarkable influence for good, not only in cases of amoebic dysentery, but also, in two of my patients, in nervous enteritis due to congestion.

Many neuropaths are affected with hypertension, with or without the early signs of arteriosclerosis. In these cases, we must apply the ordinary treatment ; but nitrite of amyl, trinitrine as recommended by Huchard,[1] thiosinamin, and tincture of crataegus oxyacantha as advised by L. Rénon, have an especially favourable effect. Rémond, of Metz, and Voivenel,[2] point out that anxiety and kindred troubles may be connected with cerebral ischaemia due to a constriction of the bloodvessels of the cortex, and they suggest attempts to modify the circulation in this part of the brain by the use of trinitrine. I have already mentioned making the same attempt on my own initiative, by giving the patients inhalations of nitrite of amyl. I have also tried Rémond's prescription, giving several drops of the solution of trinitrine. I think the results were satisfactory, although the anxiety was not so quickly relieved as by the inhalation of nitrite of amyl. The advantage of using the trinitrine solution is that it can be more readily administered for a considerable time.

Conversely, and here we come to a commoner phenomenon, a good many psychasthenics have a very low tension. Martinet, who has rightly laid stress upon the frequency of this syndrome, has found treatment by adrenalin useful, in conjunction with pituitary extract and strychnine.

Opotherapy is assuming more and more importance in the treatment of neuropaths, thanks to the growing knowledge of the importance of the ductless glands, and thanks to the increasing application of the theories of endocrinology. A good many facts seem to me to indicate that in neuropathic women there is a disturbance of the ovarian incretion, and I have therefore, in ten of these patients, tried the effect of treatment with ovarian extract. I must admit that the

[1] Henri Huchard, Maladies du coeur, 1911.
[2] " Progrès Médical," June 1, 1907.

results have not been very definite. Perhaps the treatment did contribute to the restoration of menstruation in two patients after a prolonged period of amenorrhoea, but I could not be sure of the causal sequence. The use of adrenalin seems to me to have had more definite results, and it was certainly useful in a dozen cases where the patients were asthenic and had too low an arterial pressure. In three of the cases the treatment with adrenalin had to be continued for months, for serious troubles arose as soon as the drug was discontinued. A few drops of adrenalin solution were useful in several other cases. In Adèle and Agathe the bluish tint of the hands and the feet rapidly disappeared under this treatment, to reappear promptly when the administration was discontinued. I could not observe that there was any modification of the mental condition in these patients.

The opotherapeutic medicine which I have hitherto found of most value in the treatment of neuroses is thyroid extract. I have tried this substance on thirty-five patients who seemed to me to be suffering from hypothyroidism, and I will now give a summary of the results. Some of the patients, only five, were unable to tolerate the extract ; they speedily became affected with palpitation of the heart and with flushes of heat, so that the administration had to be discontinued. I must mention that in the early days of this investigation I was using doses that were too large, $1\frac{1}{2}$ to $\frac{3}{4}$ grain, whereas I subsequently found that much smaller doses, $\frac{1}{3}$ grain, were sufficient to produce notable effects without danger. Still, some patients cannot tolerate even these small doses. Léopold Lévy and de Rothschild, who have paid special attention to disorder of the thyroid equilibrium, treated both hyperthyroidism and hypothyroidism in the same way. " Small doses of thyroid extract," they write, " regularise the secretion even in those in whom there is over-action of the thyroid." I am sorry to say that I have not been able to confirm this statement. Those of my patients who were suffering from cardiac agitation, flushes of heat, tremor, etc.—in a word, from symptoms of hyperthyroidism—got worse when thyroid extract was given, even in very small doses ranging from $\frac{1}{8}$ to $\frac{1}{3}$ grain, so that the drug had to be discontinued. Pepita, for instance, who was very fat and was suffering from intoxication, but whose pulse was apt to race, could not tolerate dosage with thyroid extract.   Patients of another group, seven in number, had no intolerance to thyroid extract when given in small doses, but the drug did not appear to me to do any good.   Intolerance in certain patients, and lack of success in other cases, must not discourage us ; but we must take the facts into account, and not be too ready to accept a glandular theory of the neuroses.

In the other patients, eighteen in number, there was considerable improvement, sometimes very remarkable improvement, under the administration of thyroid extract.   In all the cases, the circulation became regular and more active ; the chilliness disappeared ;   the attacks of migraine became less frequent and less severe, and sometimes ceased entirely ; the intestinal disturbances were less troublesome ;   menstruation became more regular.   In obese patients suffering from intoxication, thyroid extract is a valuable supplement to treatment by disintoxication and by reducing flesh.—Fe, a young woman of thirty-two, intoxicated by hyperalimentation and by alcohol, and suffering from universal urticaria, to whom small doses of thyroid extract ($\frac{1}{3}$ grain) were administered during the three months she was under treatment, improved greatly. Obviously the thyroid medication was not the only cause of the improvement, for purgatives and regulation of the diet were more important factors.—In Ie. (f., 35), however, who was also obese and was suffering from intoxication, I think that the administration of thyroid extract was the most important factor in the improvement, for all her symptoms and especially her migraine, grew worse directly the drug was discontinued.—Lema (f., 37) not only derived great advantage from the taking of thyroid extract, but she was unable to get along without this medicine.   For three years, now, she has been taking a daily dose ranging from $\frac{3}{4}$ to $1\frac{1}{2}$ grain without interruption.   Not only has she never manifested any signs of hyperthyroidism, but a great many of her symptoms have been considerably relieved.   Migraine, menorrhagia, and intestinal disorders have vanished.   The moral treatment of her phobia of fatigue has been greatly facilitated thanks to this marked improvement of her physical health.   Similar remarks apply to Cora (f., 33), whose migraine, crises of psycholepsy, and attacks of metrorrhagia, have disappeared. But this patient has likewise found it necessary to go on taking thyroid extract for years, though in much smaller doses.

Irène's case is particularly interesting from this point of view, for the patient has been kept under close observation for several years, both before and after the administration of the drug. I have already mentioned that the young woman, a typical sufferer from hysterical depression, was simultaneously affected with a multiplicity of mental symptoms and numerous physiological disturbances. I showed that it was possible to raise her psychological tension and even to increase her physiological activity by various methods which were described in connexion with the account of aesthesiogenism and of complete somnambulism. But in the chapter on treatment by excitation I mentioned that the patient was continually relapsing after a time, and that the treatment had to be begun again and again. I showed, too, that the production of complete somnambulism and of excitation were very difficult in this patient, and that often these phenomena could no longer be obtained. Just before menstruation, in certain phases of her illness, in fatigue states, it was impossible to stimulate her and to induce complete somnambulism. Sometimes several weeks' rest were requisite before anything could be done by such methods. In 1911 I began the regular administration of thyroid extract, and after various experiments in dosage I began to give ⅓ grain daily, sometimes doubling this dose for a few days, especially just before menstruation. It is now possible, after five years, to give a definite opinion as to the effect of the treatment. Speaking generally, there can be no doubt that the patient has been much better since she began to take thyroid extract. Some of her symptoms have been greatly improved, the chilliness has disappeared ; she suffers much less from migraine ; the pains which preceded menstruation, and especially the pains in the breasts, have ceased to trouble her, and the menstrual flow is no longer haemorrhagic. There can be no doubt that these improvements are due to the medicine, for if a month is allowed to pass without giving it, Irène immediately begins to suffer once more from migraine and from menorrhagia. The mental condition has not changed. The patient is affected from the same depression as of old, and this trouble must be treated in the familiar way by the induction of complete somnambulism. But I am certain that I can achieve this excitation far more readily, and that there are fewer periods in which the patient is completely refractory. No doubt, we cannot speak of an entire transformation. Fundamentally, Irène is what she was before the thyroid treatment began. The constitutional disturbance was not solely a manifestation of hypothyroidism. Still, of all the medicaments that have been tried, thyroid extract is the one which has done her most good.

Of course the cases here recorded are few in number, and extremely incomplete ; but in so difficult a matter every one must contribute such information as he possesses. Adrenalin, in a small number of cases, thyroid extract, in a larger number and more definitely, seem to have had a salutary effect in the treatment of the physiological disturbances, and sometimes in the treatment of the psychological disturbances, of neuropaths. Here we have an important indication for further researches concerning the notable part which some authorities are inclined to attribute to the endocrine glands in the neuroses.

These various methods of treatment which aim at the relief of disorders of digestion, nutrition, and circulation, do not only modify the local troubles, for they also exert an influence upon the patients' behaviour and upon the neurosis itself. They do not attack the neurosis by way of its essential symptoms, but they aim at the relief of important disturbances which may be regarded as a secondary expression of an imperfectly understood fundamental trouble. They may be looked upon as indirect ways of treating the neuroses.

3. THE SEARCH FOR STIMULANT SUBSTANCES.—ALCOHOLISM.

There are a few other methods of treatment which are more direct. They are selected because of the stimulant effect which certain agents seem to have upon the behaviour of neuropaths. In the study of these methods we shall use the same plan as before, we shall consider the spontaneous improvement which occurs in the patient under certain conditions, and the impulse which some of these patients manifest to seek for particular substances.

We know that seasonal changes, certain periods of the year, have a marked influence upon these patients. They are almost always worse at the beginning of any change of season, during the first heat of summer and during the first cold of winter. But in general they get better when the spring is well advanced, and especially during summer. There is often a fresh vital impetus at these times, which we can turn to account in order to secure greater efforts.

One very remarkable phenomenon, and one which is manifested in a very large proportion of cases, is the improvement which occurs towards the close of each day. Almost all these patients are more disturbed in the morning, more agitated, if (as we have sometimes noticed) sleep has served only to increase the quantity of their available energy without raising their psychological tension. They are more benumbed and depressed after the immobility and obscurity of the night if a rise of mental tension has not taken place. During the daytime, under the influence of light and various other excitations, they slowly become adapted to waking life, except in certain cases, when a phobia of the night or of sleep disturbs them in the evening. Generally, they improve in the afternoon, and are almost normal in the evening. How many of these depressed patients declare that they cannot do anything, and that they will not see any one, before five o'clock in the evening ! All their functions are more active in the evening, so that they digest their dinner better than their luncheon, and we may have to take special account of this fact when we are regulating their diet. Probably fresh air, light, and movement, gradually stimulate them during the course of the day. Indeed, they themselves often declare that fine weather, sunshine, and heat, have a very favourable influence upon them. Some, moreover, as I have already pointed out, say that they are better when they live in a town, even in a noisy quarter, than when they dwell in a quiet countryside. Here we have to consider various sources of excitation which are of importance.

Very often (notwithstanding digestive troubles), the taking of food, and especially the eating of a large meal, brings about a temporary disappearance of the symptoms. Whereas these depressed patients are very much out of sorts before meals— feeble, restless, obsessed with a sentiment of vacancy in the body and in the head—they are quite lively after they have eaten. But this transformation is even more conspicuous after the taking of certain particular foods. Meat, and highly spiced dishes in especial, induce an excitation which was already pointed out by Lagrange.

In the forefront of substances which induce excitation, we must mention alcohol. The ingestion of alcohol in sufficiently large quantities produces in normal human beings a complex of disturbances which have been very inadequately studied, but which pass by the name of drunkenness. In its early stages, drunkenness seems to me to be mainly characterised by a certain degree of agitation, that is to say by a quantitative excess of psychological phenomena ; whereas the mental tension, which is primarily at a high level in the normal individual, is somewhat lowered by the influence of alcohol. Sometimes we see similar phenomena in certain depressed individuals who do not tolerate alcohol well, but who very quickly pass into a state of drunkenness and into delirium. But this is exceptional, for, generally speaking, depressed persons behave quite differently under the influence of alcohol. Only with considerable difficulty is drunkenness induced in them, or it may be impossible to induce drunkenness in the strict sense of the term. One of the great objections which alcoholics always make when anyone tries to reform them is to assert that they never get drunk, that they carry their liquor admirably. A young man before coming to see me drank ten glasses of brandy " in order to have sufficient energy to talk," and he was quite free from any disturbances of speech, equilibrium, or memory. Not only does alcohol fail to induce in such patients the disturbances of drunkenness, but it often dispels antecedent symptoms and restores normal activity.—A young man of thirty noticed this for himself. " It is a very funny thing," he said. " When I ought to be drunk, I get back into normal life. It is then that I feel empowered to do what I want ; I become tireless ; I can draw up a program and follow it out ; everything goes as if upon wheels. I speak quite well ; I have a smile on my lips ; I am forthcoming with everyone I meet. I, who am always so hesitant, and am afraid to open my mouth —at these times I cannot recognise myself."—Another of my patients tells the same story. " I only become a reasonable and properly behaved man when I am drunk."—" I cannot open my mouth in a drawing-room," says Wkx. (m., 29), " unless I have had too much champagne."—The phobias of Dg. (m., 38) are checked by a bottle of wine, just as Pepita's crises are checked by a glass of absinthe. " This makes me bold, clear-minded, willing to march through fire," says Pepita. —Lydia insists, with good reason, that champagne tranquillises her far better than opium, checks her anxieties, and dispels the shocks in her head. " It absolutely bucks me up."

Moreover, alcohol acts also upon the physiological functions. After a big dinner, irrigated with plenty of burgundy and champagne, these patients digest perfectly, and do not suffer from enteritis as they do " after a mere plate of macaroni." Nay more, they sleep soundly when they go to bed, whereas they have hitherto been suffering from insomnia.—Irène checks her vomiting with champagne, and can then go to sleep.—Is. (f., 26), like many others, must drink a little alcohol when she goes to bed if she wants to sleep.—We may summarise these facts in our own terminology, by saying that alcohol in depressed patients does not merely increase the quantity of psychological phenomena. More than this, and above all, it raises the psychological tension. Thereby the patient is once more enabled to perform actions of high tension ; agitation is suppressed ; many of the morbid disturbances that result from impotence or arise by derivation are dispelled.

All these phenomena give birth to extremely important obsessions and impulses. A great many patients have an excessive desire to seek for warmth, light, and the agitations of society life ; many, in especial, are unduly fond of the pleasures of the table, of an excess of stimulating food. The bulimia which is so frequent among them does not only depend upon a sense of weakness, but also upon an impulse to experience once more the sense of wellbeing which has been produced in them on former occasions by a heavy meal. Hence arise these strange impulses to eat pound after pound of potatoes, like Bg. (m., 25) ; or pounds of chocolate, like Cm. (m., 36). Hence the manias which make these patients carry about ham sandwiches in their pocket, so that they may have something to eat before making any effort, to eat on the staircase when they are about to pay a call ; this is what makes them go about carrying a bag full of provisions, " so that I may have something to eat in these dreadful streets where there is not even a baker's shop ! " Bulimia is so closely associated with a condition of depression, that it disappears when, for one

reason or another, the mental level is reestablished.—Rox.
(f., 23), a depressed person, agoraphobic and bulimic, is continually repeating that she will go mad if she does not have something to eat instantly ; quite suddenly, she will stop these demands for food, the cessation occurring when the menstrual flow begins ; and for five days she eats reasonably like any one else ; but the bulimia recurs as soon as menstruation is over. Now that we have studied excitation by menstruation, we can understand this little instance. The reappearance of bulimia in patients who have been cured of it for a time, is a definite indication of a relapse into depression. This symptom enabled us to predict relapse in Sophie ; when she began again to eat more than usual, we could be sure that one of her delirious attacks was about to recur.

The most important of such impulses is that which leads to alcoholism and dipsomania (I do not agree that there is any real need for distinguishing between these two conditions). The problem of alcoholism is to-day a very serious one, so I think there is good reason for laying some stress here upon the true nature of these impulses, which are not, as a rule, well understood. If I mistake not, people are too ready to insist upon the poisonous character of alcohol, upon its noxious effects ; there is too much inclination to regard alcoholism as a sort of accidental intoxication which would vanish without leaving any disturbance behind if only the abuse of alcohol were discontinued. For my part, I have tried to show that in such cases there is mental disorder before the alcohol is taken, and that this disorder is to a large extent independent of alcohol.[1] I find that other authors have expressed the same view. Samuel Crothers (of Hartford, Conn., U.S.A.), Keen (of London), and Frederick T. Simpson,[2] declare that alcoholism is a primarily psychological disorder, in which intoxication by alcohol is only a secondary phenomenon. I myself, recently, wrote a paper for the Academy of Moral Sciences in which I summarised my former studies on this subject.[3]

Here are the conclusions to which I come in this paper. What is an alcoholic ? What is the mental disorder characteristic of an alcoholic ? In order to make this clear, I shall

[1] Les obsessions et la psychasthénie, vol. i, p. 529 ; vol. ii, p. 423.
[2] Alcoholism and Drug Addictions, Parker's Psychotherapy, II, i, 81.
[3] Comptes rendus de l'Académie des Sciences Morales, September and October 1915.

select from my case-books sixty-five cases of alcoholism and dipsomania of various degrees of intensity, and shall try to discover what was the physical and mental state of health of these persons before they displayed any impulse to drink ; I shall consider the conditions under which the impulse developed ; and I shall note the other disorders which developed simultaneously—for we make a great mistake when we regard the alcoholic impulse as an isolated phenomenon. Finally, I shall examine the effects of the absorption of alcohol in these patients, and shall trace out the causes of the impulse to drink.

The persons whose cases I have thus selected for consideration belong to families a great many of whose members suffered from nervous or mental disorders of various kinds. Elsewhere I have given a detailed account of the remarkable family to which Justine belonged, a family concerning which I have information regarding fifty-four persons. Studying this interesting genealogical tree, I find that thirty-four children died under the age of three ; there were three epileptics, two imbeciles, three hysterics, two criminals, seven dipsomaniacs, four sufferers from obsession.[1] In the family of Dr., a young woman of thirty-three, a dipsomaniac, whose case will require special study, we find that there were two persons suffering from impulsive obsessions, and three dipsomaniacs. These families, which I cannot now describe at length, exhibited precisely the same characters as the families of our other patients suffering from psychasthenia with obsessions. Alcoholism is one of the hereditary psychoses, as has been recognised by most of those who have studied the subject.

The patients themselves have not been alcoholics all their lives, but they were already sick persons before they took to drink. Difficult though the study of this point is, careful observation will show that before they took to drink they had exhibited multiform neuropathic symptoms. In fifty cases at least among the sixty-five, I found evidence of epileptic crises or hysterical attacks, or somnambulism, phobias, obsessions, various kinds of impulses or delusions Where precise information was obtainable, there was evidence that they had suffered from symptoms of doubt, abulia, morbid timidity, all the signs of diminution of will and attention. This fact is commonly expressed by saying that those who

[1] Névroses et idée fixes, 1898, vol. i, p. 206

succumb to an alcoholic tendency are persons of weak character. The phrasing is commonplace and kindly, but we must not let it lead us astray. What we have to recognise is that there was a definite morbid condition before the alcoholism began.

In most cases, the impulse to drink began at some particular date, in connexion with some special happening. It is easy to show that alcoholism begins under the same conditions as the various forms of mental depression. I have seen persons who for years found no difficulty in resisting the temptation to drink even when they were living in a public-house; but they became alcoholic after an infectious disorder, such as typhoid, or a slight attack of tuberculosis; others would become affected with alcoholism, just as many patients become affected with depression, after physical or mental overwork, after a change of environment, a change of situation, a quarrel, a breach of a friendship, a disappointment in love, etc.—Ag. (m., 52), for example, was greatly overworked, and became a prey to profound anxiety, when his factory was in financial difficulties. Just when the danger had been overcome and when prosperity had returned, the effects of overwork were too much for him, and it was at this time that he began to drink.—A woman of forty, Bh., has to work much too hard in the shop where she is employed. She is tormented by the fear of dismissal. " My uneasiness about this made me ill, so that I was often reduced to tears, and I took to drink."— Sadness, home-sickness, a longing for the mountain country in which he was born, brought on alcoholism in Cg. (m., 50).— A change of occupation was the cause in Fm. (m., 32).—Lav. (f., 29), who was happy in her engagement to marry, saw the name of her fiancé in the banns of forthcoming marriages at the Town Hall, and realised that her betrothed had deserted her for another. This made her take to drink.—In Ff. (m., 28), the cause was infection with syphilis, and the consequent need to relinquish the prospect of a good marriage.—Gg. (f., 30) took to drink when she was abandoned by her lover.—In Ct. (f., 25), the cause was desertion by her lover when she was pregnant.—If. (m., 32) returned home to find that his house had been plundered and that his wife had gone off with the thieves; that was why he took to drink.—Other cases of the same kind were those of Jh. (m., 27), who was jealous; Kg.

(f., 64), who was beaten by her husband and insulted by her son ; Lg. (f., 40), tormented by her husband, who was eccentric and half insane ; Mg. (f., 50), who had to live alone after the death of her children.—In most cases of alcoholism, we shall find some such cause if we look for it.

In order to understand the onset of alcoholism after troublesome happenings, we must insist upon a very important fact which is apt to be overlooked. These illnesses, this overwork, these emotions, do not simply give rise to an impulse to drink ; in most cases, unless the person concerned was already predisposed to alcoholism by previous habits, the impulse to drink develops rather slowly. They cause all sorts of troubles, sometimes akin to earlier neuropathic disorders, and sometimes to neurotic symptoms which the patient has not previously experienced. In three of my patients, there were convulsive crises ; in nine, there were phobias, such as agoraphobia, claustrophobia, the phobia of illness, or the phobia of insanity ; in eight cases, there were various algias, of the stomach, the back, or the head, with marked anxiety ; in seven cases, there were mental manias, and in especial the mania of extremism which played a part in the drunkenness of If. (m., 32), or there were tics, writer's cramp, and agitations ; in five cases there were obsessions of crime, suicide or persecution.—" I am becoming a puppet, and my husband pulls the string," said Ex. (f., 35) after the misfortunes which induced her depression.

All these patients suffer markedly from sentiments of incompleteness, which give rise to the depression, to disquietude, a sense of boredom, vacancy, dreaminess, fear, incapacity, pseudo-recognition, lack of interest, disorientation, depersonalisation, distress, death, etc. " It is sad and shameful," says Dr. (f., 33), " to feel perpetually that there is nothing in life ; nothing worth the pain of living, the pain of making an effort. It surprises me when I see people weep or annoyed about anything ; it amazes me that they think it worth while."— " All the time I feel that I am about to die," said Nol. (f., 20) ; " I am dying for lack of help."

Always, underlying these conditions, this depression, we discover disturbances of the will, incapacity for action, and especially social incapacity. The patients have grown absolutely unfitted for effort and are aghast at the thought of having to do anything.—Og. (f., 38) has become incapable

of doing her housework. She says: " My sister-in-law, who
has come to live with me during the war, complicates the situation horribly."—Pi. (m., 40), an engineer by trade and at
ordinary times a capable fellow, finds it impossible to make
up his mind to put a machine together. He thinks that this
will be horribly difficult. " Here is a new complication in
my life; I shall have to make an effort and it will be most
exhausting."—Ff. (m. 28) does not wish to live any longer
with his family. " They are too respectable, too highly
cultured. With them I always have to mind my P's and Q's.
I should like to live with people of a lower grade, so that I need
not think so much about my manners."—Qh. (m., 50) has
become incapable of any kind of activity, even of activities
which are indispensable to the provision for his son's future
career. He wants his wife to do everything in the house.—
Dl. (m., 55), intelligent and good-natured, but timid and
susceptible, grows irritated at everything, and frequently
bursts into a violent passion; he detests the society of his
fellows, " whom I cannot understand and who cannot understand me."—Vd. (m., 30), although he is a lawyer by profession,
cannot sign a paper if any one is looking at him, for this brings
on a violent trembling of the hands.—Le. (m., 41), suffering
from agoraphobia and erythrophobia, has become incapable
of saying a word to the customers who enter his shop.—This
difficulty, this absolute incapacity for social activity, whether
manifested by the ordinary signs of timidity, or else by rudeness, or else by very various disturbances which mask the
timidity, is one of the chief characteristics of the majority of
alcoholics. It depends upon infirmity of will, upon the lowering of activity, upon the psychological depression, which
in my opinion, exists in the great majority of alcoholics, not
as a result of their intoxication, but as a prelude to the
intoxication.

We note among these patients another fact which has a
most interesting relationship to the present topic. They often
exhibit other morbid impulses in addition to the impulse to
drink.—Some of them (five cases) were simultaneously affected
with bulimia; others (three cases) with erotomania.—In six
cases there were fugues, and an impulse to go on walking
indefinitely.—Ms., a woman of twenty-six, alternated between
these two impulses. For some months she had a mania for

walking, and would every day walk thirty miles on the high-road ; during this period she did not drink. Then, during the subsequent months, she gave up the craze for walking, and took to eating to gross excess, and to drinking all the alcoholic liquors she could get hold of.—Rg. (m., 37) engages in fugues in which he goes on walking immense distances for several days, and on the road he is continually drinking at every public-house he passes. At least this is what he does during the first few days. Later, towards the end of the fugue, when he has been on the go for several days, he gives up drinking.—Finally, among my alcoholic patients there are four klepto-maniacs. One of these cases, to which I have already alluded, is very simple. Oc. (m., 38) steals from his employers in order to use the money to treat chance acquaintances at a public-house. He feels thoroughly happy among these people who are drinking at his cost. I have explained how he is stimulated by the success of his thefts, and by the pride he feels in playing the part of a vulgar Amphitryon. All these impulses superadded to the alcoholic impulse are of the kind with which we are familiar ; they are all impulses to perform stimulating actions.

In view of such considerations is it not probable that the absorption of alcohol by these patients, in similar circum-stances, plays in them the same part that is played by the other stimulants ; that the alcohol comforts and cures them by the same mechanism of excitation ? It is easy to verify this hypothesis in my cases. All the neuropathic symptoms which had been noticed in such patients, disappeared after the absorption of alcohol.—In Vi. (m., 23), and in Maria, the paroxysms, the attacks of somnambulism, no longer occurred when they had been drinking.—Dr. (f., 39) is freed by drink from the enteralgia and all the other algias from which she has suffered.—Gl. (f., 45) no longer suffers from her spasmodic cough.—Ik. (m., 40) is free from his writer's cramp. " I can write very well, even in public, when I am a little drunk."—Phobias disappear.—" My terrible dread of the street, of bridges, of fire, of madness," says Uh. (m., 35), all vanish after two or three glasses of wine, and the influence may persist throughout the day.—" Before taking alcohol I cannot manage my own affairs ; but after I have had two or three glasses I become as bold as a gamecock."—" Generally speaking I am afraid of everything," says Vf. (m., 31) ; " I imagine that there are burglars everywhere. If I drink, I am no longer afraid of them and their pistols."

Finally, weakness, incapacity for activity, are cured.— " What could I do ? " says Uh. (m., 35). " When I married, I found myself quite impotent with my wife, and this upset me terribly. Now, when I drink, I am in this respect as good a man as another."—" You tell me to eat and sleep," says Fs. (f., 42), " but I find that quite impossible ; I must have a few glasses of wine before I can eat, sleep well, enjoy life."—The same is true of Fm. (m., 32) ; Pya. (m., 40) ; and Xf. (m., 40). They none of them can eat unless they have had some drink ; or cannot have sexual relationships unless they have had something to drink ; and they cannot sleep unless they have something to drink.—All these timid persons, all these social abulics, are transformed by alcohol.—Le. (m., 41) can go out, meet friends, talk to his customers without running away from them, if he has taken a few bitters or some absinthe.—Vd. (m., 30) can sign papers in public without trembling if he has privately had a few glasses of drink before making a public appearance.—Lydia can receive visitors, can play her part in social life, if she has had a half bottle of champagne to drink. Then she is bright and lively. " People are pleased with me, and I am pleased with myself."—" At any rate," says Yg. (m., 25), when I have had ten glasses of brandy, I no longer look like an idiot. Alcohol does not make me drunk ; it makes me presentable."

Here we have the essential point of the matter. Alcoholism, as a rule, is the consequence of the fact we have already pointed out, the one which these new observations bring once more to light, namely that alcohol does not act in the same way upon the normal person and upon one in a state of depression. The normal person is by alcohol rapidly brought out of his normal state and made drunk ; whereas the effect of alcohol upon one in a state of depression is to bring him out of his condition of inertia and impotence, and into the normal condition. No doubt we are not entitled to say that every one in a state of depression who is rendered normal by alcohol is an alcoholic, but such a person is already on the way towards alcoholism. He has only one more step to take. He has only to become aware that his gloomy sentiments of incompleteness, those inevitable accompaniments of depression, are transformed by alcohol; and he has only to acquire a longing for this transformation. As soon as he realises or imagines that alcohol has this power, that nothing else can exercise the same power, then he will have an irresistible craving for alcohol. Dr. (f., 33), who is suffering from a grave degree of alcoholism, gives a far-reaching explanation of the reason for her unhappy craving. She says: "Alcohol prevents my being stupid; it enables me to act; when I have had a drink I am no longer gloomy, weak, and hopeless. I have become a different person, and I want to live instead of dreaming about death. . . . Alcohol gives a value to things, and I find it intolerable to have no interest in anything. . . . When I have had a drink, I feel that I am alive, and that it is I who lives; now, I like to live, and to feel that it is I myself who lives. . . . What do you expect? If I drink it is that I may shake off gloom. It is the gloom which first takes possession of me, and then forces me to drink."

We infer from these cases that alcoholism develops when two conditions occur in conjunction. First of all, when the subject, either through constitutional predisposition or because of accidental influences, suffering from overwork or affected by profound emotions, has passed into a condition of depression. Secondly, when he has realised the stimulant effect of alcohol, and when his need for excitation has become systematised upon alcohol. This conjuncture of conditions is very characteristic in several of my cases. Uh. (m., 35) had for a long time been affected with a phobia of bridges, water and death, when, in order to cheer him up after his brother's death, some of his comrades took him to have a glass with them. Then it was for the first time that he realised that when he had had a few glasses of drink he became as vigorous as a fighting cock.—The same remarks apply to Zg. (f., 35) and to Lav. (f., 29).

This starting-point of alcoholism is especially conspicuous in a case the notes of which I have already published. A foreign medical man, aged about 40, suffering from the last stages of alcohol intoxication, told me how his terrible passion for alcohol had begun. "From youth upwards I was subject to a very painful malady. From time to time, every year or every two years, I became affected with intense gloom. For many months I would be quite incapable of doing anything, saying anything, and making up my mind to anything. The slightest activity required incredible effort ; and, above all, I suffered from horrible moral torment because of a dreadful feeling of self-contempt. It seemed to me that I had become the basest of human beings, and that I soiled every place where I was. You cannot imagine how much I suffered in these states. I had fruitlessly tried all kinds of treatment, when, one day, a number of students came to look me up. I was in one of my bad fits, but they took me with them to a university festival, and made me drink in spite of myself. The result was amazing. After I had drunk an enormous quantity of alcohol, I had no feeling of drunkenness, but I felt that I was becoming more and more normal. The veil which had covered my head was torn away. It seemed to me that I was being reborn, that I was beginning a new life. I could again speak and act, and my sense of happiness was no less exaggerated than had been the previous feeling of shame. I returned to my own rooms without difficulty, and was able to eat and sleep satisfactorily, though for a long time this had been impossible to me. When I woke up next morning I was cured. The sequel was inevitable. When the horrible sadness recurred a few days later, I hastened to seek the remedy, at first with curiosity and then with frenzy. Since that time I have never been able to pull myself up." [1] It would be easy to give, not merely a few similar instances, but fifty instances exactly like this one. I have come across the same method of development in the case of quite a number of impulses, such as the impulse to take opium or morphia, and even the impulse towards theft or debauchery, but it is especially common in the case of the alcoholic impulse.

Alcoholism will be more or less serious, and will assume different forms, according as the patient can more or less easily resist the urge, or according as he is impelled to yield by a more or less irresistible constraint. At first, and often for a long time, the patient may fly to his remedy in exceptional circumstances only.—Zh. (m., 32), an engine-driver, drinks when he has to get aboard his engine. He says : " You can believe me, this is much the best thing for the travellers in the train ! "—Pya. drinks when he goes to see his mistress ; so does Mh.—Many a woman drinks before receiving visitors ;

[1] Les obsessions et la psychasthénie, 1903, vol. ii, p. 424.

before going into the drawing-room, or " when she has to open a telegram which may contain good or bad news " ;— when her husband is away, or when she has lost her lover.— Pi. and Le. drink when they have a difficulty with their employees, and when they have to receive customers. These people drink, in a word, as they continually tell us, " when they need to buck themselves up " ; that is to say when circumstances demand that the psychological tension should be raised to the level of effort.

In this phase of development, alcoholism is not yet definitively established. It depends upon the circumstances in which the individual finds himself. Alcoholism behaves like all the impulses with which depressed persons are affected ; it diminishes when life is simple and easy, and it increases when the actions demanded by the situation are of a higher grade and more costly. Here is a demonstrative case. A journeyman tailor, a good workman, married and father of a family, had never been given to drink. Having saved a little money, he started as a master tailor, hiring men to work under him. Thereupon he took to drink, the alcoholism becoming more and more serious. Why was this ? His wife puts the matter very well, and the sufferer knows himself why it was. It was because he had to receive customers, to make commercial decisions, to pay out large sums of money. He is embarrassed, timid, uneasy, and he cannot do all these things unless he has had some drink. The change of position and the enhanced responsibility depressed this man of weak disposition ; he became an alcoholic because he had to live a life which was too difficult for his mediocre intelligence.—If the circumstances are the reverse of this, if life becomes easy, and, above all, if the depression diminishes, then the patient soon gives up drink. Lydia quickly renounces her champagne when she feels better, and when her life runs a tranquil course.

Unfortunately the patient, if left to himself, does not stay long in this stage in which alcohol is a remedy. He soon reaches the second stage, that in which, as we may say, alcohol has become to him as necessary as food. He feels impelled more and more strongly to drink. He cannot stop at the dose requisite to raise his mental level a little ; he cannot get on without alcohol in periods in which it is not really indispensable to him. Various psychological reasons play their part in bringing about this evolution, and they are all connected with the disorder of the will from which psychasthenics suffer. Manias intervene ; the mania of continuation, the mania of repetition, the mania of extremism.—" If I stop before getting drunk, it seems to me that I have not finished, that there is something incomplete ; so I have to drink some more."— " I always run to extremes ; I must always go to the very end."—The fear of relapse, the fear of suffering once more from depression, continually increases. Dr. (f., 33) feels assured when she is under the influence of alcohol that she will relapse into depressions it she stops drinking. " Horror of gloom drives me to despair. I would rather go on drinking whatever happens ; I no longer have the power to stop."—If we remember that alcohol frees these patients from intolerable torment, we shall understand why it is for them a temptation such as normal individuals never experience. Dr. said to me, in this connexion, a phrase at which I could not but smile : " Do you know what is the most horrible moral suffering in the world ? "—" What is that ? "—" To have an open bottle of whisky on the table, and not to finish it." That is why she drinks as soon as she grows agitated and as soon as she is afraid of relapsing. " Since the most trifling emotion agitates me and makes me relapse, I am continually obliged to drink."— Finally, the main cause of the development of the impulse is the continuation and the aggravation of the depression, for this lowers the will power more and more. The subject becomes more and more incapable of breaking the habit, of exposing himself to suffering ; and at the same time, he grows more and more impotent, finds that his activities are more and more often checked. The result is that he is increasingly affected with the need to be " bucked up."

At this stage, the patient is still well aware of the danger which his passion for drink entails upon him, and fully realises the sufferings which it imposes upon his family. From time to time he exhibits a desire to cure himself. He makes solemn promises, and more or less sincere efforts to pull up. Patients suffering severely from alcoholism will spontaneously go to a doctor and ask to be cured. A few years ago there was talk in some of the newspapers about a serum which could cure alcoholism. For a time a great many of my patients would ask me for an injection of this supposed serum. Even while they are drinking, the patients suffer from remorse, thoughtfulness, hesitation. It is true that they very rarely get the better of their craving, but they go on striving, from time to time at least. This characteristic has its importance as an indication of the stage which alcoholism has reached.

For, only too often, we encounter a third form. Constantly, or intermittently, the patient goes on drinking an indefinite amount without making any effort to pull up, and sacrificing everything to the gratification of his impulse. This form is the one which is commonly spoken of as " dipsomania," there being a great inclination to distinguish it from the beforementioned forms of alcoholism. The distinction was based, in the first instance, upon certain characteristics which seem to me of trifling importance. It was said that the dipsomaniac was sad, and drank in solitude, whereas the alcoholic was merry in his cups, and usually drank with boon companions. Sometimes these observations are true enough, but they lack precision, and they do not apply to all cases. When we speak of the sadness and of the cheerfulness of these patients, we must not only recognise that it is often very difficult to distinguish clearly between the two moods, but we must also take into account the moment at which the patient comes under observation. Most of these patients are sad before drinking, for they all suffer from the fundamental depression ; on the other hand, they are often merry after drinking, when alcohol has a favourable effect. All that we can say is that in the worst cases alcohol no longer succeeds in producing its stimulant effect ; or that this effect is of brief duration, and is speedily replaced by intoxication. Nor is it correct to say that all the alcoholics in the earlier stages of alcoholism drink in company. The women of whom I have spoken, those who need a bottle of champagne before they can receive visitors, drink alone and secretly, for they would be ashamed to have their need for stimulant generally known. Such a dipsomaniac as Oc. (m., 38) invites casual passers-by to drink with him, for he wants to superadd social excitation to the excitation of alcohol. All we can say is that an impulse which has become very powerful is, generally speaking, extremely systematised and very narrow ; and that the patient who has reached this stage usually thinks of nothing but alcohol. These characteristics, which are seldom of much interest, merely indicate that the impulse has grown more powerful and has become systematised.

I attach more importance to two other characteristics : that the dipsomaniac impulse occurs in crises ; and that it does not encounter any resistance. Let us consider the first point. Many of these patients do not drink constantly ; they have periods of intermission, and then suffer from alcoholic crises. After a longer or shorter period of incubation, during which the depression goes on increasing, they have a drinking bout, in which constantly, by day and by night, they consume all kinds of alcoholic liquor. This lasts for a certain time, and then they stop drinking, and will even have a horror of alcohol until the next crisis. This was the case in half of my patients. They would stay for three months or more, two years in some cases, without drinking anything stronger than water. Then, when I believed that they had been cured, they would have a terrible crisis, and would drink whatever kind of alcohol they could get hold of persistently for days or months. One of my patients, Bqa. (f., 34), exhibits a very remarkable cycle. She remains for six weeks without drinking, and then drinks for a fortnight. This cycle has continued with considerable regularity for two years.

We must not exaggerate the importance of the cyclical characteristic. It is not always present in dipsomania.— Maria, the woman of thirty to whose remarkable case I have already alluded more than once, was in the most advanced stage of the disease, for she went on drinking alcohol and ether in unrestricted quantities without making the least resistance, sacrificing everything in order to satisfy her craving, selling her dress and her petticoat in order to get a few pence to spend upon ether. But she had no intermissions, unless she was in prison or in hospital for a few weeks. Directly she was free, she began drinking again. It is no exaggeration to say that for ten years she was suffering from persistent dipsomania.—Fm., a man of thirty-two, was likewise in a dipsomaniac condition for three years.—When we see definite intermissions, periods in which the desire for alcohol is completely suppressed, this is because we have to do with a patient in whom the depression occurs in crises. Usually these are irregular and are induced by circumstances ; but sometimes they are regular, and more or less periodic, although the cause of the periodicity is not always obvious. The urge to take alcohol disappears at the close of the crisis of depression; just as the patient's obsessions, manias, and other impulses disappear at this time. Such interruptions in the alcoholic impulse do not affect the nature of the impulse, although they play a remarkable part in the evolution of the disease.

The last characteristic, the irresistibility of the impulse, which is supposed to distinguish dipsomania from alcoholism, seems to me more important, for in the study of impulses the degree of resistance is the most essential point. I have already been led to admit that impulses towards excitation are far more powerful than the obsessive impulses of over-scrupulous persons—far more powerful than what are termed criminal impulses, for instance. We must also recognise that in certain cases the impulse to excitation by alcohol seems irresistible, for it annuls even individual consciousness and memory, and is carried out in a sort of secondary personality. The dipsomaniac fugues of Rg. (m., 37), like those of Maria, are undertaken in this secondary state. The patient does not recover consciousness until towards the end of the fugue, and can only remember some of the incidents of the last days of his fugue. As regards the early days, there is complete amnesia. Although these extreme forms are exceptional, a good many patients have very little individual consciousness during the crisis. They have only one thought, that of getting drink; and no other consideration appears in consciousness to strive against this impulsive idea. Consequently, as soon as they have begun to drink, they have none of the hesitations we have spoken of as present in the before-mentioned alcoholics; and they are not checked by any consideration whatever. They will sell everything they possess, even the clothes they are actually wearing, and they will sell the possessions of other members of the family; they will sacrifice the things that they value most in the world in order to get liquor. After the crisis they cannot understand what they have done. " I know quite well that my husband and my children will leave me if I go on drinking. I love them dearly, far more than I love my own life. Why is it that I cannot think of them for a moment when I am drinking ? " Hack Tuke tells of a man who had come as a voluntary patient into a sanatorium for the treatment of such cases, where the only drink allowed was water. He noticed that the medical superintendent had given a glass of whisky to one of the boarders who had sustained a severe wound. Without hesitation he took up an axe and cut off one of his hands and then asked for a drink. This familiar anecdote serves to illustrate how the craving for alcohol can become unreflective and irresistible.

The last transformation can be explained as due to an aggravation of the before-mentioned disturbances: depression, intolerable sentiments of incompleteness, restriction of will-power, automatism. We may remark that there are super-added certain phenomena reminding us of the confusion, the restriction of the field of consciousness, and the suggestibility, of hysterics; and we may note that intoxication has as one of its effects the production of phenomena of this kind. I have pointed out elsewhere that certain sufferers from alcholic intoxication pass into a mental condition akin to that of hysterical patients. It is possible that chronic alcoholic intoxication has in these cases complicated the primary depression, and has superadded new disturbances. Such individuals as Dx. (f., 35) will experience at the outset, as the result of some slight emotion, a simple urge to raise their spirits by a glass of alcohol. But after a few years they will have a severe crisis of dipsomania when the least unpleasantness disturbs them. It is right to distinguish this new form of the illness from the forms previously described, and to speak of it as dipsomania or alcoholomania; with the proviso that we do not consider it as anything more than the final stage of the other forms; and that we are aware that fundamentally all these impulses are of the same kind, and arise in every case, if we go back far enough, out of the search for alcoholic excitation in order to escape from depression.

These studies concerning alcoholic impulses will have made it needless to give a long account of other impulses of the same kind, for other impulses have similar effects upon depressed persons. Some of the substances which play this part are tobacco, absinthe, and the various essences which form a part of this liqueur, and also those found in vulnéraire.[1]

---

[1] Vulnéraire, eau d'arquebuse, or, for short, arquebuse, is a liqueur regarded as a panacea in eastern France and Lyonnais. Cf. the special study of this liqueur and its effects by Cadéac and Meunier (see Bibliography).

There must also be mentioned ether, opium, morphine, heroin, chloral, cocaine, etc. What has been said about alcohol might substantially be repeated about all these substances. The persons who have an impulse to use them are hereditary neuropaths, who, before acquiring the drug addiction, have already had all kinds of characteristic disorders. The substances in question do not act upon such hereditary neuropaths in the same way as that in which they act upon a normal person ; they do not merely produce drunkenness, insensibility, or sleep ; they check neuropathic symptoms, do away with the depressing sentiment of incompleteness, restore the will power, relieve the patient of depression by inducing excitation.

A few examples will suffice.—Kg. (f., 64) intoxicates herself with tobacco. She takes it in the form of snuff, and also chews it, " until I get rid of the longing to throw myself in front of a tram."—Eleven patients, six women and five men, drink or inhale ether, in order to check writer's cramp and so become able to write in public, or to dispel terrible phobias, to win sleep, to check severe hysterical paroxysms, and so on.— Vc. (m., 43) used at first to take alcohol, but has now a taste for morphine, of which he takes 1½ grains daily in order to check depression, abulia, doubt, and feelings of distress. " I have such a longing to escape these horrors, and to be happy like other people."—The hysterical and delirious attacks of Sg. (f., 50) are stopped by morphine.—Duv. (f., 37), who suffers from periodic attacks of melancholia, was able in the last attack to rid herself of the melancholia by incredibly large doses of morphine.—Yp. (m., 30) an abulic, timid, over-scrupulous and affected with obsessions, used to take alcohol and absinthe to excess, but has now acquired the opium habit, drinking laudanum by the glassful like the celebrated De Quincey. A remarkable fact, in keeping with the foregoing observations, is that this patient is ordinarily prone to suffer from asthenic delusions. In former days, transforming his delusions into obsessions, he believed that he was destined to play the part of Joan of Arc, and behaved in an absurd and dangerous way. When he has had a glass of laudanum he recovers his good sense, and sets to work to undo the mischief he has wrought.—I shall mention only one other case. Om. (m., 22) has since childhood been subject to all kinds of nervous symptoms, circulatory disturbances, severe attacks of muco-membranous enteritis, abulia, various forms of impotence, sexual inversion, phobias, complicated by the sentiment of incompleteness, erotic obsessions, and sexual impulses. When he finds it impossible to satisfy these sexual impulses, they give rise to severe fits of hysterics, with abundant and often haemorrhagic ejaculation ; sometimes, this disturbance is accompanied by an epileptic fit. He has been addicted to all kinds of drugs, such as laudanum, veronal, ether, morphine, cocaine, adalin. The last-mentioned drug transformed him for a time, giving to him remarkable cheerfulness and self-confidence. Cocaine, he said, enormously magnified his energy, and raised his spirits immensely. But he has given up all the others in favour of heroin, of which he came to take enormous doses, as much as 13 grains daily by hypodermic injection, the effect being marvellous. Nearly all the symptoms were suppressed for eighteen months. His digestion became normal ; a feeling of wellbeing and warmth replaced his attacks of anxiety ; his sentiments were once more normal ; his sexual impulses vanished, and thereafter the hysterical paroxysms and the epileptic seizures completely disappeared.

It has often been noticed that such patients have tried all kinds of poisonous substances while paying very little attention to their physiological effects, being simply inspired by the strange urge to take some unusual and dangerous drug. It is said that they are merely toxicomaniacs. This is quite true. Among my own cases, there was a woman of sixty-two, who had successively tried five different poisons. Another of my cases, a young woman of twenty-six, a doctor's daughter, was successively addicted to alcohol, ether, chloroform, opium, morphine, codeine, atropine, hyoscine, and thiantine, until, finally, she was put under restraint. These patients are not content with the physiological excitation produced by the chemical substance ; they are in search of a more complicated excitation, one of a psychological kind. Some of the women who are drug addicts have their spirits raised by the fact that they are performing a strange action, one which other women do not perform. This factor sometimes plays its part even in the simple opium habit. When Emma is delighted at smoking opium in a Chinese opium den, and when she declares that this fills her with beautitude, " as if the soul, liberated from the body, were living alone and in freedom," the effect is only to a minor degree due to the opium, for the greater part of it depends upon vanity and swank. In the toxicomaniacs, there is also the lure of danger, and the desire for new sensations ; these add their stimulant action to that which is proper to the drug. We have recognised a similar complication in cases of bulimia and of alcoholism, when we have seen alcoholism complicated with kleptomania, and when we have seen Mc. spend days and nights consuming coffee and stolen rolls, in order to add excitation by food the excitation derived from forbidden articles of diet and from stolen foods.[1] The substitution of one of these excitations for another is most interesting, for it shows that such phenomena have an underlying kinship. Eh., a woman of thirty, who had been subject to depression and to hysterical paroxysms, had long been treated by hypnotism and by aesthesiogenic excitation which relieved her of her symptoms, but which had to be repeated very frequently. When circumstances deprived her of the care of her doctor, it occurred to her to try hypodermic injections of morphine, and she found that these produced the same effect. Such complications and substitutions remind us of the existence of other excitations due to mental and moral agents, but they do not suppress the fundamental fact that certain poisonous substances can produce excitation. When a subject whose mental condition has been raised by one of these poisons, is deprived of it, when he is no longer under the action of the drug, he relapses into his condition of primary depression, the symptoms and the sufferings which had been temporarily suspended return. Furthermore, he exhibits the physical and moral symptoms of the intoxication peculiar to the drug, these being superadded. The morphinomaniac in a state of deprivation is pale, cyanotic, drenched with cold sweat, tortured by frequent diarrhoea, cramps, attacks of anxiety, syncopal attacks. It is natural that he should ardently long to escape from these tortures, and that he should crave for the hypodermic injection which will relieve him. This urge varies in accordance with the degree of depression and in accordance with the duration and the intensity of the intoxication, ranging from a desire kept within bounds by considerations of health and money, up to an utterly unreasonable and

[1] Névroses et idées fixes, 1898, vol. ii, p. 194.

irresistible impulse. There are morphinists and morphino-maniacs, just as there are alcoholics and alcoholomaniacs.

In an earlier chapter we saw that the mental condition, and in especial the psychological tension, could be modified by the performance of certain actions. The studies we have just been making, aim at disclosing another psychophysiological phenomenon, namely that the ingestion of certain substances can produce the same effect. Herein we have a notion which is of great importance in psychotherapy.

4. DIRECT METHODS OF TREATING NEUROSES.

These impulses to take stimulating poisons serve to warn us of a danger, but they also give us a therapeutic indication. Unfortunately, as regards both these points, I can only give a few brief hints.

Stimulating drugs do not merely induce excitation ; they have secondary effects which are extremely injurious. No doubt depressed persons are more resistant to intoxication than normal persons, and some of my patients, like Yg. (m., 25), never seem to become intoxicated. In the end, however, most of these patients present disturbances akin to intoxication, and even more serious than intoxication. A moment arrives when the psychological tension is no longer proportional to the quantity of psychological phenomena, the result being agitation, incoherency, and delirium. In many of the patients whose cases I have been describing, the agreeable phase of excitation ends in delirium.

When the absorption of alcohol or some other toxic substance is frequently repeated, and when the dose is continually increased in order to intensify the excitation, secondary effects connected with the intoxication tend more and more to appear. It may be said that at the outset the introduction of a poison into the organism puts all the functions on guard, and, like the beginning of a war, leads to the mobilisation of all the energies of the organism, so that the general activity and consequently the psychological tension are raised. But if the ingestion of the poison is continued in increasing doses, if the war lasts too long, the resources of the organism are exhausted, intoxication and invasion occur, and the depression becomes so great that nothing can overcome it. These hypothetical explanations of phenomena which have never been adequately analysed, may perhaps furnish us with an image which will help us to see how the mechanism of physiological excitation by a poison is akin to that which we have already considered in connexion with psychological excitation by simple and familiar actions. At the same time, the image may enable us to understand how these excitations have limits beyond which it is dangerous to go.

When we have to do with an alcoholomaniac or a morphinomaniac, it is obvious that we are primarily concerned with a person in a state of intoxication, and our first care must be to disintoxicate him. We must suppress the poison by a strict supervision of the patient, by complete isolation; we must suppress it more or less gradually; we must prescribe a special regimen, perhaps purge the patient, or use other measures which will promote elimination; and we must do everything we can to sustain the patient's strength during the distressing period of elimination. These are well-known facts. I have already indicated the general lines of treatment by disintoxication, and it would be superfluous to give a detailed account of demorphinisation. But, if I mistake not, this is but the first part of the problem, since our main trouble is that we have to do with an individual who is intoxicated because he had a need for an intoxicant. It does not suffice to concern ourselves with the poison, to attach all the troubles to the presence of the poison. I have already criticised those who, when they have to treat alcoholism, think only about the alcohol; those who think that they will suppress alcoholism by putting a heavy tax upon alcohol, while forgetting to consider the alcoholic individual who has created alcohol and who will replace it by some equivalent if alcohol is kept out of his reach. We must, then, in the second place, concern ourselves with the depression which has induced the need for the poison before ever intoxication has occurred, and which will make the same need show itself once more after the fullest possible disintoxication.

The case of Om. gives an excellent demonstration of the part which depression and its oscillations can play in the course of disintoxication, in the treatment of morphinomania. This young man, quite unbalanced, and ordinarily in a state of profound depression, nevertheless (like so many of these patients), passes through periods in which, for various reasons, his psychological tension is more or less completely re-established. Sometimes one of these periods of excitation will last for six weeks or two months during the summer heats in July and August. If, by chance, the attempt at demorphin-isation coincides with this period, it is perfectly successful. If the patient be sent to a sanatorium during one of these periods, he tolerates a rapid diminution of the drug, and soon the use of heroin can be completely suppressed. The doctor secures a triumph. But when the patient has returned home, within a few days the first symptoms of depression reappear. Despite all his efforts, he begins to use the hypodermic syringe again, and soon he gets back to the original dose of heroin. Now the attempt will be made to demorphinise once more, but since by this time he has entered the phase of depression, matters do not run the same course as before. The diminution of the drug promptly leads to the appearance of very serious symptoms, attacks of anxiety, enteritis, genital impulses, hysterical crises with ejaculation, epileptic fits, etc. The symptoms which had been suppressed by the heroin returned as soon as the dose of the drug was diminished ; it was necessary for the time being to give up the attempt at demorphinisation.— Similar considerations apply to alcohol. There are times when we can readily cut off Lydia's champagne and Dr.'s whisky ; but there are other times when the suppression is extremely difficult and when deprivation induces severe bodily and mental disturbance. Even if we do succeed temporarily in disintoxicating these patients, should we fail to treat the underlying depression there is a grave risk that within a few days they will return to the use of the same poison or of some other intoxicant.

Apart from certain particular measures rendered necessary by the state of intoxication, the treatment of dipsomaniacs and toxicomaniacs must, therefore, be on the same lines as the treatment of the general impulse to seek excitation. We must fight against the exclusivism of the impulse, must seek out other sources of excitation, must make the patient feel that there are excitations of a mental order as well as physio-logical excitations, and above all we must diminish the need for excitation by reducing the depression, by raising the psycho-logical tension in every possible way. These are difficult problems, the multiform solutions of which have again and again been considered in the present work. Dr. was hypnotisable after an aesthesiogenic sitting, she experienced the same excitation that could be induced in her by alcohol. She was a woman who needed guidance and whose mental and moral expenditure was lessened when she felt herself to be under strict direction. In three months it was possible to free her from an alcoholic impulse which had affected her for years. In other cases, I used the method of rest, that of the simplification of life, that of excitation by work, etc. The treatment of toxicomania requires, over and above the special treatment proper to this or that form of intoxication, no very special methods. The difficulties we have to face are the ordinary difficulties attendant upon the treatment of depressed neuropaths.

Putting aside this particular problem, the existence of such impulses discloses to us the stimulating effect of certain substances. The utilisation of this notion would demand studies which seem to me to be as yet in their infancy, studies concerning drunkenness, or rather concerning different forms of drunkenness. Such studies were begun in the days of Moreau de Tours ; they were continued by subsequent observers, and especially by the exertions of Charles Richet ; but I regard them as still in a larval condition. French psychiatry, which has unfortunately forgotten its traditions and is inclined to tow in the wake of foreign metaphysics, would do well to return to these matters, and to resume the observation of concrete facts. The study of the different forms of drunkenness, of the direct and remote action of this or that substance in different individuals whose mental state before taking the drug has been carefully examined, would be extremely fruitful. It would reveal important phenomena which might be turned to the greatest possible account in psychotherapeutics.

To-day we are still very ignorant about all these matters, and we can only grope our way, cautiously applying the little knowledge we have concerning the properties of certain substances. When we have to do with patients over whom we can exercise thorough control, in whom we can study the psychological effects of the drugs, and in whom we can stop the administration whenever we please, we can make an excellent use of these stimulant substances. To take the most delicate case first, it seems to me that doctors, in their kindness of heart, are too reluctant to talk about alcohol. Generally speaking, if the doctor says anything at all about wine or spirits, it is only in order to forbid their use absolutely. It is not always wise to suppress a habitual stimulant suddenly without asking by what it can be replaced. Consider the case of Rh. (f., 58), obviously predisposed to neuropathic disorders, and readily depressible, but intelligent and extremely active. Since she was suffering from certain gastric troubles taking a hypersthenic form, her doctor examined her diet and found that for years she had been nourished largely on meat, and that she had drunk wine regularly, a good deal of it, though not to marked excess ; and that she also had the habit of drinking coffee. He explained to her, probably with good reason, that all this was very dangerous to her stomach. The patient took fright, and, perhaps overstressing the matter a little, she put herself upon a strict regimen of water and farinaceous food. Thereupon, not only did her physical energy suffer, but in addition her mental and moral energy rapidly declined. She became affected by doubts, phobias, and obsessions. " I no longer exist, I only live to do foolish things." Shall we go far wrong when we put her back upon the earlier regime, when we allow her some wine and stimulants which will rapidly bring about improvement ? Lagrange has made similar remarks regarding coffee.[1] " Stimulant drinks like tea or coffee, may," he writes, "occasionally favour sleep in overworked persons. I have seen harvesters, who, after a terribly hard day's work, could not sleep unless they took coffee when they went to bed. At ordinary times, the same men would have been kept awake all night if they had permitted themselves the same indulgence after a day's rest." Thanks to my own observations on the peculiar effect of these substances in depressed patients, I have advised a dozen of my patients to take a glass of champagne, a little spirits, some coffee, or sometimes some kola, in order to check attacks of anxiety, crises of self-interrogation, or morbid impulses. I have allowed my patients to go on drinking a half bottle or sometimes a bottle of champagne daily, while insisting from time to time

---

[1] Les mouvements méthodiques, etc., p. 439.

upon a week's or a fortnight's intermission ; and in this way I have helped them to get through difficult periods without suffering from unpleasant symptoms. Alcohol is a drug, and must only be used as a drug ; but we need no more be ashamed to prescribe wine or spirits than we are ashamed to prescribe strychnine. The ordinary stimulants, if carefully used, can do us good service.

Alienists are more accustomed than neurologists to make use of opium, which was also recommended by Esquirol,[1] and which is given rather freely in melancholic states. It may be useful in most forms of depression, although its action is irregular, and some patients hardly seem to notice any stimulating effect. The use of morphine in the treatment of the neuroses, which at one time was widespread, had unfortunate results. It created a great number of morphinomaniacs, the reason being, in my opinion, that the patients were allowed to dose themselves too freely and without proper supervision. Unquestionably this drug is dangerous when it is left in the patient's hands ; or if the doctor does not regularly supervise the oscillations of the mental level, and does not take care to vary the stimulant he uses. He must, therefore, avoid prescribing it when these conditions cannot be fulfilled. When he does use it, he must do so as far as possible without his patient's knowledge, for the invalid should not always know what drug is used in an injection ; and the doctor must avoid administering it regularly for long periods at a time, and must frequently substitute other drugs for it. But if used with care it may do much service to the psychiatrist for a time. It will check the crises of anxiety, and very often the delirious agitations from which the patient suffers ; it will facilitate the use of suggestion, and will favour the inauguration of various forms of psychological treatment, which, as soon as they take effect, will enable us to suppress the use of opium. Being myself extremely cautious in these matters, I have used the drug in a very small number of cases only, and for brief periods ; but, thus administered, the results have been satisfactory ; and I think that in days to come, when we have a fuller knowledge of excitation by opium and its derivatives, we shall be able to use these substances more frequently.

In addition to the drugs which are well known to the public,

[1] Des maladies mentales, vol. i, p. 153.

and notorious for the frequency with which they give rise to
a drug habit, there have been discovered various other substances which influence the quantity or the tension of psychological phenomena, and these likewise have been turned to
account in psychotherapeutics. I cannot enumerate them all.
It will suffice to mention a few of them, in order to show that,
psychotherapy must on no account ignore them.

The bromides seem to reduce agitation. They appear to
act by lowering the intensity of the reflexes, by increasing the
difficulty of awakening tendencies, and by diminishing the
number of tendencies in a state of erection and ready to become
active. Although the psychological mechanism of the action
of the bromides has as yet been little studied, I believe that
these drugs act in the same way as certain illnesses or certain
paroxysms which exhaust the patient's energies and tranquillise
him by weakening him. It is probable that the bromides do
not directly induce a rise in the psychological tension, but
rather that they diminish the quantity of available energy,
and thus reestablish a satisfactory relationship between
quantity and tension. For these reasons, the various bromides
are the most interesting among drugs which affect the mental
condition. Apart from the symptoms which are properly
called epileptic (in which, despite certain contradictions, they
have a well-recognised action), the bromides can play a useful
part in the relief of a good many neuropathic symptoms. I
have noted in a great number of cases that large doses of
bromide have had a marked effect upon spasmodic symptoms,
and in anxiety states and obsessions. In one remarkable
instance, bromide in doses ranging from $1\frac{1}{2}$ to 2 drachms per
diem, given for only a few days, cut short serious crises of
blepharospasm with photophobia, lachrymation, and intense
rhinorrhoea, in a youth of seventeen, in whom these crises had
continued for several weeks, and had induced a very serious
condition. But we must not generalise. A good many patients
suffering from similar disorders do not seem to me to be benefited in any way by the prolonged administration of bromide.
Most probably we must distinguish more clearly in these cases
between disorders of psychological quantity and disorders of
psychological tension. Our stumbling-block is the inadequacy
of our psychological study of the patient.

Gilles de la Tourette used to recommend in the treatment

of convulsive crises and various kinds of agitation the use of chloroform in small doses, as given during childbirth. " It always has a powerful effect," said he ; " and since the drug is a disagreeable one to inhale, there is no risk of a drug habit arising." The last statement is incorrect. I have known two patients who had acquired a mania for chloroform. Any drug may lead to a drug addiction unless the patient is carefully watched. Except in certain cases of contracture, when chloroform may be a useful aid to diagnosis, I think its administration for the relief of neuroses is fruitless and dangerous. It would be better, when anything of the kind is indicated, to give a few whiffs of ether, or still better to inject ether, for this is valuable in convulsive crises and in fainting fits. Magnan advised the use of hyoscine hydrochloride to tranquillise patients suffering from maniacal agitation, and he declared that the drug might almost be looked upon as a specific. But we know still less about the action of this substance than we know about the action of the bromides.

Much more attention has been paid to tonic drugs which may exercise a stimulant action. A good many authorities, such as Axenfeld, Huchard, Féré, and Brissaud, used to recommend iron as a stimulant for neuropaths. To-day it does not seem to be supposed that this drug has a stimulant action. Phosphoric acid was rendered fashionable by the studies of Joulie and Cautru. In twelve cases in which I administered this drug by itself, I thought that it had a useful effect in relieving the patient's mental depression. Arsenic and its derivatives, although their value has perhaps been exaggerated, certainly do promote vitality, and thus exercise a valuable stimulant effect. Jean Lepine has had satisfactory results with nucleinate of sodium, a drug of which I have had hardly any experience, but it would seem to deserve a place in the list. Toulouse has published some very interesting experiments upon the stimulant effect of hypodermic injections of oxygen. The principle underlying such investigations is a fascinating one, for there can be no doubt that in these states of depression there is a diminution of oxidation, as evidenced by a fall in carbonic-acid production. It seems likely that here we have a valuable guide for future researches.

Doctors whose practice lies among neuropaths have made

a trial of recalcifying drugs, being perhaps led to administer these by a study of the results they have had in the treatment of tuberculosis. I think such attempts are very interesting, and for some time I have myself subjected some of my patients to a regimen akin to that which Ferrier advised for tubercular patients. We must take dietetic precautions to avoid decalcification, and must give the patient phosphatic and calcic preparations. The results secured within a few months in thirteen cases have been encouraging, for it has seemed to me that the treatment acts simultaneously upon the agitation and the depression. We have to remember that calcium phosphate, calcium glycerophosphate, calcium hypophosphate, and the similar magnesium salts, have long been advantageously administered to neuropaths. In a certain number of cases, chloride of calcium has seemed to me especially useful, above all in patients suffering from disorders of the circulation.

The stimulant drug most in fashion to-day is strychnine sulphate. For a long time this has been prescribed in the majority of nervous disorders. Some authors report success from the use of strychnine in dipsomania as a substitute for alcohol.[1] Hartenberg, in his work on the treatment of neurasthenia (1912),[2] proposed a modification and an extension of the use of this drug. He showed that the dose can be considerably increased without danger, and that, in large doses, strychnine is a real nervine tonic. Whereas, with exaggerated caution, most doctors are content to prescribe doses not exceeding one-sixtieth or one-thirtieth of a grain per diem, he declares that as much as one-fourth or one-third of a grain of sulphate of strychnine can be given daily, either by mouth or hypodermically. These large doses may give rise to slight intoxication, and may be followed by a little stiffness in the masseter muscles, or in the muscles of the legs, for half an hour ; but the symptoms are transient and unimportant. When they have passed off, the patient experiences a marked sense of wellbeing, and a greatly increased activity can always be secured by the treatment. Recently Martinet has also referred to strychnine as a drug competent, in smaller doses (ranging from one-thirtieth to one-tenth of a grain) to raise the intravascular tension, which is often much lowered in neuropaths.

[1] Tolvinsky, Popoff, Traitement de la dipsomanie, "Vrach," 1912.
[2] See Bibliography.

For a good many years I have myself given strychnine by hypodermic injections, in doses ranging from one-twentieth to one-twelfth of a grain. Since reading the recommendations of Hartenberg and Martinet, I have tried to increase the dose in some of my patients, and have studied the effects of this treatment. Some of them bore the increase of dose badly. It is difficult to exceed one-fifteenth of a grain in Wkx. (m., 29), for he becomes affected with a moderate amount of vertigo, and grows alarmed thereby, so that his phobias are intensified. I noticed the same thing in a young woman of twenty-six, Kx, for the continued administration of such large doses gave rise to kindred symptoms. But these two cases were exceptional. In most of my patients I could raise the dose up to one quarter of a grain by mouth, or one-sixth of a grain hypodermically, without notable symptoms of an overdose. In some cases I could often give as much as one-third of a grain by mouth without any obvious ill effect. Beyond these doses, if we transcend the limits of individual susceptibility, there occur attacks of vertigo, muscular stiffness, and alarm ; and in my cases these disturbances lasted from half an hour to three-quarters of an hour. I, too, have noticed, especially in two of my patients, that these disturbances were followed by a sense of wellbeing, and by an obvious increase in the intravascular tension, which might last for several hours. There is here something unquestionably akin to the effects of champagne or spirits, and it is probable that if this influence were better known to the general public we should soon have to deal with cases of strychninomania just as now we have to deal with cases of alcoholomania. Some of the patients who were treated in this way were obviously and lastingly benefited, but there can be no doubt that in these cases the strychnine was not the only cause of the improvement. Still, these experiments have been encouraging, and they show that in strychnine we have a valuable addition to the drugs which the patients' own appetites have already shown to be useful— to the drugs which, under conditions that still require more careful study, can induce a valuable excitation.

Several of these drugs, such as cacodylate of sodium, glycerophosphates, and strychnine, can be given by hypodermic injection ; and the method is valuable, for it safeguards the digestive organs and ensures more satisfactory assimilation. Jules Chéron, in former days, and de Fleury more recently, believed that the injection had, per se and simply qua injection, a markedly stimulating effect. Various artificial serums have been recommended, as a means by which we can take advantage of this stimulant effect of hypodermic injections. The action certainly seems to be a real one in a few cases ; but it is not very powerful, and is comparatively unimportant. Where it occurs, I think the excitation can be explained as due to a physical irritation of the nerve terminals. If this be so, we are concerned with physical rather than chemical effects, but they are none the less interesting.

In former days, considerable importance was attached to hydrotherapy in the treatment of neuropaths. The superficial shock caused by the action of cold water was supposed to stimulate the functioning of the nervous system. " Cold water," writes Marro, in his book on puberty,[1] " accustoms the body to react promptly. This habit does not merely modify the peripheral circulation ; it also affects the mental condition, and is the best way of treating fear." I agree that this is true in many cases, and I have frequently had occasion to note remarkable changes in the condition of certain depressed persons after a cold douche. It is especially valuable in doubters, in persons who are continually questioning themselves regarding their personality, and who are perpetually asking " Is it I who feels, is it I who hears ? " Such persons no longer feel the slightest doubt as to their individuality when they are under the cold douche ! Unfortunately, at any rate in the cases I have myself studied, this excitation is fugitive ; and it is often followed by a depression due to fatigue. We must be on our guard against the fatigue resulting from the cold douche when the reaction is neither speedy nor readily induced. Hot douches, or mixed douches, do not produce the same unsatisfactory results. I have noticed that local douches may do good in disturbances of sensation or movement. Especially valuable have been hot and long-continued vaginal injections (Luxeuil's method) in women suffering from disorders of menstruation. Prolonged warm baths have a well-known effect in states of agitation ; they often tranquillise the patient better than any other method. It is true that hydrotherapy was at one time practised to excess ; but that is no reason why, by an exaggerated recoil, we should now deny that it is of any use.

Great hopes were also founded upon the electrical treatment of neuropaths. It seems very probable that electricity may have a powerful effect upon the working of the nervous system. The valuable experiments of Leduc upon the electric sleep, show that the electric current can profoundly modify the activity known as sleep. Various interesting observations have been published concerning the tranquillising or stimulating effect of currents of electricity, or of static electricity, upon neuropaths. I have myself been able to note very remarkable results ; but I am still inclined to believe that suggestion, which is more marked in the case of electrical treatment than in the case of any other kind of treatment, had a good deal to do with the results achieved. Some day, perhaps, electricity will be one of the most valuable among the agents that can modify and stimulate these patients ; but as far as our present knowledge goes, it must be regarded merely as a useful adjuvant.

Various authorities, such as Bardet, Gilles de la Tourette, Lagrange,[1] and Peterson,[2] following in the footsteps of Charcot,[3] have been inclined to attach considerable importance to a method of treatment in which use is made of the influence of vibrations. Such vibratory massage is said to have had an excellent effect in certain neuropaths. I myself made use of this treatment at one time, and I hoped to perfect it by modifying in various ways the frequency of the vibrations, and by adapting the frequency to the patient's special condition. I even had special forms of vibratory apparatus made. It did not seem to me that the results justified the continuation of these difficult researches. We are still too far from anything like precise knowledge as regards the frequency or speed of certain elementary psychological processes. Vibro-massage facilitates the treatment of certain spasms and contractures, especially abdominal spasms and contractures. Furthermore, as Dubois (of Saujon) has pointed out, when applied to the head it may benumb the patient a little, may fix his attention, and

---

[1] Les mouvements méthodiques, etc., p. 432.
[2] " Medical News," January 1898.
[3] " Semaine Médicale, July 20, 1892.

may predispose him to accept certain suggestions more readily. It is difficult to say any more in favour of the method than this. Light, climate, and high altitudes, may also exercise a certain effect ; but, inasmuch as exact psychological studies upon these matters are still lacking, it is not easy to arrive at precise indications for their use.

The foregoing account of the psychophysiological methods which may play a part in the treatment of nervous and mental disorders has been cursory and incomplete. My aim merely was to show that psychotherapy must not ignore such methods. I wish to insist that we must recognise them to be important additions to our armamentarium. It is a matter for regret that our studies concerning the treatment of vasomotor disturbances, concerning the modifications in the activity of the endocrine glands, and concerning various forms of intoxication, are still in an elementary stage. When we know more of such matters, we shall certainly be able to turn them to valuable account for psychotherapeutic purposes.

CHAPTER SIXTEEN

MORAL GUIDANCE

ALL the special methods of psychotherapeutics we have been studying under the names of suggestion, moral disinfection, rest, isolation, reeducation, and excitation, were successive outgrowths from the general methods of religious and moralising treatment whose importance was expounded in the first part of this book. Are we to suppose that these newer methods of treatment have completely exhausted the therapeutic influences which belonged to the older methods of moralisation ? May it not be that these earlier methods contained a residue which has not yet been properly analysed, an important therapeutic influence which has not yet been isolated ? It is possible that we shall disclose a residual effect of this kind when we study the moral guidance of our patients.

I. HISTORY OF MORAL GUIDANCE.

When studying the earlier methods of mental and moral treatment we noted how important a part was played by the individuality of the psychotherapist. His success did not depend to a notable extent upon the psychological method he employed (and employed in a very vague way) ; for it depended mainly upon the essential fact that the method, whatever it might be, was used by a particular individual, always for each case the same individual, who acted upon the subject throughout a considerable period. In our analyses of the various methods, both of excitation and of suggestion, we were considering the essential character of the psychological phenomenon which the psychotherapeutist was attempting to produce, without paying any particular attention to his individuality. It is now proper to point out that a good many authors have been exclusively interested in this personal point of view, that they have made this individual action of the doctor the foundation of a special therapeutic method.

In the organisation of religious houses, a great place has always been allotted to the personality of the Superior ; and the old systems of morality, such as Stoicism, recognised the importance of the director of the conscience.[1] The Catholic faith was not content with instituting the confessional, for the Church advised the faithful to avoid constantly changing their father confessors, and it perfected the notion of the director of the conscience. Ignatius Loyola, Francis of Sales, Bossuet, and Fénelon (from whom in an earlier work I have quoted freely)[2] were well aware of the importance of continuity in the treatment of over-scrupulous persons, who were much better guided when in the hands of a confessor who had had them under his care for a long time.

In an earlier work [3] I analysed the remarkable phenomenon which the magnetisers described under the name of " magnetic rapport." These forerunners of psychotherapeutics allowed for the importance of the personal factor in the guidance of their somnambulists, but they expressed their recognition in a rather strange way, using the terminology of their theory of fluids. They were familiar with the phenomenon of electivity ; of the sensibility, the ready obedience, which the subject displayed towards the one by whom he had frequently been magnetised, and they attributed this peculiarity to a special fluid proper to the magnetiser, a fluid which had permeated the subject. They expressly forbade the mingling of influences and of fluids, and a good magnetiser would not allow any one else to make passes over his chosen subject.[4] They knew by experience that in the treatment of these patients a serious difficulty would often arise when it became necessary to change the magnetiser of a subject who had been impregnated by the fluid emanating from that magnetiser. We must not be too ready to laugh at the simplicity of this terminology. In our own practice to-day, we shall come across kindred facts, although we shall describe them in other terms.

---

[1] Constant Martha, Sénèque directeur de conscience, Les moralistes sous l'empire romain, 1864.
[2] Les obsessions et la psychasthénie, 1903, vol. i, p. 707.
[3] L'influence somnambulique et le besoin de direction, Névroses et idées fixes, 1898, vol. i, p. 423.
[4] Deleuze, Instruction pratique sur le magnétisme animal, 1825, p. 109.

The moralisers who, like Paul Dubois, seemed to attach importance only to reason and to the inculcation of a stoical morality, have in practice availed themselves also of their personal influence. They recommend that the doctor should attend his patient regularly in order to understand the patient better, and in order by prolonged association to develop the sympathy which is indispensable to the treatment. Dejerine was merely adopting Dubois's ideas and expressing them with greater precision when he said : " For me the foundation, the only foundation, upon which psychotherapeutics rests is the beneficent influence of one human being upon another. We do not cure a hysteric, we do not cure a neurasthenic, we do not change their mental condition, by reasoning or by syllogisms. We only cure them when they come to have faith in us. I am, in fact, convinced that in the moral domain no idea finds acceptance when it is cold, that is to say, when it lacks the emotional stress which leads the conscience to accept it and which arouses conviction." [1]

In some of my earlier books, those published from 1896 to 1903, I insisted in various ways upon the personal influence of the doctor, and upon the part which this influence plays in the treatment of nervous disorders. " We must transform this guidance into a profession which is consciously practised ; and which was practised unwittingly in former days by those who came into contact with the patient, or else was reserved for the use of his religious directors. . . . It is one of the characteristics of our own day that this task of moral guidance is sometimes incumbent upon the doctor when the patient does not find enough natural support in his customary associates." [2]

Ideas of this kind, moreover, are to be met with in most works on psychotherapeutics. De Fleury insisted upon the need of a tutor for the mind, " a moral tutor, like the material tutor [stake] requisite for certain plants ; " and he insisted that we must meticulously regulate the use which our patients made of their time,[3] Putnam, in his lectures at the Lowell

---

[1] Dejerine, Les manifestations fonctionnelles des psychonévroses, 1911, p. ix.
[2] Le traitement psychologique de l'hystérie ; L'influence somnambulique et le besoin de direction, Congrès de Psychologie de Munich, 1896 ; " Revue Philosophique," February 1897, p. 113 ; Névroses et idées fixes, 1898, vol. i, p. 423 ; Les obsessions et la psychasthénie, 1903, vol. i, p. 708.
[3] De Fleury, Introduction à la médecine de l'esprit, 1897, p. 281.

Institute in the year 1905, said very aptly that the habit of obeying an authority, always the same authority, helped the patient to rid himself of the dangers of hesitation and doubt. " The doctor," said Deschamps, " has only one essential thing to do, to make himself the friendly and loyal guide, the impartial director, of the neurasthenic, to teach the patient to know himself and to make the best possible use of the defective instrument with which nature has endowed him." [1]   In another work the same author speaks of treatment by confidence and sympathy. ": The doctor must exercise influence by all possible means ;   above all he must understand each patient, and must have the tact which will enable him to do his best for each patient. The patient needs this guidance that he may be helped to complete the psychological operations of which he feels himself incapable." [2]

Grasset wishes the doctor to guide the neuropath's whole life. He even aims at the prophylaxis of the neuroses, for this is to be achieved by arranging that the doctor shall supervise marriages, shall guide sexual unions and births, so that in this way a social defence against nervous disorders shall be organised.[3] Lewellys F. Barker, in his book *On the psychic Treatment of some of the functional Neuroses* (1906), tells us that, while we may begin our treatment with the medical absolutism which does not leave the patient any freedom, his own aim is in most instances, and by degrees, to cultivate in the patient a certain amount of "self-direction " ; but he does not hesitate to admit that in some cases the medical guidance of the patient must last throughout the latter's life. It would be easy to multiply quotations of this kind, for the idea of the medical guidance of neuropaths has found general acceptance in recent works on psychotherapeutics.

Nevertheless, it is easy to see the inadequacy of such conceptions. The doctor wants to replace, as far as these patients are concerned, the natural head of the family, or the priest. He does so, simply because he believes himself to understand rather better the morbid symptoms of the disease. But does that suffice ? Is the doctor also equipped with the principles and rules according to which this guidance can be

[1] Deschamps, Les maladies de l'énergie, 1908, p. 314.
[2] Deschamps, Le rapport psycho-moteur, " Paris Médical," June 1912.
[3] Grasset, Prophylaxie individuelle, familiale et sociale, " Revue des Idées," 1906, p. 161

practised in different cases ? Such a contention is open to doubt, for the doctor must, as Deschamps says, appeal to "tact," that is to say, to an acquired but unformulated experience, which is supposed to come to his aid under the inspiration of the moment ; he must appeal to sympathy and to devotion. All this is not very reassuring for the patient, for it seems that the head of the family or the priest could do the same thing just as well. It would be better if the doctor could rely upon an exact psychological knowledge of the phenomena of guidance—but unfortunately this pscyhological knowledge can hardly be said as yet to exist. Here we reach the crux of psychotherapeutics, which can only acquire superior rights in this matter of guidance when it can base the claim to such rights upon science. The science in question is still embryonic. In the hope that I may contribute my quota to this psychology of the future, I here give a few summary observations upon the results and the nature of the moral guidance of neuropaths.

2. Chance Guidance.

Here, once more, we must take as our starting-point the improvement of the cure which is brought about accidentally by certain circumstances in which the subject is temporarily placed, and also the impulses which drive the patient to seek the influence which he himself feels to be requisite.

One detail has struck me when I have been recording the pathological history of persons suffering from psychasthenic disorders. A great many of them, after having suffered from serious symptoms in early youth and up to the age of twenty, exhibited a marked remission, an apparent cure, towards the age of twenty-one, and during the years spent in military service.—A man of thirty-five, who at the present time has been suffering from a remarkable phobia, " the dread of his wife's eyes," and who at the age of sixteen became affected with agoraphobia, then with the phobia of isolation, the mania of forebodings, etc., himself declares that the only time his mind was really tranquil was when he was with his regiment at the age of twenty-one. " There can be no doubt that military discipline suited me, for I was quite at ease in the barracks. I dreaded nothing there, and I never incurred any reprimands.

The improvement actually lasted for some time after my term of service was over, and I believed that I had been delivered from my follies. But before long, when I was living a free life once more, the troubles recurred."—Almost exactly the same remarks could be made in the case of Vd. (m. 29), suffering from severe abulia, morbid timidity, and all kinds of phobias. The trouble began when he was still in the higher school, with crises of stammering and erythrophobia ; but he was perfectly well during his term of military service, being then free from disorders of the will, stammering, and phobias.— Ak. (m., 32) is at the present time suffering from the phobia of fatigue, and he had had the same trouble at the age of nineteen ; but he is amazed to recall that he was free from this symptom for several years. " It is a strange thing. I was able to make long marches when I was with the regiment. I suppose it was because I was marching in the ranks with the others."—Jc. (m., 26), over-scrupulous and phobic, who when he is left to himself can never walk along the roadway, but must clamber along the bank at the side or even in the ditch (because he is troubled by all sorts of strange thoughts), could walk straight ahead without difficulty when he was with the regiment, and was then not afraid of anything. He was extremely distressed when his term of service was over, and hastened to a seminary " in order to have chiefs once more, and to be subject to discipline." We are astonished to learn that persons who are undecided, timorous, and hypochondriacal, were in their time excellent soldiers, who never objected to any duty however fatiguing. This improvement in the general activity during the period of military service, which is recorded in my notes on fourteen cases, seems to me very characteristic. It takes us by a short cut into the study of guidance, inasmuch as it shows us the favourable effect of discipline.

I have just referred to the case of a psychasthenic who, when he had to leave the barracks, took refuge in a seminary, and continued to feel fairly well there. It seems probable that if we had accurate information concerning the mental life of the dwellers in convents, we should find that in former days a great many sufferers from severe psychasthenia found a refuge in these religious houses, and were comparatively well there. Indeed, we have evidence of this to-day in the lamentations of some of our patients who have left convents.—

Az. (f., 31), who was five years in a convent, found the place very much to her taste, and felt well there. " I do so like to have fixed hours for everything, so that there is no change from day to day. It troubles me to have to settle things for myself. What I need is a Mother Superior who decides everything for me."

From time to time, though rarely I regret to say, there become established in the ordinary world associations between a patient and a healthy and energetic individual, who undertakes the guidance of the patient and who keeps his associate in order. This is what happens in a great many families in the case of the younger children. Often enough the onset of the neuroses is checked by the beneficial influence exerted by one of the parents. That is why we so frequently see such troubles arise after the parent's death. Unfortunately this guidance, this moral direction, by the father or by the mother, grows more difficult when the son or the daughter reaches the age of twenty or more ; but in some cases the influence continues long after this age.—Ah. (f., 37) was still under her mother's guidance at the age of thirty-five, and the patient did not become obviously psychasthenic until her mother died.—The same thing happened in the case of Fg. (f., 36).—I have seen it in many other patients who had remained little children in relation to the father or to the mother, and who did not break down until after the parent's death.

We often see the same thing in married life. It is true that marriage to one of these neuropaths is apt to be disastrous. The healthy member of the pair grows disgusted and runs away ; or becomes exhausted, and is contaminated in his or her turn (as we have seen in a foregoing chapter), although the patient derives no particular advantage. But in certain cases, and where special circumstances are operative, things run a different course. For some years, the healthy member of the pair seems to have sufficient energy to impose a discipline, and then, unwittingly as a rule, he cures the partner. No doubt in the cases that come under our observation, things have turned out badly in the end, for the patient is not brought to us unless the guide has lost his power or has abandoned his task. But we must not forget the years during which the patient secured tranquillity and happiness under this influence .

and we must not forget that there must be a good many cases that never come under medical observation, the reason being that an adequate balance is maintained throughout life.

It would be well to study some examples of this conjugal guidance.—In the household of Wo., the husband kept his wife well in hand for four years, and was able to check her crises of over-scrupulousness. After that, the wife needed medical care for a year, but then the husband was able to resume her guidance without much difficulty.—In the Fv. household, the wife, who had always been weakly and inclined to phobias, was guided fairly well as long as her husband was vigorous, and her symptoms only became serious when the husband grew old and became himself affected with cerebral troubles. "I can hardly say that I loved my husband," said this woman ; "but he was good, and kept me in order. He was indispensable to me. Before I married I was under the domination of my mother, and from that I passed under the sway of my husband. I needed guidance. When he was away for a little while, I counted the hours with despair. Now he has failed me, and I feel myself in the void like an uprooted tree."—Similar remarks might be made in the case of a good many other married women.

In the Ka. household, on the other hand, it is the wife who, with a great deal of difficulty and after a struggle which lasted for years, has gained the dominion over her husband, who is abulic, unstable, restless, and jealous. She has made life tolerable to him to this extent, that he can no longer get on without her.—Gac. (m., 27) has lived happily for years under his wife's guidance, and it is only because she has left him that he has relapsed and is once more good for nothing.— Ui. (f., 45) sadly relates how she found it necessary to transform herself, to gain will power, and to manage everything in the household. "I did this because I saw that my husband was afraid of everything. Now, I have myself broken down, but I was able to manage him for many years."

Sometimes, of course, we find a similar association in the group formed by a lover and his mistress. Consider, for instance, the remarkable case of Gri. This woman of thirty is now in a very poor condition. She is a morphinomaniac, a cocaine addict, obsessed with ideas of suicide and a prey to manias of interrogation, inert and loose-living. In youth, she was in a similar condition for a time, and a medical student rescued her from a sordid place where she stupefied herself with absinthe in order to forget her dread of death. He made her his mistress, but he took a serious view of his part and showed himself " tender and exacting." He cut off the poisons, and organised her life for her. " Everything went on perfectly for five years. I lived properly, was happy, was good for something, for he was satisfied with me." When her lover was compelled to leave her, all her troubles began anew.— Tkm. (f., 39) had been the mistress of a man " of a high type and a tyrannical temperament." This man played a great part in her life. " For six years, he made it impossible for me to think of anything but himself." When she had to separate from him, she lived a disorderly life and became troubled with thoughts of suicide.—Vh. (f., 45) had to conceal her liaison with a lover whom she adored. " The situation was complicated and difficult. He was a master, and made me suffer, but how much I regret my lost sufferings." When her lover died, she did not know how to live without him and became affected with all kinds of hypochondriacal obsessions.

Bs. (m., 41) has been admirably guided by his mistress, who has not only been able " to make him experience sensations, which no other woman had succeeded in doing," but has also been able to make him throw off his inertia, do some literary work, believe that he had a certain literary value. It is a pity that she took a dislike to this profession of psychotherapeutist, and that she wanted a rest, for since then he has no longer been able to " feel anything," but has become afraid of everything ; and he spends his life in a state of despair, continually exclaiming " I am alone ! alone ! alone ! "—We see exactly the same thing in the case of Nl. (m., 30). His parents made a grave mistake when they compelled him, a young fellow of weak character, to withdraw from a liaison with an intelligent and capable woman, in order to marry a young girl who, like himself, was of weak character, and who had had no experience in managing men. The result is that he has become depressed and is affected with all kinds of algias, digestive troubles, enteritis, etc. He is perfectly aware what remedy he needs, saying : " I would rather go back to my mistress than have to spend years in sanatoria."—Ji. (m., 32) appears to be suffering from a strange disorder. For several months at a time he will give full satisfaction to his family because he works intelligently, is good-humoured, and in excellent health. Then he suddenly passes into a state of depression, which may last for several months, being now tormented by phobias and incapable of doing anything besides treat his enteritis. His doctor talks gravely of " cyclothymia," and is well pleased with himself for having discovered a name that explains everything. For my part, I think that this fine term does not apply, for I am in the patient's confidence, and I know the real root of the mischief. He has a love affair with " a little woman who will sometimes care for her big baby, and sometimes grows tired of him."

We encounter similar phenomena in other sorts of association than these sexual partnerships. Often enough, in contrast with what may be regarded as the natural law, we find that a son or a daughter may be the prop of one of the parents. The case of Madame X. is amusing. She is fifty-three years of age, but says " I have never been able, and never shall be able, to live without my son." She had her first grave crisis of depression when the son was called up for military service, and she recovered her reason when he came back. Every time that he has to go away for a few months she has a serious relapse. Furthermore, at these times, her bodily health suffers no less than her mental health, so that she becomes extremely emaciated when her son is away ; but she can get on with her ordinary work and grows fat once more as soon as he comes home.—The history of Zy. (f., 45) is exactly the same.—Lh. (f., 46) used to live with a nephew whom she had adopted, " on whose behalf she made an effort to live." When her nephew had to leave her it became necessary to send her to an asylum.

In other cases, as in that of the Xl. family, we find that the patient receives the necessary guidance from a sister.—The case of Léa and Lydia, to which I have repeatedly had occasion to refer, is extremely interesting in this connexion. They are twins, and both suffer from psychasthenic depression, but Lydia is much worse than Léa. As I have already related, a grave mistake was made in marrying off Léa before Lydia, and in suddenly breaking up their intimate association. In spite of immense difficulties, it was found absolutely essential for the two young women to run a joint household, so that, although they were married, they could continue to live to-gether. Even now, though Lydia is forty, she cannot get along without the constant aid of her sister.—Similar is the case of Ig. (m., 36), who falls sick if he is separated from his brother, although these brothers are not twins.—To the same category belongs the case of Km. (m., 30) who used to be guided by his sister and who succumbed to an obsession of jealousy when she married.

In certain cases, as in that of Aj. (f., 37), I was able to note that a priest, to whom the patient confessed frequently, was able to guide successfully for several years a patient who without this aid would have been very difficult to manage. Such instances must be common, for there can be no doubt that psychasthenics are numerous among those who go regularly to confession. Abbé Eymieu's writings show that in his priestly work he has acquired a certain amount of experience of these patients.[1] Nuns, schoolmistresses, nurses, and masseuses, often find it necessary to play this part of guide, and in a dozen of my cases I find that such persons had been able to guide the patient very successfully for years. In most of these cases, the patients' parents had been greatly distressed by the situation. They regarded it as abnormal, and they were afraid that the patient, a young woman, being subject to " undue influence," would hand over all her fortune to the schoolmistress or other guide. Such fears are not unfounded. The danger certainly exists in cases of chance guidance ; and I shall have to return to the topic presently. But it is none the less true, if we look at the matter purely from the medical outlook, that the guidance is an excellent thing, and that the discontinuance of it may give rise to serious disturbance. Be-sides, the danger in question occurs in other circumstances.— Ba. (m., 50) passed completely under the influence of an able practitioner of Christian Science. It was not, as might be imagined, a domination effected through the influence of love. The woman's only interest was in talking to her patient about philosophical problems, occupying his mind, setting him to work, and, above all, persuading him that he was a great man whose genius had remained unrecognised. These things sufficed to relieve his sufferings and to dispel his delusions ; but it also enabled the Christian Science practitioner to plunder him

[1] Eymieu, Le gouvernement de soi-même, 2 vols, 1906 and 1910.

shamefully, and to ruin him—to the despair of his wife and his
children, whom he abandoned without any prick of conscience.
—A woman of forty-five passed wholly under the influence of
the nurse who had cared for her when she was staying in a
sanatorium and who became her companion when she left
the institution. The influence exercised by this sometime
nurse was dangerous no doubt, but it had its beneficial side.—
A good many patients, like Clarisse, were transformed for
years through the companionship of some particular nurse,
and relapsed when the nurse had to leave them.—Similar
associations sometimes exist between two friends. Cxc.
(m., 30) lived for years in a condition of comparative tranquillity
in intimate association with a friend " who guided him without
being aware that he was doing so."—Daniel (m., 41), tormented
by all kinds of doubts, superstitions, and mental manias,
passed his days regretting the period during which a young
man in whose company he spent most of his time, had dis-
coursed to him about the positivist philosophy and had dispelled
as if by a miracle all his apprehensions. " Why cannot I
again find a friend who can have the same power over me."—
Emma, to whose case I have frequently referred, was directed
for a long time by an old lady who had conceived a friendship
for her. It was when this lady became disquieted by some
of Emma's symptoms, and was afraid to assume responsibility for the patient any longer, that the latter's illness grew
serious.

The most remarkable of all such cases is when the association is between two patients who seem, in real life, to
illustrate the parable of the blind man and the paralytic. I
have notes of three such couples.—I have already published
that of Ai. (f., 43). She was abulic, a sufferer from doubts,
and affected by the phobia of contact, so that she was no longer
able to touch any of the toilet requisites, and was therefore
exceedingly uncleanly. When she was about thirty years
old she met a sometime schoolmate, who was likewise depressed
and abulic, the trouble in this case taking the form of obsession
with thoughts of death and suicide. The two women ex-
changed confidences, each of them inclining to make good-
humoured fun of the other's fancied miseries. As a result they
both had their spirits marvellously raised, and were tranquillised for several days. This experience led them to set

up a joint household, and for ten years they lived together with considerable success, each being a support to the other. Then the tittle-tattle of some servants made them uneasy about the purity of their relationship, and they decided to break off the connexion. Thereupon they both of them became so seriously ill, that the only thing I could do was to dispel their scruples and to persuade them to join forces once more.

When we carefully study the whole history of a patient who comes to consult us because of some serious neuropathic trouble, we shall usually find that there have been periods when the patient improved greatly, and it is our business to study such periods no less carefully than the periods when the patient was very ill. We must not be content to say of a patient whose illness is periodic that, of necessity, he or she is restored to health now and again in virtue of a " periodic law." The notion of periodicity does apply to certain cases, but much more rarely than doctors are apt to suppose. We make a great mistake, if we allow this theory, like the old geological theory of cataclysms, to save us the trouble of searching out causes—and causes still at work. Among the causes which have played a notable part in the evolution of neuropathic disorder, we must always give the first place to social causes. Very often, as we have seen, society, the intercourse with habitual associates, will be a cause of grave relapse. But we must not overlook the converse cases, in which improvement, and even what is tantamount to a cure for a long period, may be the outcome of social influences, and in especial of domination or guidance. No doubt in many of these cases such domination or guidance has been accidental, involuntary, and sometimes unwitting—but it may have been most efficacious none the less.

3. OBSESSIONS OF GUIDANCE.

We have seen that in certain cases our patients' obsessions and impulses appear to be the expression of needs, morbid no doubt and badly interpreted, but nevertheless real ; and we have realised that such obsessions and impulses can furnish us with useful indications. In this connexion, where guidance is concerned, we encounter all kinds of extremely characteristic obsessions and impulses. We are brought back once more to obsessions of love, to the need for being loved, which we have again and again had to consider, since it plays so large a part in the sufferings of neuropaths As far as this matter is concerned I must be content to refer the reader to what has already been said about such obsessions, and shall merely consider them in connexion with the need for guidance

The simplest of the obsessions we have to deal with among the obsessions of guidance are the obsessions of regret which trouble patients who for a long time have been benefited by guidance, and who have then lost this guidance. Such disturbances arise after the death or the departure of parents, a husband, or a child, when one or other of these has played the part of director.—We think of the lamentations of Bs. (m., 41), who cries : " Alone ! alone ! alone ! "—Or we think of the lamentations of Ci. (f., 60) after the death of her husband : " Alone I can only do stupid things ; but my husband used to prevent my doing them, or would put things right when I had done them.   How can such a woman as I possibly live alone ? " —To give another example, I may refer to the distressing condition of Noémi during the war, when her husband had been called to the front.   No doubt her husband, when he was with her, did not seem to play a very important part, for she was already tormented by numerous obsessions and did not appear to notice his presence much ; but when he had been called away she realised how important he had been to her. She became absolutely incapable of doing anything ; she neglected her children and her household, and lived in utter disorder. She was perpetually thinking of the dreadful risks run by her husband ; her mind turned always to scenes of massacre, and to images of his death.   She pondered what she would have to do when she had been widowed.   She exhausted herself by impotent efforts, and was constantly weeping and wailing.   " I simply cannot get on without my husband ; it is impossible.   Already I had noticed that I felt completely lost if he were away for only a few days during the holidays.   How could I possibly go on living after his death.   He is the only person who understands my strange, fantastic, wayward, and affectionate nature.   He only can treat me like a child, and enable me to live.   I know that I should get well again at once if he should come back."   The serious character of the symptoms showed how important guidance had been to her, how much aid her husband had really given her.

We may class under the same head the " disillusionments of guidance," an understanding of which will enable us to explain certain forms of the " pathology of conjugal life." Eia. (m., 49) was for years sustained by his wife's devotion. When the wife died, he completely lost his moorings for a time, but he soon recovered when he became filled with the hope of replacing her.   He fell in love with a young woman of twenty-five, and was convinced that she could give him the moral guidance that he had lost.   On her side, this young woman, being herself a neuropath and extremely depressible, imagined that Eia., so much older than herself, would be the good director whom she needed.   When they married and came to live together, both were speedily reduced to despair.   " This man is absolutely no help to me," said the young wife.   " He can only repeat everything that I say.   If I smile, he smiles ; if I frown, he frowns.   He will not take any responsibility. He runs after me all the time ; but I cannot live near him, it will drive me crazy."   In actual fact, she grows frenzied, is intensely agitated, and has severe fits of hysterics.   The husband, for his part, is terrified by this young woman.   " She is no use to me at all in my difficulties.   She increases my responsibilities instead of diminishing them.   She frightens me by her fits of hysterics and fills me with remorse.   I must get away from her as soon as possible.   I must feel assured that I shall never see her again, for otherwise I shall go absolutely out of my mind."   Thus both became seriously ill, and each of them began to suffer from obsessions and delusions relating to the other.   The illness was the result of the lack of guidance, and of the regret at having failed to find what had been hoped for.

Other kinds of obsession may develop when the patients still have their director, but are afraid of losing him or her.   This is one of the causes of the obsessions of mono-polisation and of jealousy which we have studied in con-nexion with the need for excitation.   To the examples already considered, we may add that of Cora (f., 35), whose jealousy was concerned more with this matter of guidance than with love properly so-called, or with the need for excitation.   " It is not that I am so passionately fond of my husband. In many respects he is indifferent to me. But I am incapable of acting by myself and without his aid. As soon as he is away, when he is not there to say to me ' do this or do that,' I do nothing at all. I move restlessly about the room, which no longer seems to be my room ; after a time I go out and roam about the streets until he comes back. He is indispensable to my life ; that is why I am filled with terror when I think of how he may become interested in some one else, and leave me all alone. I must have some one to look after me, must have a good watch-dog."

A girl of thirteen, daughter of a man who is himself hereditarily tainted, manifests at this early age serious psychasthenic symptoms, and is terribly jealous. " Do look at me, Mother. When you look at another girl, you are not interested in me and what I am doing. How can you expect that I shall go on doing it ? Do look at me, Mother ! " The study of these various needs for excitation, for guidance, the study of doubt and disquietude, will enable us to win more accurate knowledge of the psychology of the various forms of jealousy.

Even more interesting obsessions arise in patients who have no guide, and who are perpetually tormented by the longing to find one. " I need to be ruled, sustained ; I do not want to be left to act freely."—" I need to obey some one, I need to be guided, to be ordered about as one orders a servant, to be driven like a machine."—" I want the help of a friendly will ; I am quite at a loose end ; I need moral support."— " I am continually wanting to talk to some one, to confide in some one, to be guided by some one."—" I am always like a child which has not learned how to stand upright ; I still need to have a mother that I may ask what dress I ought to put on."—" I need to live in the shade of some one."—" I feel the utmost need of strong direction, a thing I have always lacked. If I had been religious-minded, and had had a good confessor, I should have got along well enough."—" Here I am, old enough to be a grandmother, and yet I am still a child, needing to be chided and guided by some one."—Such phrases are familiar in the experience of those who have to do with patients of the kind.

These patients go still further. They tell us in precise terms what they need. They want the guidance to be effected

in a particular way ; it must be accurately defined and firm ;
but at the same time it must be gentle and skilful.—" These
people think they can guide me, but they do not know what
guidance really is, how clear and definite it must be. When I
am taking food, what I need is that some one should say :
' Eat this ; eat that ; now you have had enough.' When I
am offered potatoes, what I need is that some one should say
to me : ' These are potatoes.' When I ought to drink, some
one must say to me : ' Now then, it is time to have something
to drink.'—" It is not enough simply to give me orders. The
orders must be given with firmness and energy. Here, people
are not strict enough with me, and that is why they cannot
do me any good."—" It is no use being strict with me. I
only accept guidance when people are gentle with me ; they
can do nothing with me unless they are gentle and are interested
in me. I must be guided tactfully ; must be given orders
without being annoyed, and without my being made to feel
that I am being ordered about. I need that the one who is
to guide me shall realise my half-formed wishes, shall try to
make me do what I myself really want to do, and not try to
constrain me to do something I am reluctant to do. Why
should I be deprived of the pleasure of doing something on
my own account, or at least of fancying I am doing it on my
own account ? How clumsy these people are."

It is obvious that if all these demands are to be satisfied,
the guide must have remarkable qualities. Our patients
are well aware of the fact.—" If the person who directs me has
no more energy than I have myself, we shall get nowhere,
and it would be futile for me to give myself up to his guidance.
I want an ideal friend, a profound philosopher who will have
sufficient authority to be a moral guide ; he must also know
how to guide me when I am amusing myself. He must,
therefore, have very varied qualities."—" I am in despair
because I am alone in the world like a dog without a collar.
I have not only lost my shadow, but have lost my very self.
I can only exist as the reflexion of an imposing personality."—
" What I need is a man of genius as my guide, some one of
outstanding intelligence and inexhaustible energy ; some one
who is sincere and who is disinterested ; some one who is
actually in my life and not outside it."—Many of these patients,
above all when the need for guidance is not intense, add that

they wish to be loved for their own sakes, and this, as we have
already learned in an earlier chapter, means that they do not
wish to pay anything in return for the services rendered. But,
in many instances, this is nothing more than an appearance.
What they really want is that they may be delivered from the
effort of having to make any return, that they may rest assured
that the guidance will be continued even if they do nothing
to deserve it. But in practice they are too much afraid of
being abandoned, and they make all sorts of efforts, many of
them absurd efforts, in order to gain or to keep the master
they have chosen.

That is the origin of the impulses to attract attention,
the attention of some particular person ; and that is the origin
of the various manias of coquetry. The patients try to arouse
interest by all sorts of grimaces, prayers, and flatteries. " I
became a little medicant, begging for affection, reproaches,
and orders." This, likewise, is the origin of the mania for
giving presents, and the mania for devotion, whose effects
upon the associates we have previously discussed. " I should
like to be some one's good angel." But these manias are somewhat different from the others we have just been considering.
The devotion is no longer perpetual and general ; it is solely
addressed to one particular person, who is apt to find it a
nuisance.

Impulses that appear to be religious have the same origin.
A genuine religious sentiment, the worship of a superior being
who is at once chief, father, and the ideal object of love, is
closely akin to these needs for being guided and loved. I
hope some day to publish a more detailed study of a remarkable
ecstatic whose case I have already described under the name
of Madeleine.[1] I shall then endeavour to show how psychasthenic doubts and scruples have, in this patient, induced a
religious mania. But the study of the case now would take
us too far from our present topic. Enough here to mention
the patients who go from one church to another in search of
" an ideal confessor " ; or those who think they have found such
an ideal confessor, and who plague the unfortunate priest
with their exactions. I have notes of six such cases. One
woman actually entered a convent in the hope of finding in

[1] Une extatique, ' Bulletin de l'Institut Psychique International,"
1900–1901, p. 209.

the Mother Superior some one who would be simultaneously gentle and firm, and who would support her mind effectively. " But," said the patient, " the Mother Superior is a great lady who is quite unapproachable, and who sends me to the confessor ; and he is so stupid as to fancy I have no vocation." This woman persecutes the Mother Superior, declaring that it is the latter's duty to guide the nuns.

Sometimes, the patients go even further. Although they are, in general, of a miserly disposition, and are full of dreads for the future, they will make expensive presents, will sacrifice their fortune and the fortune of their relatives, in order to keep with them at any cost a music mistress, a maid, a governess, or a masseuse. This is the starting-point of these dangerous impulses, so much dreaded by the patient's relatives.

In many cases, such impulses have a deceptive appearance, making us believe that there is considerable sexual excitement. Numerous errors arise in this way. Young girls who are continually dreaming of caresses, and who spend their lives in awaiting " the footstep of a lover on the stair," are not always true lovers.—" What especially troubles me is the emotion of being alone, the sentiment that I am not under some one's protection. I have so great a need to lean upon some one, I feel such a sense of vacancy in life, and that is why I am always waiting for love."—In such conditions, a great many patients make ridiculous marriages, or give themselves to lovers, or behave in an altogether shameless way (so it seems).—A young woman of nineteen, being in despair because a headmistress to whom she was greatly attached had gone away, flung herself into the arms of a young man, and simulated a violent passion.—Many such women, though they seem utterly shameless, must not be confounded with those who, like Pepita, are really in search of sexual excitation and sexual adventures ; they have no strong sensibilities, are little interested in love affairs, and are afraid of risks.—" But how else can I manage to secure that some one shall take an interest in me, shall give me the impression that he is a superior being ; how else can I find some one to whom I can entrust my soul, since I cannot entrust it to myself ? "

In my first study concerning the need for guidance, to which I refer the reader, I gave various examples of dangerous situations into which the patient was precipitated by this need for a master. At the close of that study I mentioned the remarkable case of a patient who, although she remained sane, had all her life a fixed longing to be cared for in an asylum, under the observation of an alienist. She was continually trying to get herself put under restraint, and feigned madness so well that she succeeded in the end. "Here," she said, "I know quite well that I shall not be allowed to do anything stupid. Consequently, I no longer bother myself about such matters, but sleep soundly and am happy. I need to be strictly guided. I need to be behind bars."—Others, instead of trying to take refuge in an asylum, will accept, will seek for, the most debasing slavery, in the most abominable places, simply in order that they may feel themselves constantly "subjected to a powerful influence."—In the same category we may class the manias for hypnotism which were especially frequent at one time. A good many women (I have five such cases among my notes), sacrificed everything for years in order to be again and again hypnotised by a person of doubtful character, but on whom they had become absolutely dependent. "I am lost unless there is some one who is interested in me in this way." Thus the need for guidance will assume a different form at different times.

I need not lay any more stress upon obsessions of this kind, for I have frequently described them before, and they are closely akin to the other varieties of obsession with love. The starting-point of all such obsessions and sentiments, however diversified they may seem, is a phenomenon analogous to the vertigo that seizes certain people in mountainous regions. One who is subject to vertigo can, in reality, walk readily enough, but he must not deviate from the path, must not take any false step. Being overwhelmed by the dread of deviating from the path, by the dread of taking false steps, he finds himself, in the end, unable to walk at all. But if there is a solid parapet beside the path, or a strong bannister of the staircase, such a person can walk well enough, and is free from vertigo. For the sort of patients I have been describing, the husband, the friend, the director, plays the part of the bannister, whose presence relieves them of the sense of vertigo which affects them in life. That explains the power of this urge for guidance. Furthermore, these considerations show that the feeling is not an absurd one. A strong bannister enables us to go freely up and down the stairs, and we can readily infer from a study of the foregoing cases that guidance was often extremely useful to these patients.

4. STATES OF INFLUENCE.

It is important to note, strange as the fact may seem, that kindred phenomena can often be witnessed during psychotherapeutic treatment. We must not imagine that such methods of treatment always run a regular course. Their effect is constantly modified by some influence foreign to the therapeutic method per se. The effects are modified by the influence of the operator, and by the influence of the time for which the operator has acted upon the subject. These facts gravely affect psychotherapeutic practice, and make it very different from any physical therapeutic method. Sodium sulphate always purges the patient, whoever has prescribed it or administered it. On the other hand, the suggestion to walk will cure a paralytic if it be made by Dr. X., and will have no effect at all if it be made by Dr. Y. The reason why many observers refuse to admit that such practices have a scientific value, is that they do not make a proper allowance for personal influence. A law is not invalidated by the fact that its applications are conditional. If we want to learn exactly how the law works, we must make ourselves fully acquainted with the conditions ; that is all. Personal influence plays a part in all psychotherapeutic methods. If we wish to understand it, we must see how it works in this or that treatment, in suggestion, in aesthesiogenism, in treatment by excitation. Elsewhere, in my study of somnambulist influence and the need for guidance, I have given a detailed description of some of these phenomena.[1] Enough, here, to summarise what I said in that book, and to adduce a few additional examples.

Although we have abandoned the ideas of the magnetisers concerning the potency of the fluid they supposed themselves to emit, we know perfectly well that certain persons can readily hypnotise predisposed patients, whereas others are unable to hypnotise them. What is clear is that an individual who has frequently been hypnotised by some particular person, will pass into a hypnotic state at the slightest hint from this

[1] Névroses et idées fixes, 1898, vol. i, p. 423.

person, and will nevertheless resist for an indefinite time attempts made by another person to hypnotise him. It may well be that we are concerned here with particular suggestions (the matter will have to be discussed), but the fact has great importance none the less.

Let me remark, first of all, that we see similar phenomena in connexion with suggestion without hypnotism. Suggestion is not an immutable phenomenon, which can be induced at will, simply because the subject is suggestible. Save in exceptional cases, and in persons who are seriously ill, the effect of a suggestion will vary enormously according as one person or another makes it. I am not speaking only of experimental electivity, when the hypnotist is able to secure an obedience which a stranger cannot secure ; I am speaking of therapeutic suggestions conveyed under the best possible conditions. In the present book we have studied the effect of suggestion in a remarkable case of contracture of the trunk. No. (f., 40), who had been cured twenty years earlier of extreme contracture of the abdominal muscles, would still fall ill from time to time, once or twice a year, after fatigue or emotion. She then invariably adopted the same attitude that she had adopted at the outset, the only difference being that the contracture became more and more extreme in successive attacks, so that in the later attacks she was completely doubled up, with her knees in contact with her chin. Even when I had not seen her for more than a year, I could cure her in a trice by the repetition of certain phrases which were always the same, and by rubbing the abdominal muscles a little. She uttered a few cries, laughed spasmodically, and then straightened herself perfectly. However severe the symptoms in any particular attack, and however long it had lasted, I could cure her completely in a minute. I have mentioned this as one of the most typical instances of the therapeutic effects of suggestion in a subject who has been well prepared for its use. But if the symptoms came on during the vacation, when No. could not find me at the Salpêtrière, she would ask some one else to do her the same service, and would confidently expect a cure. One of the senior students, who had seen me treat this case, uttered the same phrases and made the same gestures, but the result was quite different. He had to go on for hours, and make the patient come again and again. In the end, he relieved the contracture to some extent, but she was still partially doubled up so that she could only walk with difficulty ; and thus she remained for a month until I came back. This personal element in suggestion, especially where we are concerned with subjects to whom suggestions have long been conveyed by some particular person, is a familiar fact. It would be needless to give additional instances.

This particular influence is also well marked in the production of aesthesiogenic phenomena. There is no doubt that such modifications cannot be obtained by the first comer, even though he be familiar with the method employed, and even though he be dealing with a subject who has already presented such transformations several times. I described, in the chapter on aesthesiogenism, how difficult I found it to bring about in Marceline the changes which my brother had been easily inducing for several years. We should see the same thing in Irène to-day if any one but myself tried to influence her. The favourable transformation which I induce in her by the excitation of memory cannot, indeed, be always obtained. We have seen that its induction depends upon the existence of a particular state of health in the patient. But when the circumstances are favourable, it is enough that I should lead the patient to undertake a few efforts of attention, and that I should induce sleep for a few instants. Then she passes promptly into the second state. But I am certain that no other person could bring about a similar modification in her. Were it not for my intervention, Irène would be just like Marianne, whose case I have described. She would be one of those patients who suffer from periodic depression, and in whom we have to await the end of the crisis without being able to modify it.

This special influence of a particular person does not merely modify the outward attitude, for it likewise gives rise in the subject's mind to feelings and thoughts which crop up in a fairly regular way. It is interesting to compare these feelings and thoughts with the need for guidance, which as we have seen, spontaneously arise in some of our patients.

During the period of reestablishment and of activity which we have termed the " period of influence," the subject frequently preserves in a remarkable way the thought of the hypnotiser, and continues to hold a confident belief in his beneficent action. I might add numerous examples to those which I have already recorded, but a few of my patients' utterances will suffice.—" For a week," said Cora, " it seems to me that I am with you, it seems to me that you are following me about, and that appears to me very quaint. During this period I find myself unable to give myself up to my ideas of jealousy."—" I no longer have my crises, which used to come on every day. The reason is that I feel your presence near me, like a shadow that follows me about all day."—We find, as I have already shown, this feeling of " companionship," of " presence," in a great number of patients, who, after the sitting is over, continue to feel that their guide is with them, and who go on conversing with him in imagination. These are facts which should be carefully analysed, in view of the light such an analysis can throw upon many interesting psychological phenomena. In especial, it will help us to explain the famous feeling of divine protection and the feeling of the divine presence of which the mystics talk, which are as a rule so imperfectly understood. During the period of influence, our own patients sometimes compare their feelings to those of the mystics, as we see in the following remarkable letter from Qi. (f., 40) : " Although I have myself never had any religious faith, I seem to behave just like a religious person. I am like one of those true believers who go to seek comfort in the churches, and I carry my own comfort about within myself just as the true believer carries his god. These scrawls which I send to you, and which you probably throw into the waste-paper basket without reading them, do me just as much good as prayer would do to any one who believes in prayer. I, too, have my guardian angel."—Sometimes this remarkable phenomenon is exaggerated, and gives rise to more or less complete hallucinations, closely akin to the hallucinations which occasionally warn or check mystics. Some of our patients hear the voice of the hypnotist checking them when they are about to commit a folly. In an earlier work I recorded a very remarkable instance of such an illusion in a patient who, in a fit of bad temper, had planned to escape from the Salpê-trière, and had actually succeeded in getting out of the institution unseen. " I had not walked ten steps," she said, " when by a strange chance I met you. You asked me what

I was doing there, and you made me go back." [1]   Monitory hallucinations of this kind are produced here almost experimentally, although they are not the direct outcome of suggestion.   Thus they can be carefully studied.   It would certainly be well to become thoroughly acquainted with them before light-heartedly undertaking the study of the monitory or prophetic visions which people are too apt to regard as mysterious and occult.   We have seen that during the periods of partial cure this condition of influence is rarely lasting, for it is soon interrupted by a more or less serious relapse. The relapse gives rise to a new condition which precedes the return of the patient to the hypnotist, a period which we have named the " period of the somnambulist passion."   The name is justified because this period is characterised by an intense urge to return to the person who has previously hypnotised the patient ;   and the longing speedily assumes the impulsive form which we have detected in all our studies of excitation.   During this period the patients continue to think a great deal about the hypnotist, and are perpetually asking for him ; but the thought has now different characters, for it is no longer automatic and potent, and no longer does them any service.   The subject no longer has an internal conversation with his guide, and he has no hallucination ; he has lost the feeling of the director's presence, and any fresh troubles that may arise are no longer checked by the evocation of the director, which he vainly tries to achieve by an act of will.   He feels himself to be abandoned and neglected, just like the mystics in their periods of aridity, which are so like the periods of somnambulist passion by which hysterical patients are affected. " I feel myself to be alone, isolated, friendless.   It is a shame to have abandoned me like this."   They grow angry with their director, and heap abuse upon one whom a little while before they were comparing to God.   I have elsewhere drawn attention to this sense of abandonment, and to the serious disturbance it may induce.   A patient in this condition, when he is waiting for a somnambulist sitting, is very like a morphinomaniac whose hypodermic injection is due.   Just as the morphinomaniac can only be tranquillised by an injection of morphine, and by the dose to which he is accustomed, so our patient can only be satisfied, can only get back into the state of influ-

---

[1] Névroses et idées fixes, 1898, vol. 1, pp. 449–450.

ence, when he has been rehypnotised by the same person and in the same way as before.

Such phenomena occur in an exaggerated form in hysterical and hypnotisable patients, but it must not be supposed that they exist in such patients only. As soon as we recognise the essential characteristics of these various phases and of these successive sentiments, we shall be able to detect them in many other neuropaths who undergo regular series of psychological treatments at the hands of one and the same physician.

During the happy period which sometimes follows a sitting, patients who have never been hypnotised or subjected to any form of suggestion, will feel towards their director sentiments closely akin to the sentiments of " presence " which we have been describing in hysterics. This is shown by the expressions they use when returning thanks after their exaggerated fashion. —" It seems to me that you have taken over the responsibility for my poor little self, so that I no longer feel alone."—" I constantly turn towards you as a believer turns towards the priest who discloses God to him."—" Into my darkened spirit there has broken a light which does not leave me."—" I feel I am being aided and urged onward by some one who stays by me ; I no longer feel any desire to chatter to all and sundry about my fixed ideas, for I can constantly talk to you about them ; it is enough for me to think of you, and I feel reassured." —" I am full of confidence during the days after I have seen you, for I feel a great need to be accompanied by some one. You dominate all my thoughts. It seems to me that you are constantly keeping watch over me. From time to time you scold me. This both pleases me and annoys me, for, substantially, you order me about as if I were a little dog."— " When I am far away from you I am terribly afraid of doing something which will displease you. This is another way of feeling myself to be near you, and that makes me behave properly."—" To entrust my whole being to another being (God, man, or woman) so greatly superior to myself that I no longer need to guide myself in life ; to find someone who will take the trouble to guide me ; that has always been my dream. At the hospital I have found what I needed, something that always goes with me, a rule, a domination."—" I had a great need to be taken in hand, and this is what has been done for me."—The ten patients from whom these phrases are quoted, have been chosen haphazard from among a hundred of the same kind, for such expressions are often used by them during a certain phase of the treatment. We might almost say that the phraseology is characteristic of the disease at a particular stage in its evolution.

Not only do the patients use such expressions with regard to their director; but their behaviour towards him, and their way of thinking about him, are typical. They want him to intervene in all the actions of their lives, and therefore they tell him everything they do; or else, like Nadia, they write to him several times a day in order to let him know all that they do and everything that has been said to them. Thus it is that they tell us with a wealth of details the stories of all the members of their family, or of all their friends—displaying in this an amazing indiscretion. Noémi goes even further, for she wishes to implicate me, not only in her present life, but also in her past life. She thinks out romantic combinations in order to prove that I played a notable part in all the happenings of her life, even during the days before she had made my acquaintance. This remarkable phenomenon may be paralleled by the retrospective delusion of persons suffering from mania of persecution, and it helps us to understand that particular form of mental disorder.

We must not put too much confidence in these fine sentiments, for they are as fugitive as they are exaggerated. After a while, the scene changes. By degrees, or suddenly, after some strange feelings—"that of a cloud which comes down, or that of a wire breaking in the head with a noise as of breaking glass"—the patients relapse more or less completely into their depression. Now their feelings towards their director are entirely changed. Their letters no longer contain any affectionate or grateful expressions, but are full of complaints and reproaches. In especial, the patients make claims, eagerly demand that the director should again devote attention to them, for they await with more or less confidence the same comforting action.—" I need once more to have a talk with you. Perhaps you will do me a certain amount of good, although I have almost lost faith in doctors as well as in confessors."—" I want to see you again, for I am like a locomotive which needs coal ; the engine wants stoking."—" Again I need a prop, a support, a hand to guide me. For a moment I had the illusion that you held me in a firm grip, but you were only holding me by a hair. It was really rather stupid of you when you were trying to save a drowing person to be satisfied with seizing a single hair."—" You must keep a tighter hand upon me. Why did you give me back this liberty which terrifies me and of which I can make no good use."—" It is no longer your presence that I feel near me, but once more that of the demon ; you must try to exorcise him."

The patients have lost their old enthusiasm. They are simultaneously tormented by the urge to confide themselves once more, and irritated by their humiliation. They want to see their director, and are annoyed with themselves for having the desire. That is to say, in relation to this particular act they have relapsed into their customary indecisiveness and contradictions.—" I have always needed to be bucked up by some one, and this infuriates me. I want some one to be concerned about me, to be interested in me; and yet I regard myself as so inferior and so puerile that if I were to see my double I should detest him. How, then, can I expect any one to be interested in such a creature ? "—That is why, when they call to see us again, they are so cold and disagreeable in their manner—a manner which seems strange to us after the enthusiastic and adulatory expressions of the previous days. We have to go through the work with them once more ; and then, just as with the hysterics who exhibited the phenomena of aesthesiogenism, the cycle begins over again.

The succession of the feelings which these patients exhibit towards their director is, in fact, absolutely identical with that of the hysterics who are periodically transformed by aesthesiogenism. It would be superfluous to stress the analogy between the feelings observed during treatment by suggestion or by excitation, and those which we have just been describing in cases of chance guidance and in impulses to search for guidance. In all the cases alike we have to do with an influence exercised by a particular person. Sometimes this influence is real and active, so that the subject recognises its good effects ; but sometimes the influence is no longer exercised, and the subject, who deplores the lost benefits, passionately desires its revival.

5. PSYCHOLOGICAL INTERPRETATION OF THE PHENOMENA OF
INFLUENCE.

The psychological interpretation of these phenomena of influence has already been expounded in a fairly complete manner in an earlier work. It will suffice here to summarise the conclusions to which I there came, and to insist upon certain points which seem to me to deserve closer attention to-day.

It is plain that we have to do with complex psychological phenomena, with phenomena which are the outcome of numerous factors. Many writers have pointed out that there is good reason for assigning a certain part to suggestion or to kindred phenomena. The reader will understand that when I use the term " suggestion " I always do so in the precise sense previously explained, and that I do not denote by this term any indefinite psychological phenomenon, for this would lead us nowhere. It cannot be denied that this or that phenomenon of electivity, as exhibited by certain somnambulists, may be connected with the more or less involuntary and maladroit suggestions of the doctor, or with ideas spontaneously conceived by the subject, which play the part of suggestions because they are seed falling on a specially prepared soil. Hypnotised persons, both because of the modifications which they undergo and because of their predisposition to a restriction of the field of consciousness, are naturally inclined to pay exclusive attention to the hypnotist, and to all which they regard, rightly or wrongly, as dependent upon him.[1] This is the essential fact, and it is easy to understand how it can give rise to very various ideas or suggestions. The results of these suggestions may be reproduced more or less completely during the waking state, may play a part in the phenomena of the period of influence, and even in some of the phenomena of the period of somnambulist passion.

The relationships between suggestion and influence are even more interesting if we consider, not the actual phenomena of suggestion, but suggestibility, that is to say a predisposition to exhibit such phenomena. It is obvious that suggestibility

[1] L'automatisme psychologique, p. 283 ; Influence somnambulique et besoin de direction, Névroses et idées fixes, 1898, vol. i, p. 424.

towards a particular individual is much greater during the periods of influence, whether these are induced accidentally or deliberately; and that it diminishes during the periods of need or of somnambulist passion, to reappear when the influence is renewed. In this connexion I have made experiments concerning the duration of suggestions after hypnosis, and I have found in a certain number of cases that this duration is approximately the same as that of the period of influence.[1]

There is, then, a close relationship between the two phenomena, but we must not for this reason assume the phenomena to be identical. In actual fact, the phenomena of influence are far more extensive than those of suggestion, and even those of suggestibility. They occur in subjects who have never before shown that they had any ideas concerning phenomena of this kind. We see them in patients, and especially in psychasthenics, who are very little suggestible, and in whom we can never detect the automatic realisation of ideas, for such persons are apt to find it extraordinarily difficult to realise ideas. Finally, in influence we note a great many phenomena which are far more comprehensive than any suggestion which can have been made. Some of these phenomena are even opposed to the suggestions that have actually been made, those especially aimed at increasing the durability of the influence. We have always suggested to the patient to get well once for all; and the customary relapse, far from being an outcome of suggestion, is in conflict with suggestion. In this case, as in all the others, suggestion does not explain itself. Why are these subjects so suggestible in a particular phase, and not suggestible in the subsequent phase? Above all, why are they so greatly influenced by the words of one particular person, while refractory to all other persons? If, in certain cases, one of the two phenomena we are considering is dependent upon the other, I am inclined to say that in the majority of instances the suggestion varies with the influence, and is dependent upon the influence.[2]

Another, and no less interesting, explanation of these phenomena probably contains a large measure of truth. This is the explanation put forward with a certain amount of

---

[1] Influence somnambulique, etc., p. 443.   [2] Ibid., pp. 445 and 456.

exaggeration by Freud and his followers, who connect the phenomena of influence with normal manifestations of human affection, and especially with the emotion of sexual love. Here, once more, it is essential to take the same precautions, and to come to an understanding as to the meaning of the terms we are using. If we agree, once for all, on the ground of preconceived theories, that all social relationships, all the tendencies which draw human beings together, are sexual phenomena, there is nothing more to argue about. Then, all the phenomena of influence, all the urges which lead us to draw near to any definite person, are manifestations of love. But this would be a purely verbal convention, and would teach us nothing as to the real nature of the phenomena. It would be much better, at any rate in the early stage of our psychological studies, to reserve the definite term " sexual love " to denote the desire for sexual relationships with a specific person, and not to assume apriori that all the social sentiments, whatever their kind, are of the same nature as this desire.

Having made these reservations, and summarising an argument which I have already expounded, we have to admit that in a certain number of instances the attitude and phraseology of the patients is practically identical with that of lovers, so that it seems likely that there is an analogy between their feelings and those which are inspired by sexual love. Besides, it is plain that, in some of our patients, affectionate sentiments of this kind, true sexual passions, are mingled with the desire for influence. We see these needs for guidance in persons who are lovers ; in a lover abandoned by his mistress, who simultaneously lacks guidance and sexual gratification. In the foregoing chapter we learned that erotomaniac impulses can play a great part among the impulses which take the form of a search for excitation. They are all the more likely to play a part here, inasmuch as the search for excitation is an important element in the search for influence.[1] Moreover, there is nothing to surprise us in such a mingling of sentiments, for sexual love is one of the most deep-seated and the most active of all our feelings, and it readily comes to play a part in most of our actions.

Must we infer from this that the phenomena of influence can be wholly explained in such a fashion, and that they

[1] L'état mental des hystériques, 1892, vol: i, p. 159.

contain no other psychological elements ? I think such a view is most exaggerated. In many cases the feelings aroused by influence do not culminate either in desires or in actions which can properly be termed sexual. The subject who asks for orders in order that he may escape the need for having to come to a decision on his own account, or who fishes for compliments in order to deliver himself from a sense of self-abasement, must not be forthwith confounded with an erotomaniac, whose only desire is for the sexual act properly so-called. On the other hand, I have before pointed out that in certain subjects we may observe the coexistence of a need for guidance by a certain person with amorous longings towards another person. I have given an account of patients who were equally sedulous in keeping their appointments with the doctor for treatment, and their amorous assignations with another person, never confounding the two. This shows, at least, that in their minds there was a distinction between the two psychological phenomena. Finally, I may add that the strange evolution of these phenomena of influence is hardly paralleled by that of love sentiments, for the latter do not appear regularly at an appointed hour, to disappear regularly after a brief and determinate period.[1] In their totality these sentiments seem to me distinct from amorous sentiments properly so called ; and I am inclined to say, as I said before, that the phenomena of influence are more general than the phenomena of love in the strict sense of the term, so that, far from depending entirely upon these phenomena, they rather contain them as one of their varieties.

We must beware of exclusive explanations ; and to the before-mentioned phenomena of suggestion and love we must add a great many other phenomena which have an influence upon the distressing depression of neuropaths, and which have given rise to the various methods of treatment studied in earlier chapters. In these appeals to the influence of one particular person, we often discern a natural desire for treatment by rest, for treatment by the simplification of life, or for treatment by excitation—methods of treatment whose importance has already been recognised.

The patient is a fatigued, exhausted person, who has an

---

[1] Influence somnambulique, etc., op. cit., p. 457.

urgent need for rest and for the economising of energy ; but
he does not know how to rest, and he continually allows himself to become involved in activities which exhaust him still
further. His obsessive ideas, which are like " a gimlet boring
into the head," his repetitions, the resolutions he forms, his
doubts, his interrogations, his desperate but fruitless efforts,
keep up and increase his exhaustion. " I am terrified when
I think of the tremendous amount of work which I shall never
really be called upon to perform ; I dread the persons whom I
meet, and I wonder what they will ask me to do ; I worry
myself in advance, and I am constantly trying to do a number
of things which no one asks of me : this is what fatigues and
depresses me. I spend all my time in riveting a costly slavery
upon myself." The patient is " attached " upon some little
problem which life has raised ; he is persistently confronted
by the same action, which he is never able to complete, but
which he is continually trying to do and thus exhausting himself ; he is always running his head against a wall. The actual
life in which he has to take part presents complications, or
situations which he believes to be complicated. He wants
to be fully informed about all the details, he discusses the
various motives for the action, he gets involved, hesitates,
and in the end can neither come to a conclusion nor to a
decision. He begins the same deliberation over and over
again, being equally unable to perform the action and to
renounce the attempt to perform it. " I cannot cross the
threshold of this house, and yet I cannot go away from the
door." When the patient's life is simple, he complicates it
for himself by his impulse to domination, to teasing, to back-
biting, to the mad search for love, to dangerous adventures
which disturb his social environment. These perpetual
attempts and these diversified efforts, give rise to an unceasing
expenditure of energy in one who has little energy to spare.

The sitting with the doctor, whatever its kind, whether
it is concerned with hypnotism, suggestion, the dissociation of
ideas, the simplification of life, or education, saves the patient
much of this effort and expenditure. Obsessions, manias, tics,
are checked ; actions are simplified ; resolutions are taken ;
situations are liquidated ; interminable deliberations are
brought to a close by a simple decision. No doubt the work
has been done by another ; but it has been done, and the efforts

:ease. The patient has learned to perform practical actions
vhich save him from "attachments," phobias, and anxieties ;
ιe learns to behave thriftily, he discovers the art of resting.
3esides, the main expenditure for the ensuing days is econo-
mised thanks to the doctor's orders, which regulate minutely
he patient's use of his time, and save him from having to come
o decisions from moment to moment.[1] The saving is obvious,
ιnd it has been effected thanks to the doctor's guidance.

So true is this, that simple treatment by rest in bed is not
eally efficacious, and cannot be properly applied, unless in
ʻirtue of the constant influence of the doctor and the nurses.
t is the regular visit of the doctor which enables the patient
o stay quietly in bed, and which by degrees leads him to
ιdopt an attitude of rest. The other methods of treatment,
ʼy gymnastics, by education, by physiological procedures,
annot be applied to abulic neuropaths as they can be applied
o ordinary patients. These subjects, who are incapable of
ιccepting an action, and above all incapable of continuing
ιn action for some time, if it be a little disagreeable, cannot
ʼerform exercises, or follow a regimen, or even take a medicine
egularly. Nothing but the persistent influence of the director
ιan secure a certain consistency in the application of any
method of treatment.

In other cases, the patients feel incomplete, impotent,
lissatisfied, because all their actions are incomplete, unfinished,
vithout unity, and without joy. But after we have succeeded
n making them pronounce certain words, make certain efforts
ʼf attention, after we have been able to awaken old-time
ιctivities, after they have achieved some real success, have
leserved compliments whose substantiality is apparent to
hem, they feel inspired for a time with greater activity ;
ιnd when they associate with a person who has known how
o stimulate them suitably, they rediscover self-confidence
ιnd the joy of life.—" My ideas were in a tangle. They needed
ombing out. . . . My brain, which was no longer mine, is
oming back into my own possession. Nothing but emotion
ιan enable me to act, and I no longer felt any emotion. But
ιs soon as I am able to weep once more, I become a person
ιgain."

Does not this suffice to account for the way in which the

[1] Influence somnambulique, etc., p. 470.

patient is attached to the person who has rendered him these services, so that he continually thinks of that person, cherishes that person in his memory? That is why he feels himself to be "accompanied and supervised," during the period in which this uplifting of his mind continues. The feeling of "presence" in neuropaths, just as in mystics, depends upon certain dispositions of mind which they feel developing in themselves. One of the most important laws of social behaviour is that we do not act in the same way, we do not adopt the same attitude, when we are alone, and when we are in the presence of our fellows; we do not have the same attitude, we do not behave in the same way, towards different persons; we are capable of having special attitudes, clearly distinguishable one from another, towards certain determinate persons. These differences of behaviour are the origin of all distinctions between persons, and give a significance to proper names. The patients have assumed towards their director a special and somewhat complicated attitude, which is, among other things, the attitude of obedience, security, consolation, excitation, the attitude of "being understood," and so on. When, after the sitting, even after the director has gone away, the subject becomes aware that he has once more adopted this peculiar attitude, when he feels himself to be just what he was in the presence of his director, he ought to say: "I feel as if I were in his presence." But he forgets the "as if"; in his enthusiasm he has the full sentiment of the director's presence; and he even has, in cases where his belief is quite uncritical, a more or less complete auditory and visual hallucination of the director's presence. It is obvious that the same reflections would easily explain the sentiment of the divine presence experienced by mystics whose spirits are sustained by the thought of divine guidance.

When, after exhaustion or emotion, or thanks to the simple passing of time, the psychological tension is once more lowered, and when the old symptoms reappear, these attitudes are completely changed. The subject is again abulic, full of doubts, incapable of acting and believing. Now, therefore, he has no reason to believe himself to be accompanied, for he no longer feels himself to be what he was in the presence of the director. He goes on saying to himself, like Bs. after his mistress had left him: "What drives me to despair is that no one is interested in me ; that no one says to me, ' Where are you going ? What are you doing ? ' I feel so terribly alone." All these patients speak in the same sort of way : " Some kind of emotion affects me, and in a twinkling you have vanished ; I am alone, and am filled with despair." [1] To all the troubles of the will, the attention, and the memory, and sometimes of sensibility, there are superadded regret, and the perpetual evocation of the person who formerly guided them and restored them.

Regret is the incomplete activation of a tendency which is continually awakening, which rises up to the level of desire and of effort, and which is repressed by the thought of the disappearance of its object. During the period of influence, the psychasthenic mingled the thought of his director with all his actions. Now he tries to act as he did then, mingling as before the thought of his director with the actions. But he is obliged to repress the attempts as soon as the desire grows definite, for the disappearance of the director makes it impossible for him to perform the actions in the old way. These renouncings and perpetual repressions necessitate a great expenditure of energy. The result is exhaustion and increasing depression, which are characteristic of the period of the somnambulist passion, and of the period of " the need to be loved."

In a word, those who associate with the patient are capable of acting upon his mental condition in order to induce rest or excitation. Inasmuch as the patient has a great need for both rest and excitation, inasmuch as he has impulses to seek them by all possible means, he is also inspired with sentiments and impulses towards these persons who have been able temporarily to procure for him rest and excitation, and who, he believes, can still procure him these things.

The foregoing studies, which I have expounded elsewhere in almost the same terms, seem to me, according to my present lights, to leave obscure one important point, the part played by the personality of the director. We have learned why a psychotherapeutic sitting does the patient good, and why, when the patient relapses, he ardently longs for another sitting of the same kind ; but we have not learned why he insists

[1] Influence somnambulique, etc., p. 473.

that the psychotherapeutic sitting must be held with the same psychotherapeutist. The morphinomaniac who wants a hypodermic injection, accepts this injection (provided, of course, that the dose in sufficient) whoever gives it him ; but the neuropath who wants suggestion or excitation is by no means satisfied unless he has the familiar operator. It is not enough to say that these persons seek for a social action ; that they want to be commanded, supervised, amused, stimulated, by another person ; that they need " to have faith in another's faith." This does not always explain why they need some specific person to command them, direct them, stimulate them, whereas, to all appearance, plenty of other persons could render them the same service just as well.

Let me point out, first of all, that it is not true that every chance-comer is equally competent to play this part. A certain measure of intelligence is requisite in order to perceive the needs and wishes of the subject ; a certain energy is requisite in order to impose upon him the solutions, even when he desires them, or to inspire him to perform actions which he cannot conceive for himself. A certain delicacy and a certain self-confidence are requisite in order to console or to praise. Not every one who wishes can be a flatterer or even a consoler. Finally, we must realise that there is requisite a certain competence in order to be able to explain, to make suggestions to stimulate the sensibilities or the memory, etc. These reflections bring us in contact with the great problems of sympathy and antipathy. We have seen that congenial persons are those whose presence and words, instead of rendering the actions of others more difficult and more complicated simplify and facilitate these actions, thereby giving rise to an excitation which irradiates the whole mind. A congenial person is one who, far from being costly, renders an assistance which he knows how to conceal. He cannot do this unless he has suitable qualities, a high psychological tension, and a considerable measure of skill. If all this be true, is it not natural that the patient should seek out such a person, and should prefer his aid to that of another ?

There is some truth in these considerations, and the subject who has often difficulty in discovering such a congenial person will naturally, when he has found one, continue to turn to this person for aid. Nevertheless there still remain a good many unexplained phenomena. The qualities of which we have been speaking are fairly common, and a great many persons are capable of being congenial in this fashion. Why, then, are they not all acceptable to the patient? The skill requisite for making suggestions or for hypnotising is very small, and plenty of people are competent to do these things. Why are they not all equally successful? I can say without vanity that I practised hypnotism and aesthesiogenism on Marceline with quite as much skill as my brother, perhaps with more, and certainly with far more experience of these methods—and nevertheless for a year I had very little success with this patient. Nay more, it sometimes happens that highly skilled guides, persons who take the utmost pains to fulfil their duties, will completely fail in particular cases; whereas some casual person, a member of the family, a lover, or a nurse, quite unskilled, will be extremely successful with the very same patients. Those who succeed easily with one person will completely fail with another person, even though they take far greater pains in the latter case. After I had treated Marceline for a few years, I could do anything I liked with her, for she would respond to the most trifling signal, or to words which might be ill chosen; but at first I failed to influence her, though I took the utmost care and adopted the very best methods. We must not suppose that the patient's director must always be a person of great worth; for though these patients are apt to clamour for persons of genius, they are often content with something very much less. The high qualities of the director are, no doubt, among the factors of success, but they do not wholly account for it. Love does not go by desert; and in the case of guidance as in the case of love, other elements than desert play their part.

One special condition which must often play an important part is an accurate knowledge of the patient and of the procedures which have an effect upon him. We know, for instance, that a hysteric is readily drilled, and easily acquires a number of habits which often assume a very precise form. Mrb. (f., 26) had been managed in a strange and ridiculous way by her first hypnotist. It was necessary to touch a particular spot on the forehead to put her to sleep, and to pull the lobule of the right ear in order to awaken her. When she had contractures it was necessary to pull the lobule of the left ear in order to dispel them. By pressure upon the right breast she could be made to speak when she was mute; and by pressure upon the left breast her breathing could be regularised when she was suffering from breathlessness; and so on, and so on. Everything was meticulously regulated so that this woman had come to resemble a complicated piece of mechanism with a number of knobs which had to be pressed on suitable occasions in order to make the mechanism work. Obviously such a patient will prefer to remain under the care of the person who is thoroughly familiar with the machinery, for any one who should wish to awaken her and should pull the lobule of the wrong ear would get quite a wrong response! Something analogous to this happens in the case of many depressed and susceptible persons. Any one who trys to act upon them must be forewarned as to what they are capable of, as to what they can speak of sensibly, as to what they can say nothing about; he must have carefully noted what humiliates them, what wounds them, what flatters them, what consoles them. He must know how, with one person, to avoid a particular topic of conversation which may be an extremely suitable one with another person; he must be competent to adapt his attempts at excitation to the patient with whom he was to deal. This special and individual competence is, in many cases, more important than the general competence to which I referred above, and it explains a great many successes which seem almost inexplicable at first sight.

But here, likewise, difficulties arise. A person who, as my own experience has taught me, has played the part of director, or one to whom the patient has wished to allot the role of director, has not always been one who was well acquainted with this particular individual, not always one who knew perfectly how to manipulate the mechanism. In this matter it is as with love; for, as we have just seen, we are really concerned with a sort of love, although sexual phenomena play no part in it. The lover endows the object of his affections with qualities that do not always exist. Love is an effort to verify the preconceived image of the well-beloved, and the essential thing is the imagination which endows the beloved object with wonderful qualities. In the problems connected with social relationships, we must never forget that there are at least two persons in any social relationship; and we must never forget that the social phenomenon under observation depends upon the relationship between their respective psychological states. It is not enough to consider the action of the director, and to attribute the whole efficacy to this ; it is equally essential to understand the attitude of the person who is under direction.

Obviously, then, the person subjected to guidance has towards the guide a peculiar attitude, and exhibits a peculiar mode of behaviour, these being characteristic of the phenomenon of influence. Formerly, when describing the mental condition of hysterics, I referred to this attitude of hysterical patients, which has not always been fully understood. I wrote : " The person who is interested in them is no longer, in their eyes, an ordinary human being. He assumes a preponderant position, one which overshadows that of all other persons. For his sake they will try to do anything, for they seem to have taken once for all a resolution to obey him blindly. But, on the other hand, they are extremely exacting. They want their doctor to be wholly occupied about their affairs, and to pay no attention to any one else. He must be continually coming to see them, must pay them very long visits, and must be profoundly concerned about their disquietudes." [1] The same sort of attitude is adopted by all the patients whose cases we have just been studying, and it is precisely because they have this peculiar attitude that we have been led to detect and to study the phenomenon of influence. In the life of such patients, this peculiar attitude plays a very important part, for it forms the substratum of a great many special kinds of behaviour. As I have so often said, it is probably one of the essential factors of suggestion, or of that systematisation of suggestion which makes the subject so suggestible in relation to one particular person, while less suggestible or not suggestible at all in relation to other persons. Not only does the subject not resist the realisation of the idea suggested by this favoured person, but he goes even further, for he does his utmost to encourage the development of this idea. That, likewise, is the explanation of the credulity which we encounter in certain psychasthenics side by side

[1] Les stigmates mentaux des hystériques, being vol. i of L'état mentaux des hystériques, 1893, p. 158 ; Influence somnambulique, etc., p. 446.

with their everlasting doubts. " It is absolutely essential that I should believe some one," says Lydia, " for I cannot believe myself. I always believe you, for I made up my mind to do this a long time ago, and I cling to this decision as my safeguard."—" I am so terribly afraid of being left to myself," says Cora, " and that is why I always make such great efforts to obey you and to believe you."

In relation to this same director, they are not only docile ; they are also and above all excitable. The compliments or the criticisms of the director arouse violent reactions ; his words are the starting-point of great efforts of tension, leading to profound changes. This, too, is the outcome of the attitude they have adopted, far more than of the actual power of the words used by the director.—A young woman of twenty-two had for a long time been talking to all comers of her scruples, and of her fear that she would kill her mother ; and a hundred times she had been told that these notions were absurd. But now her actions are governed by her dread lest I should regard her as an imbecile. " I am less troubled with ridiculous ideas, for when I have them I must tell you about them, and that makes me ashamed."—Nadia does not wish any one to tell me of the follies she has committed ; she wants to tell me about these herself, no doubt toning them down in the process ! " I have decided not to show myself up in too bad a light."— Most of the artificial excitations we have been considering exhibit these elements of collaboration on the part of the subject, who explains his efforts and his successes.

We must not fancy that we have to do here with a reflective and voluntary type of behaviour, which comes into force for each action every time the director issues an order or pays a compliment. If that were so, this behaviour would not display so much regularity as it actually does ; it would be impossible at a moment when the subject is incapable of an effort of will and attention, that is to say when he is depressed, precisely when such behaviour is useful. It is an automatic form of behaviour, which, luckily, can recur at the desired moment without the need for a fresh decision. Patients whose state of depression puts them in an unfortunate humour, sincerely believe that they will not listen to a word that is said to them, that they will not believe a word ; and they are themselves surprised to find that, as usual, they listen to and believe the words of their director whatever these words may be. They have a well-organised and stable tendency to react by this special form of behaviour, by suggestibility and susceptibility to stimulation, in response to the words of one particular individual, whether this individual has or has not at that moment any special merits. Those who are not subject to the influence of a director, those who are not transformed by such an influence, are not always persons who have failed to come across a competent director ; they are those who have not as part of their equipment a preorganised tendency to the reaction of influence in response to a particular individual.

What is the origin of such a tendency ? How is it that it thus exists ready-made in certain minds ? No doubt we have good reason to say that it is a very special form of various other tendencies which existed already in the mind of the subject long before the illness. Freud and his followers have rightly pointed out that we are concerned here with one form of those primitive tendencies which induce a little child to follow his parents, to obey them, to seek refuge with them and protection at their hands. "' You must forgive me if I stick to you like a limpet," said Nadia (f., 33) ; " I cannot help it ; I was born with this disposition, and I think that I shall always be hanging on to some one. Formerly I used to cling to my mother's apron-strings. Now she is dead, and I cannot get on with my father, so that I feel utterly forsaken. In many respects it seems to me that I am like a little child of six years old abandoned by its parents. I assure you that I am not mad ; but I have so urgent a need for protection, that it makes me hang round some one's neck." As we have already seen, moreover, the sexual tendencies play a certain part in this disposition, if it be only by the natural inclination of every individual to react in a particular way to orders issued, criticisms made, or praise uttered, by a person of the other sex. Although there are doubtless many explanations of the fact, we may say in general terms that a woman is more readily guided, in the manner we have been studying, by a man than by another woman. Finally, it is obvious that we must allow for the simplest social tendencies, for the tendencies of hierarchy, obedience, even servitude. It need not surprise us to find that, in the disposition to accept and to seek for this special guidance, there reappear all these

primitive tendencies, for we know that in every kind of excitation there are appeals to this sort of deep-seated tendency.

It is, however, obvious that the foregoing explanation does
not explain everything. First of all, the tendency to become
subject to the influence of the director is not exactly the same
as the behaviour of a child towards its parents, nor is it
exactly the same as the behaviour of a mistress towards her
lover. There is something very special about this behaviour
It is not the pure and simple activation of one of these elementary tendencies, for it is a new combination realised in relation
to very special circumstances. Furthermore, these primitive
tendencies of the child, the slave, or the loving woman, exist
at the bottom of all human hearts ; and if they were the whole
explanation of this phenomenon of influence they should
perpetually manifest themselves, should perpetually give
rise to the behaviour characteristic of influence. But we
know as a fact that this behaviour characteristic of influence
frequently fails to manifest itself, notwithstanding the latent
existence of such primitive tendencies. In influence, therefore, there must be something over and above the primitive
tendencies.

We have to assume that at a certain moment in their treatment the patients have formed in their minds this special
tendency towards a specific person, towards the person who was
specially interested in them. We can speak of this moment,
of this remarkable action, as an " act of adoption " ; and we
can point out that, if it plays a great part in direction, the
act of adoption also plays a great part in many other forms
of behaviour, in the organisation of hierarchies for instance,
and in love properly so called. Whether we have to do with
love at first sight, or with love which gradually comes to life,
there must always be at the outset of the passion such an act
of adoption. In the case of this action, as in the case of all
our new actions, the same thing happens. The action comes
about through the mingling of numerous earlier inclinations
of a more or less kindred kind, synthetised in a peculiar way.
The deep-seated tendencies of which we have just been speaking,
the sentiment of a present danger and of the weakness of the
will, the more or less skilful behaviour of the person considered,
the frequent repetition of encounters and of sittings under

favourable conditions—all these play their part in the synthesis which has been happily effected in the minds of certain subjects.

In cases of deliberate guidance, in cases of medical direction, it is easy to discern the moment when, in such subjects, the tendency to accept influence comes into being. As a rule this takes place after the treatment has lasted for a certain time ; but occasionally, as I have shown, it appears rapidly and suddenly. The subject's attitude towards the doctor is modified. Instead of exhibiting towards the doctor a generalised kind of behaviour like that exhibited towards various other associates, the patient adopts a form of behaviour exhibited only towards the doctor. This behaviour can be expressed satisfactorily by the idea the patient forms of his doctor, for the ideas we have of a person are nothing other than a greatly abridged summary of our behaviour towards that person. Whereas, prior to the change, the patient regarded you as just like any one else, as one doctor among many, as an individual who was just as good for numerous other persons as for himself, the patient now begins to look upon you as exceptional in one way or another. He declares that you are the only person in the world able to understand him ; the only one who is really trying to do him any good.—Nadia, an incredibly obstinate woman and a despot in her family, wrote to me one day after she had been treated by me for two months : " I thought myself the most obstinate person in the world, one who would never obey any one. I am astonished to find that you are more obstinate than I am, and that no one, not even myself, can resist your will." I need hardly say that Nadia's idea concerning my obstinacy and my energy of will has no relationship to the facts, and that she is obviously a poor psychological observer ; but nevertheless, her idea upon the matter has made her admirably docile for ten years, and has saved her from madness.

Many neuropaths, after having repeated for an indefinite number of times that no one could ever understand them, seem all of a sudden to discover that there is one person at least who does understand them. This idea of " not being understood " or " being understood " plays so large a part in their talk, that we must look into the matter more closely. When we ask them what they mean by saying that we understand them, they find it very difficult to explain. " You do not make fun of my strange ideas. You know that I am not really stupid, although I say stupid things ; that I am really kind-hearted, although I seem selfish ; that I am good, although I may seem bad. Finally, I feel that you understand me, and you cannot imagine how much good that does me. If only I am understood, everything is well with me." Here is another strange illusion. It is by no means certain that we do understand them. A few superficial observations do not enable us to get to the core of a mental condition. My perpetual recurrence to the theory of suggestion, my complicated explanations of impulses, will have shown the reader that I myself am far from feeling that I understand these patients. No matter ! Certain patients have told me of their conviction that they were understood by persons who had studied them less, and had understood them less satisfactorily, than I had. It is not certain that we do not make fun of them. Sometimes such raillery may be useful, and they accept it willingly from one who is their director. It is by no means certain that we have so favourable an opinion of them ; and they are ready to accept very severe criticism from us. In reality they have a very hazy idea of what they mean when they talk of " being understood."

This notion of " being understood " merely corresponds to a special form of behaviour which they adopt towards the person who, they believe, understands them. When they have arrived at this conclusion, they will thenceforward be able to express to that person their feelings and their ideas, whereas ordinarily they have been unable to express themselves clearly, and have sought refuge in jesting and irony. When they say that we take them seriously, they mean that they themselves have made up their minds to talk seriously. They do, or try to do, whatever this chosen person tells them to do. They say that is because the director knows their strength and does not ask them to do the impossible ; but in reality they have become stronger thanks to their trust in the guidance and the assistance given them, so that they feel able to carry out certain orders. " All right ; this time I feel that you have understood me. I have the trust of a child that begins to walk, a child that feels itself supported, if only by a corner of its pinafore. I give myself up to your guidance. You will see that I can put my will into this obedience." What

I have just said with regard to " being understood " might be repeated as regards all the ideas which the patients have of their director. We are invariably concerned with a special form of behaviour towards him, a form of behaviour which is organised in the patient's mind, and which is more or less correctly expressed by such ideas.

The director must not give way to pride because of the flattering opinion expressed by his patients. When the patient, in his good moments at any rate, declares that his director is a quite exceptional being, one superior to all others, this is not the expression of a justified appreciation, for these patients are incapable of anything of the kind. The phrase is merely a conventional affirmation, an expression of the act of adoption. The behaviour we have termed " behaviour of influence " is a special form of behaviour which only exists in relation to a particular individual. It is natural that the patient who adopts such a kind of behaviour towards a particular individual should regard that individual as exceptional. It is because you have become the patient's director that the patient regards you as admirable—just as a writer who has been elected an academician becomes an " immortal."

To sum up, human beings are continually acting upon one another; and social influences are among the most potent causes of health and disease, of depression and excitation. After having studied the social influences which are dangerous and depressing, we have been endeavouring to understand the social influences which are protective and stimulant. There are many such influences, they are of many kinds, and we have studied a number of them in the foregoing chapter. In order to summarise here the characteristics of direction, we shall do well to compare with direction another influence which is in some respects analogous to that of the director, the influence of one who looks after the patient, the influence of the nurse.

The action of caring for or nursing a patient is likewise a social, protective, and useful action. It is thanks to the nurse that the patient, who is incapable of protecting himself and of following unaided the doctor's advice, avoids dangerous actions, carries out the treatment, rests at appropriate times, and undertakes some of the useful efforts which have been prescribed. This action of the nurse exhibits important psychological characteristics ; it has to be continuous, for the effects of the nurse's action are transient. The action of the nurse upon the patient only exists, for practical purposes, at the moment when it is exercised. The nurse prevents the patient from getting out of bed, and a moment later she has to do the same thing over again. The transient character of this influence shows us that the nurse induces in the patient psychological phenomena which are of a comparatively low grade. The extension of human actions in space and time is proportional to their elevation in the psychological hierarchy. The nurse, in fact, only acts in virtue of resistances which give rise to perceptive actions, or by simple orders which give rise to extremely elementary intellectual phenomena. Finally, the action of the nurse is of a generic character. Material resistance, the issuing of simple orders, can be the work of different persons ; it is not essential that the nurse should be one particular individual. The majority of social influences are exercised in a generic fashion. Parents are, before all, parents ; characterised by the role they play, independently of their personality. A woman acts upon a man in virtue of her sex, because she is a woman, before she acts upon him specially because she is this woman or that. The leader, the priest, the professor, the doctor, each one of them has a generic superiority which is the same for every one of the class. The nurse acts in the same way, inasmuch as she is a nurse, and not in virtue of her individual characteristics.

Direction is obviously in certain points identical with the action exercised by the nurse ; it is useful, in like manner, in that it checks hurtful actions, induces attitudes of repose, organises methods of treatment, leads the patient to perform stimulating actions. But these results are achieved in a very different way ; the action of the director is far more efficacious ; and, above all, it need not be continuous, for it is not merely instantaneous. It takes effect by giving rise to actions of a much higher psychological grade, and having a much greater extension. It gives rise to resolutions, beliefs, efforts ; in a word, it acts mainly by inducing excitation. What distinguishes even more this influence of the director from the influence of the nurse is that the director acts far more in virtue of his own individuality. In the phenomena of influence we saw at the outset that there are certain generic social actions, of extreme importance. But at this stage, I think, we have to pay attention to a social influence of a peculiar kind; I mean, the directive and stimulant influence of the individual qua individual. Since there occurred a development of forms of behaviour, and of ideas relative to individuality, to personality, and to liberty, men have come to attach great value to the individual, to the penetration of the individual, to the conquest of the individual; they have invented intimacy, that is to say special relationships determined by the peculiar character-istics of two persons in association, " because it was he, because it was I "; and these delicate and perfected relationships are among the most potent stimulants which society can offer us. Neuropaths, who are always in search of sources of excitation, realise this, in so far as they are intelligent and subtle. All their lives they dream of a personal friend, one perfectly suited to them, one who will understand them, and whom they will understand. I need hardly say that they are usually incapable of achieving such an association, for it is extremely difficult to achieve. But when, by chance, or thanks to artificial help, they do succeed in achieving it, and when the act of adoption has been made, they derive great benefit therefrom. Direction is the therapeutic utilisation of this particular form of the social action which human beings exercise on one another.

6. CONDITIONS UNDER WHICH MEDICAL GUIDANCE OCCURS.

Our study of the phenomena of influence has shown us that we have to do, in this case, with complicated and delicate psychological phenomena which cannot be easily produced at will, and cannot readily be made use of whenever we wish. It is not enough that the patient should need guidance, nor is it enough that he should demand a guide; it is not enough that the doctor should be competent to play the part of director and that he should try to play it. These circumstances do not suffice to establish between doctor and patient the peculiar relationship which is required; they are not enough to organise a useful and durable influence. When we think over the conditions upon which the occurrence of these phenomena depend, we see that these conditions are not easy to bring into being.

There is no need to insist upon the conditions which the director must realise. As I have already stated, they are less important than is usually believed. Some day it is probable that the advance of psychology will be so great that any one whose ambition it is to guide the minds of the sick will have to be master of the whole science of the human mind ; but to-day, unfortunately, the amount of useful psychological knowledge at our disposal is small, and can speedily be acquired. It is enough to have a certain taste for psychological analysis, to have some sympathy for moral suffering, a little power of observation, and a certain strength of character, to be able to fulfil this role as well as it can be fulfilled at present. We have seen that a good many persons whose previous education might seem to have equipped them very ill for playing the part of guide, have nevertheless succeeded perfectly. The main difficulty, as I have again and again declared, is an accommodation between the time at the disposal of the director and the time which it is necessary to give to the patient. But, more often than might be supposed, both men and women are capable, in this way, of rendering great services to persons whose minds are debilitated. It is not from the side of the director that the main difficulty comes.

The crux of the problem lies with the patient. It is the patient's situation, the patient's mental condition, upon which the possibility or impossibility of guidance depends. We may ignore points of minor importance. Appearances to the contrary notwithstanding, the sex, the age, and the previous education of the patient, have very little influence upon his situation from the outlook at which we are now placing ourselves. Although it is true that in the cases I have reported there has been a preponderant number of women, this is because nervous disorders susceptible of treatment by guidance are commoner in women than in men, and because women more than men have time to spare for treatment of this kind. Men who are suffering from the same sort of disorders, have the same needs as women, and often benefit greatly by the same sort of treatment. No doubt among my cases there is a very large proportion of fairly young patients, persons at ages ranging between twenty and thirty-five years, this being the age at which curable neuroses most often come under our notice. But persons above thirty-five may exhibit the phenomena of influence very satisfactorily; as we see, for instance, in the remarkable case of Madame Z., who was sixty-five years of age. The most that we need say about age is that comparative youth in the patient and comparative age in the doctor are helpful in the early stages of guidance. As regards suggestion, we have already considered Bernheim's contention that suggestibility is especially manifest in persons who have been poorly educated, and in those who are accustomed to the role of passive obedience. An inclination to accept influence depends much more upon a morbid state than upon the patient's education, and may be conspicuous in persons of very varying social stations. It is, however, perfectly true that intelligent and well-educated persons are apt to be more critical of their directors. A man of fifty, noted as a writer and as a moralist, said to me sadly : " I am constantly being advised to put myself under some one's authority ; I am told that if I submit to some one's influence my doubts will be dispelled. But it is really very difficult to follow this advice when, with the best will in the world, I find that my director is too stupid. You surely would not wish me to accept my gardener as the director of my conscience ? " This patient's criticism is open to objections, for the superiority of the director is not a purely intellectual matter. Still, we may admit that a certain intellectual superiority makes it easier for the director to establish his influence over some of his patients. We may conclude that the practice of psychotherapeutics demands from the doctor a more general education than the practice of other therapeutic methods. To sum up, the patient's condition as to sex, age, and education, though it must not be entirely ignored in this connexion, is really of little importance.

Social conditions are, I think, of more moment. I refer now to the conditions that comprise the patient's environment. We might suppose that a patient who is isolated and independent, one who has no family to act upon him in various ways, would be in the most favourable condition. Patients of this kind continually repeat that they are alone, forsaken, and that they need some one on whom they can rely. Actual experience, however, does not fully justify the inference in question. A young woman of twenty-three, who had lost her mother and whose father paid little attention to her, was suffering from psychasthenic depression, and lamented her isolation. " I have nothing to sustain me ; I am, as it were, hung up in the air ; I have no interest in anything or anybody ; I am like a piano that is out of tune, so that I need a tuner." She was continually trying, as her whims might guide her, to discover the desired " tuner " in one person or another.— I have notes of five similar cases in which patients complained of their moral isolation, and for years, having full liberty of choice, vainly endeavoured to find among doctors and priests a director with whom they could be satisfied.—Among such patients, whose family, position, or fortune makes them too independent, we often find types analogous to what Charcot used to speak of as the " Wandering Jew " ; persons who consult all the doctors in the neighbourhood one after another, without ever being influenced for good by any one of them, seeing that they invariably change their medical adviser too soon, and before the phenomena of adoption have had time to manifest themselves. The cause of this disorder is the difficulty of the act of adoption, which needs persistent effort, especially in depressed persons of an inert type. Every kind of psychotherapeutic procedure is a slow business ; it must be practised for a considerable time by the same person. Patients in independent circumstances must impose regularity and continuity of guidance upon themselves, they must deliberately subject themselves for a considerable time to the influence of the same person, before they can gain any advantage. Nevertheless, their illness makes them incapable of regular and prolonged action. If left to their own devices, they will never succeed in organising the guidance of which they feel the need. When there is a family which can insist upon the patient's choosing a doctor ; when there are relatives who are able to understand the need for a certain regularity of treatment, and who can insist upon it ; then, obviously, we have conditions favourable to the inauguration of guidance. At a later stage, once adoption has been achieved, the patient will himself be willing to continue the treatment.

On the other hand, the patient's associates may raise difficulties. The entourage may consist of vacillating and unstable persons just like the patient, persons who are incapable of understanding the need for continuity in treatment of this kind. Often enough the relatives, through excess of devotion, call in one doctor after another, arrange for a number of consultations between these doctors, are never content unless several doctors are treating the patient at the same time. A great many Parisian practitioners will recall the celebrated case of " Mignonne," whose treatment was never successful. Even in general medicine, it is only in special cases that joint consultations are desirable ; in cases of mental disorder they are almost always disastrous. Here the division of responsibility and of influence is especially liable to eventuate in inaction. Influence cannot possibly be established unless the doctor who plays the part of director is left alone in his treatment of the patient for a considerable time.

Apart from these difficulties relating to the choice of the doctor and to the doctor's freedom of action, the patient's associates may complicate the problem of guidance in various ways. In many instances parents, a husband or a wife, friends—all of whom may themselves be more or less neuropathic—exhibit the authoritarian characteristics we have frequently had occasion to study. Although they are incompetent to exercise a real and effective guidance, they wish to maintain authority over the patient, or at least to keep up the semblance of authority. All the more do they want to do this in proportion as the patient manifests a need for guidance, an instinct of obedience, and in proportion as these authoritarian persons find in the exercise of authority over the patient gratification of their secret longings to dominate. Often enough such persons are filled with jealousy when they contemplate the influence exercised by the doctor. Whilst openly, and more or less sincerely, they express the wish that the doctor shall guide a sick mind, and thus relieve sufferings which they themselves have not been able to relieve, below the surface, and perhaps unconsciously, they do all they can to thwart the doctor's influence. This remarkable attitude is one which I have often seen in the mother, the sister, or the daughter of a patient ; and in these cases the masked struggle has made it impossible or difficult to exercise the requisite influence.

In other cases the position is even more delicate, for one of these authoritarian relatives will be found to have acquired a genuine influence over the patient. We have had occasion in this book to study many cases in which neuropaths are living under the influence of a parent, a lover, or a nurse. As long as the influence is effective, and suffices to sustain the patient, there is no reason to complain. But in many cases the guidance is incompetent and inadequate. The patient's condition sometimes makes it necessary to seek medical aid, and yet all the time the patient remains in large measure subject to another influence than that of the doctor. The one who is playing the part of guide knows well enough that he is playing it badly; but he does not wish to abandon his position, perhaps from affection for the patient, and perhaps from some interested motive. In such circumstances the doctor will find it difficult to do any good. The patient is torn this way and that through being subjected to two opposing influences; he is disturbed and wearied to no good end.—In the case of a young man of twenty-two, who was suffering to an ever more marked degree from asthenic delusions, the despotic and clumsily exercised influence of his mother rendered successful treatment impossible.—A woman of thirty-seven could not be subjected to any valuable guidance because she was under the influence of a nurse who was interested in maintaining, and succeeded in maintaining, her own influence over the patient.—When we have to study the mental condition of a patient, we must be careful to ascertain all the influences which are acting upon him. Unless we can free him from these influences, it will be useless to attempt to cure him by moral guidance. The outcome of these reflections is the inference that the patient's associates play a considerable part in connexion with such methods of treatment. In some cases they may render the treatment difficult or impossible; in other cases, if they are intelligent and self-sacrificing, these associates may enormously facilitate the treatment. There is nothing that need surprise us in such facts, seeing that the neuroses are, before all, social maladies. Their first appearance, their development, their treatment, and their cure, depend in large measure upon the subject's moral environment.

Among the conditions that influence treatment by guidance, even more important are those which relate to the morbid condition itself, and to its intensity. We must not suppose, as so many people wrongly imagine, that medical guidance can be effective in all forms of mental disorder. We should do wrong to forget that the state of influence is nothing other than the more or less automatic development of a tendency which has come into existence in the patient's mind at the outset of the treatment ; and that the formation of this tendency, the act of adoption, has necessitated an important effort on the patient's part. But many patients are incapable of performing this preliminary work, are incapable of the act of adoption. They cannot organise, in relation to their doctor, a special tendency, a tendency which is new in certain respects ; and for that reason they cannot make their doctor into their guide, and cannot subject themselves to his influence. For example, when asthenic dementia is far advanced, the lowering of the psychological tension is so great that any new act of adaptation has become impossible. Such patients are indifferent to all the happenings of their actual life ; they live in the past, for they exhibit nothing more than the functioning of tendencies formed long ago ; they cannot add any new tendencies related to the present. They know nothing about their environment. In the new entourage they form neither friends nor enemies. It is obvious that in these conditions they will not acquire a guide. I have frequently referred to the case of Agathe. She was continually clamouring for some one who would be interested in her, who would shake her out of herself, who would keep a tight hand upon her, who would make her do something. Nevertheless, although she has seen me at regular intervals for years, she has never given me any important position in her mind, and has never shown the least inclination to obey my orders. Her depression was already far advanced when she first came under my care. In these cases of asthenic dementia we sometimes note an even more distressing development. At the outset of the illness, when the depression is less severe, we may find that these patients will adopt the doctor as guide even though imperfectly, and will subject themselves to his influence in an encouraging way. The malady, however, continues to run its course. Not only does it render impossible the formation of new tendencies, but it makes more and more difficult the activation of recently acquired tendencies which have not been firmly established. By degrees, the influence which has been established with so much difficulty, wanes. This is one of the most distressing terminations of guidance, and it is a matter to which we shall have to return.

We see the same thing, although to a less marked extent, in crises of asthenic delusion, or in the severe phases of depression and obsession. Patients who are completely overcome by hypochondriacal delusions, or by delusions of blameworthiness ; uneasy patients who can think of nothing but themselves ; abulic patients in whom all social actions have become arduous—adapt themselves with great difficulty to a new direction. In less severe cases, they seem to welcome the doctor, they speak to him, they appear to understand him. But their perceptions and actions are superficial and fugitive ; no memories, or practically none, are left. No new tendency is originated. I have seen patients, like Irène at the outset of her treatment, who were unable to describe my face, and were unable to say whether I was dark or fair, after seeing me daily for four months. In such circumstances, it is obvious that no adoption has been made, for adoption mainly consists in preserving in the mind a more or less accurate representation, solidly built, of the doctor's personality. The patient must have towards the doctor a special and individual attitude, quite different from the same person's attitude towards every one else. In the case of such patients, we must content ourselves with the simpler methods of treatment previously described, such as suggestion (if this be possible), treatment by rest, isolation, excitation, physiological methods, etc. Perhaps, in favourable circumstances, these methods will raise the patient's tension to a degree at which adoption becomes possible and the method of guidance can be utilised.

Are we to infer that the establishment of guidance will only be successfully effected in those whose illness is not severe, and therefore only in those who have little need of guidance ? This would be an erroneous statement, for one of the conditions of influence, so far as my experience goes, strange though it may seem, is important. It is not easy to treat by influence a subject whose illness is not yet serious, one who is in the early stages of the disease, one whose only troubles are tardiness of action, doubts and trifling scruples which disturb his relatives far more than they disturb himself. Such a patient will not realise that there is any need for treatment, especially for a treatment which will necessitate an effort on his part. When, on the other hand, neuropathic symptoms, owing either to their kind or to their gravity, have given rise to real moral suffering, the patient becomes alarmed, applies for aid, and is inclined to make a certain amount of effort in order to secure relief.

Thus it is in the intermittent phase of the illness, before it has given rise to serious delusions, or else in the remissions, when the patient has regained a certain amount of energy, that the establishment of a valuable guidance can most easily be effected. This fact was obvious in many of the cases I have recorded. To take one example only, that of Irène, the phenomena of influence only began to appear towards the fifth month of treatment, when the main delusions had already begun to pass away. As soon as adoption had been effected, the influence became powerful, and it was possible to treat the patient by the aesthesiogenic methods which have already been described. In Irène, the influence was durable, and was extremely useful in her numerous relapses, for it was always possible to check these in the early stage, and they never became so severe as the first crisis. If this phenomenon could be established as a general one, it would suggest an interesting reflection concerning the treatment of neuropaths. Psychotherapeutic procedures must not be undertaken in these cases only in the worst phases ; they must also, and especially, be undertaken in the periods of remission and improvement. It is then that we must do our utmost to acquire an influence over our patients' minds. Once we have gained the necessary influence, we shall find only too frequent an occasion to turn it to account.

These brief reflections anent the conditions under which guidance can be organised and can become effective, show that treatment by guidance cannot be employed indiscriminately in every case. This is not a serious matter, for other treatments remain available when treatment by guidance is impossible. But in this matter of guidance, we can look forward to advances in psychotherapeutics which will enable us, some day, to formulate definite methods of treatment applicable in specific cases.

7. DIFFICULTIES IN THE WAY OF GUIDANCE.

The complete study of the guidance of neuropaths would comprise an examination of the various phases of guidance from its beginning to its close, with a mention, at each period, of the difficulties and dangers encountered. Such a complete study is impossible to-day. I can only deduce from my case-notes certain observations regarding the various phases, observations which may be useful, and may become the starting-point of new researches.

Problems of the opening Phase of Guidance. The foregoing studies have already illustrated the essential conditions of the establishment of influence in the opening phase of guidance. It will be enough, now, to point out certain circumstances which, in my own cases, have seemed to constitute obstacles to the initiation of guidance; and to refer to certain practices which have appeared to me to have a favourable influence.

Most neuropaths have suffered a great deal from the ambiguous and rather absurd character of their illness. They are often robust and intelligent to outward seeming, and yet they are incapable of acting, or they behave like imbeciles. Their parents and their friends have long since become aware of this paradoxical character of the invalid's behaviour. Sometimes these associates of the patient completely fail to recognise the reality of the illness, and sometimes they think that the trouble can be cured by making fun of it. In war-time, such invalids are treated as " shirkers ; " in peace-time they are regarded as sufferers from imaginary illness. The precautions they find indispensable, the persistent economising of their energies, even their sufferings, are turned into ridicule. A great many of these patients have told me how they have been filled with despair and anger when they have consulted a doctor, only to find that this expert has joined in the chorus, and has said more or less amiably : " You are very silly to be ill ; your troubles would soon vanish if you only wanted them to." One of the important factors of guidance is the patient's conviction that the guide will always " take him seriously." We cannot at the outset of guidance lavish too much pains to inspire this conviction.

The psychological examination of the patient must at first be performed with due discretion, for I have seen cases in which clumsy or hasty investigations have interfered with the progress of the treatment. Emile (m., 18), who was suffering from asthenic delusions of timidity, was for a long time cared for by an excellent doctor who had absolutely no influence upon the patient. To start with, this doctor had applied Jung's method of association, which was then fashionable, and told the young man that the asking for associations to the recommended list of words would disclose his secret thoughts. "By this means I shall be able to discover everything that you have in your mind." Emile, who had hardly any thought of concealing his obsessions, and who would have made no secret of them in ordinary conversation, was terrified by the new method of enquiry, and remained obstinately secretive. I need hardly say that Jung's tables revealed nothing at all, for these tables, like most of the well-known laboratory methods, only reveal what is already known to the experimenter ! We must be extremely careful at the outset to do nothing that will needlessly alarm the patient.

It is equally important to avoid making him uneasy by asking too much effort of him, and by speaking too much of the exercise of his will, for then he will take fright at the thought of the tasks which are about to be imposed on him. A young woman of twenty-six, in search of moral guidance, went to consult an able practitioner, who, at the first interview, told her that success would depend upon the voluntary efforts she made. But the young woman, over-scrupulous, and extremely abulic, was obsessed by the thought that she had no will power at all. She was reduced to despair when she was told that the only way in which she could be cured was by an appeal to a will power which she no longer believed herself to possess. The result was that she became tortured by thoughts of suicide.

Finally, a great many of these patients complain that they have been deceived, and lose all confidence, because they have discovered, or have fancied that they have discovered, a contradiction in their doctor's words. It is difficult to realise how ingenious neuropaths are in this matter. However disorderly their thoughts may seem, they are continually on the look-out for trickery, bear it ever in mind, and, when they believe that they have been duped in any way, become incurably suspicious. It is a terrible, though very common, error to treat an asthenic like a dement. However difficult the problem, it is almost always a good thing, when we have ascertained the degree of the patient's intelligence, to speak to him as frankly as possible, and to tell him in plain terms the little that we know about these strange disorders of the mind, about the dangers attendant upon them, and about the prospects of improvement.

Conversely, one of the best ways in which the doctor can establish his influence, is to have a precise knowledge of the patient. It is impossible to lay too much stress upon the importance of the study of the patient's past life, of his education, of the incidents of his youth, of the sentiments he has experienced, of the efforts he has made in former days. We must write down all these details, con them at leisure, and glance through them just before we see the patient again, so that we can allude to them and avoid needless repetitions. We must amplify the patient's confidences by those made to us by other patients, for there is a remarkable resemblance between all these neuropaths when they are at the same stage of the disease. It is just as well to show the patient from time to time that we are aware of his sentiments before he expresses them, that we are familiar with the ideas which have passed through his mind. Doubtless we must be careful to avoid an attempt at undue accuracy ; we must not make the mistake of formulating obsessions which still exist only in the germ. With regard to obsessive ideas, just as with regard to hysterical symptoms, authorities have often and justly insisted that we must not fix troubles which are still vague. Obviously we must behave differently towards a child of fifteen who is just beginning to suffer from neurotic symptoms, and towards the patient who has been chewing the cud of his mental manias for ten years or more. These are problems of tact. Unfortunately, however, the patients who come to consult a specialist have, almost always, well-established symptoms, and there is very little we can teach them. In a word, the treatment of a neuropath must be adapted to the individual case ; it must not be a generalised and commonplace treatment supposed to be suitable for all cases alike. A knowledge of the patient's life and individuality, will give him the important feeling that he is " understood." The development of influence presupposes that the subject will have a tendency and a special form of behaviour adapted to your own personality. Now, if you wish him to adapt himself to your personality, begin by adapting your own personality to his.

One of the difficulties we encounter in the establishment

of influence is the change of guidance. If the doctors previously consulted have only given casual consultations, if the guidance has not been really inaugurated by any other person, we are faced, as it were, by an uninfluenced subject, by one who will adopt his new adviser more or less rapidly, the time varying with the patient's character and his powers of adaptation. But if some particular physician or other person has cared for the patient throughout a considerable time and has exercised a personal influence over him, and if the guidance has then been interrupted for one reason or another, we are concerned with a patient in a very different condition. No doubt he has been made aware of the advantages of guidance, and is accustomed to experience states of influence ; we may put these facts to the credit side of the account. On the other hand, he has systematised his tendencies to suggestion and excitation ; he is accustomed to react in a specific way in response to a particular person, who has special attitudes, special modes of expression, and special methods of approach. We must not suppose that this change will be a trifling matter to the patient. We have to do with one of a class of persons to whom every change, and, above all, any change which is connected with psychological tension, is a serious matter ; and the change of directors necessitates an entirely fresh adaptation, involving effort and the expenditure of energy. The mere fact that our patient has lost his customary director, that the familiar visits to this director have been broken off, has already depressed the patient, and has induced in him a condition ill-suited for the new adaptation.

Despite all our precautions, such a change is invariably a difficult matter, and will be very apt to give rise to relapse. I have elsewhere described the difficulties with which I had to deal when I undertook to treat Marceline, taking the place of my brother who had had so powerful an influence over this woman. I encountered similar difficulties in the treatment of an asthenic who had been very carefully guided for several years by my esteemed colleague Magnin. After his death, the patient had a serious relapse. Another patient, a married woman of thirty-two, who had been for a long time successfully guided by a priest, became very ill when he went away, and it was difficult to establish an influence over her. To her preexistent troubles there were now superadded various scruples, and self-accusations of inconstancy. " It seems to me that I am committing sacrilege when I pass from one person's hands to those of another." In these cases we note strange phenomena in the matter of the patient's thought of the director, which, as we have seen, plays a considerable part in guidance. The idea of the previous director crops up among and mingles with the phenomena of the somnambulist passion ; then it alternates with the thought of the new director, and combines with it. During this period the subject is unhappy, and is very ill. A considerable time must elapse before he can recover peace of mind, for this does not ensue until the thought of the new master has completely effaced the thought of the old one.

Special precautions are needed throughout this period. If possible, we must make ourselves acquainted with the methods used by the previous director ; and, to begin with, we must imitate these methods closely, modifying them only by slow degrees. In such patients, and also in patients who have not previously been subject to influence, we must, during the phase when influence is being established, make use of all the economising methods at our disposal ; we must treat the patient by rest, isolation, and simplification of life. Thus we shall enable him to accumulate the energy requisite for the adaptation we wish him to make.

The essential point in all cases is that the sittings shall occur at regular and short intervals, and that they shall be continued for a considerable time. Throughout this period, we must turn to account all the previously described methods of psychological treatment. If the patient is favourably situated, he will by degrees become enabled to perform the act of adoption. Then we shall have more influence over him, and the efficiency of any methods of treatment we have been applying will be considerably enhanced.

Disorders connected with Guidance. It would be needless to dwell once more upon the characteristic phenomena of influence, such as have already been studied and explained. We need not particularise the improvement, the rise of mental tension, in the patient thanks to the influence of the guide ; we need not say any more concerning the relapses which almost invariably follow the departure of the guide ; we need not speak of the peculiar impulse which leads the patient to seek once more to see the former guide. Treatment by guidance is based upon the therapeutic utilisation of these fundamental phenomena. But in actual practice we encounter difficulties, and it is the difficulties that it now behoves us to study.

We must not fancy that the influence of the director will at once make it easy to modify the subject in any way he pleases. The most suggestible hysterics, who can easily be induced to realise indifferent suggestions, display a marked resistance when we try to dispel their fixed ideas. Asthenics, who to all seeming allow themselves to be readily comforted, are refractory to advice and explanations where their obsessions or delusions are concerned. If we insist, we note oscillations and protracted hesitations. At one moment it may seem that the patient wants to obey the director blindly, at another he is refractory. In the end, after hours of discussion, nothing is done.

These resistances give rise to multiform agitations. Certain subjects, even when hypnotised, will have attacks of major hysteria because the director demands prompt obedience, or simply asks for a pledge. The fact is familiar. Bad temper, reproaches, fits of anger, doubts, continually return in similar circumstances, lessening or completely suppressing the well-being of the period following the sitting.

These resistances and agitations are not, as a rule, dangerous; but they become very important when they threaten the essential power of the director. In such cases, hesitation and doubt relate to the word and to the worth of the very person who ought to inspire a confidence which will do away with hesitation and dispel doubt.—" I ask you to be perfectly frank with me, but now it seems to me that you are trying to humbug me."—" There are contradictions in what you are saying to me. How can you expect me to believe you ? "—" Do you really understand my case ? Once more it seems to me that I am not understood."—" You must dominate me in such a way that all I need is to render an easy obedience. I never really know what I want ; I love to yield before a definite and firm will, which imposes itself upon me. But the least hesitation, the least sign that one who ought to dominate me is merely groping his way, inspires me with distrust."—" There is no longer any one who holds me in hand,

and I am so terribly nervous when I am not properly guided."—
" Once more you seem to me far away and unknown."—Above
all, they doubt the worth, the superiority, of their guide ;
they are overwhelmed with distress at the most trifling failure,
or at the slightest word of criticism which has been breathed
into their ears.—" I, who have always been on the look-out
for some one of overwhelming superiority, was lost when I
heard a critical phrase which deprived my idol of his halo."
" It seems that there is no one who can guide me as I should
like to be guided."—" I need a genius as director. I am
much less distressed by anything which seems to detract
from my own worth, than by something which lowers my
esteem of the worth of the person to whom I have entrusted
myself. I am always ready to obey instantly a person
who manifests true superiority."—This last was a polite way
of saying that I did not exhibit true superiority, this being
the reason why my patient did not instantly obey me.

In such cases, naturally, there develop in the patient's
mind all sorts of more or less deserved criticisms of the director.
He is not the " ideal friend " whom the patient had hoped to
find. " A friend, a true friend, does not write notes about
one's moral sufferings, nor enjoy them as a subject of study ;
he does not keep one's intimate private correspondence among
his medical papers. Such a friend is not a person whom one
can only see at appointed times, and under conditions in which
frank and free relationships are impossible. One knows
something about his daily life, and he reciprocates one's
confidences. . . . It has always been my dream to be loved
for my own sake, and not to be subjected to a remote and
transient professional influence."—These doubts are increased
by the following reflections. " Substantially, I do not know
you at all, and I am not sure of my judgment about you. . . .
I am an unfortunate wretch, utterly miserable. I find everything an effort, everything a tension, even belief."

In these circumstances, the discontented patient watches
his director, making demands of this worthy which become
manias closely akin to those with which the patient is accustomed to torment his relatives. He shows himself exacting
in the matter of the sittings. He wants to regulate them,
they must always be exactly alike. He tells us that if there
is the slightest change in the details they will not do him any

good. When the patient experiences the phenomenon of the somnambulist passion, or feels the need for guidance, he wants a sitting instantly, and he is furious if the doctor is not always and immediately at his disposal. "How can anyone refuse my request, when he knows that such a refusal makes me ill?" Zoé becomes stubborn and ill-tempered if she cannot get her way at this moment. She is like a fury. She drives all her associates crazy. She begins once more to cry out that no one understands her. Such fits of anger are especially serious when we wish, as we must, to have a reasonable interval between the sittings. "To adjourn me for a fortnight like a tiresome law suit! It would be less hardhearted to refuse bread to a destitute person." We shall have once more to consider these difficulties in the spacing out of the consultations when we come to study the closing phases of guidance.

When he is with his director, the patient is very apt to be affected by a mania of questioning, closely related to his condition of doubt, and, naturally, systematised upon the person of the director. He prepares numberless questions, or repeats the same question over and over again under different forms, worrying about the existence of God, the fatality which governs the world, or the microbes which infect a teacup. Sometimes we see a mania for teasing or sulking. The patient, in heartrending tones, will make reproaches which he knows to be undeserved, simply because he wants to see the effect of his feigned onslaught; or from moment to moment he will make as if to break off relationships with the director, in order to see the effect of this simulated rupture.—"It is futile for me to write to you, for you do not even read the pages it has given me so much distress to pen."—"What is the use of my coming to see you at the hospital? I reveal to you the depths of my heart, and all you doctors care about is to laugh at us, and make your unfortunate little patients tremble."—Or, on the other hand, there may be a mania for devotion. "I should like to regard you as my son, to complete your education, so as to render you worthy of my affection."—"I should like you to have a thoroughly happy life, thanks to me."—These same patients will try to arouse jealousy by stringing out a list of persons who have more influence with them than the director; and in many cases they themselves suffer from jealousy. There is no occasion to give detailed descriptions of such moods for they are described at length in the books of the old magnetisers, and I have myself given descriptions of them in earlier works. In these writings there will be found accounts of the jealousy exhibited by hysterical patients who have been hypnotised, their jealousy of other patients treated in the same way; of the rivalry between somnambulists, a rivalry which played a distressing part in the quarrels between the factions of magnetisers, and, more recently, in the erroneous teaching at the Salpêtrière. Similar remarks apply to neuropaths who have never been hypnotised. Very often, as soon as influence is established, the patient becomes authoritarian, exacting, and jealous. It is difficult to treat two persons of this kind who belong to the same family. Lise and Adèle grow more ill when I pay as much attention to their sisters as to themselves. We must often exercise care to avoid inflaming such jealousy.

Like most of the symptoms from which neuropaths suffer, these disorders can be complicated by giving birth to phobias, to obsessive ideas, accompanied to a greater or less extent by impulses connected with the phenomenon of influence and with the patient's relationships to the director. We have already studied the obsessions and the fears relating to the efforts which the director is likely to expect from the patient, and which, the patient believes, will give rise to exhaustion; and those relative to the danger they believe that they will incur by getting under the influence of so exacting a person.— " This doctor makes a speciality of treating nervous and mental disorders. I, therefore, must have a mental disorder. What a dreadful thought ! It is he who reawakens my fear of going mad. His mere presence, the thought that he is coming to visit me, upsets me and arouses the most appalling anxiety."—In other cases, the patient's doubts concerning the capacity or the sincerity of the director become magnified into obsessions. " The doctor said to me one day : ' I am sure that you will get well ' ; and another day he said : ' I am nearly sure that you will get well.' The two statements are not identical; there is a contradiction. My life in the world to come, the life which is to compensate for the miseries of this earthly existence, will be compromised if I allow myself to be guided by such a liar."—Even more frequent are obsessions which take the form of a fear of forfeiting independence, of remorse for exhibiting a degrading obedience. Here are some characteristic utterances illustrating this important obsession, culled from the notes of a score of my cases.—" The Salpêtrière alarms me and fascinates me. I think too much about you. You dominate all my thoughts. It seems to me that you are continually watching me. This is absurd, and I am losing the liberty which I value so greatly."—" Shall I not be dominated and exploited, if I allow any one to rule me in this way ? Will not my liberty completely disappear ? "—" I am always thinking about you. You make me do whatever you like. That seems to me ridiculous. I am revolted by the thought of this foolish attachment; it infuriates me."—" I constantly have the feeling of being caught in the act of some offence, and this irritates me."—" I am afraid of losing my reason, of forfeiting my individuality, when I make any one a confidant and relate all the trifling things that I do."

We are sometimes astonished to find, in these same patients, obsessive feelings of the very opposite kind, fears of not being guided by a sufficiently firm hand, fears of escaping from domination, fears of becoming once more free, too free.— " Now I am afraid that you will not have enough influence upon me. It seems to me that I am becoming incapable of attaching myself, subjecting myself, to the person who is guiding me ; nor can I fix my thoughts upon him. Take care lest I escape you. You do not drive me with a sufficiently tight rein. You do not scold me enough."—" I am afraid of getting too fond of you, and at the same time I am afraid that I am not sufficiently fond of you. These are two different aspects of the same thing ; the same obsession dressed differently on two successive days."—" What would happen if I took a dislike to you, if you could no longer encourage me ? How dreadful it would be ! "—" I have made attempts to break away, and I then find myself forsaken and in the void. I realise how earnestly I desire guidance ; and this revelation, no less intense than distressing, has reduced me to despair."— " I feel scruples about the influence to which I am subjected, and yet it is indispensable. Should I not fall if I were alone ? "— Thus the patient oscillates between two obsessions. He is equally distressed, equally unhappy, whichever of the two is dominant.

Superadded, of course, are all the scruples of morality.—
" If I obey you too strictly, you will deprive me of my ideas
of duty and of the remorse which seems to me essential, for
these ideas and this remorse are right. I shall behave badly
through forfeiting my independence. I certainly want my
doctor to have an influence over my body, but it is too much
that he should have an influence over my mind "—" It is
immoral to develop in me these ideas of surrender and humility.
That will give me ideas of inferiority which conflict with a healthy
morality."—" You have not the same religious ideas as myself.
That is what makes my obedience immoral.   When two people
do not agree in their thoughts about religion, one cannot give
himself up wholly to the other's guidance."—Others go even
further, and are disquieted about differences upon political
matters.   They will suffer from scruples at obeying any one
who does not share the views of their own family upon methods
of government.   Sometimes we see obsessive scruples of an
economic kind.   The patients reproach themselves on account
of their personal expenditure upon the treatment, or upon
the cost to the family.   In many patients, finally, especially
in women, we encounter scruples regarding sexual morality.
There is a dread of " lapsing into sentimentality."   These
scruples are natural enough, seeing that the development of
such sentiments of influence closely resembles in certain cases
the development of the love sentiment.

Such obsessions, of course, induce corresponding impulses,
which lead the patient to try to escape from the director, to
strive against the influence which is regarded as dangerous.
Struggles of the kind will supervene even in patients who seem
to be most completely under influence. I described them in
the case of Marceline, who was affected by them in times of
serious relapse. She then declared that it was necessary
for her to emancipate herself from me, and that I, for my
part, had not the time to spare for her. Henceforward, she
declared she would live without any support. The result was
that she spent whole days and nights asking herself : " Shall
I go ? Shall I not go ? " In many patients these impulses
give rise to resistance, or to a fugue, or to the beginning
of a fugue.

In cases which, happily, are rare, the foregoing obsessions
may be intensified to become true delusions ; and, as I have

previously pointed out, the same thing may happen in the case of the majority of psychasthenic obsessions. Far more often than is usually believed, delusions of persecution, and delusions of influence, are genuine psychasthenic delusions; that is to say, they arise in connexion with psychasthenic disturbances and preserve the essential characteristics of psychasthenia. Usually, these delusions arise in family life, in the social entourage of the patient, and concern the ordinary relationships of social life. Often, they concern the patient's immediate associates, those in whom the patient is particularly interested, those of whom he is especially fond, and those whom he wants to love him. The delusion of persecution is a frequent sequel of the obsessions of loving and of being loved. In the cases with which we are now concerned, the delusion develops under more definite conditions, in the course of psychotherapeutic treatment by guidance, and the object of the delusion is the director.

In my first study of influence,[1] I reported an instance of this delusion in Me., a woman of thirty-seven. She suffered from hypochondriacal obsessions. No more than a very incomplete hypnotic state could be induced, but in this state it was possible to counteract a grave fixed idea of consumption. In that respect, rapid improvement took place. The patient seemed to forget her hypochondriacal ideas and her suicidal impulses. The influence exercised upon her appeared to have satisfactory results. But, after a few sittings, she began to speak of another fixed idea. She complained that she was continually conversing with me, that she never ceased seeing me, that she was persecuted by my influence, which was exercised upon her through walls. She was kept under observation by me from a great distance. . . . In a word, she constructed upon the foundation of the ordinary phenomena of influence a delusion of persecution, of which, happily, it was possible to rid her speedily.

Since that time I have seen two closely similar cases, and I need not record them here. I think it well, however, to refer to the case of Uw. (m., 45), for it affords an interesting example of the relationships between the delusion of persecution and the psychasthenic state. Until he was about thirty-five years old, his only trouble had been psychasthenia, with

[1] Névroses et idées fixes, vol. i, p. 450.

disorders of the will, sentiments of incompleteness, typical doubts and obsessions. We could already detect in him manias of questioning, manias of explanation, and especially that craze for systematisation which is so common in psychasthenics. The power of criticising systems, the power of taking advantage of experience in order to confirm or to invalidate our hypotheses, the resignation and the disinterestedness which enable us to abandon our systematised ideas when they conflict with observed facts—these are complicated and late acquisitions of our mental development. They are the first to disappear in all forms of mental degeneration, and whenever the psychological tension is lowered. A systematised explanation is an inferior type of explanation, a primitive type ; it often persists in isolation, and plays a great part in such minds. But in Uw. this craze for systematisation, which was already conspicuous, exercised itself at first upon religious and moral ideas, and had little effect upon the general course of the illness. From the time he was thirty-three years old, ideas of persecution made their appearance as an expression of the inadequacies of his social activity, and as an explanation of his sentiments of incompleteness and of his lack of success. Thus, he was always timid in sexual matters, and he had already before this time been affected by phobias and hypochondriacal ideas relating to the sexual life. Now he began to give expression to these disorders by saying that " some one " made him fail to keep his appointments ; that, in a mysterious way, " some one " was ruining him. This, he said, was " some one's " vengeance. In that way he explained all sorts of symptoms, and especially those which were induced by his phobia of professional responsibilities. The craze for systematisation was superadded to these explanations, making them more coherent and less easily modified by experience. I shall not lay stress here upon this mode of origin of the delusion of persecution, which I hope to study some day more fully. I merely wish to mention a transient incident in this patient's illness, a result of treatment. Uw. is, like many psychasthenics, extremely sensitive to moral treatment; he is easy to guide; he is very glad to feel himself under a directive influence. He seems to undergo rapid modifications. He accepts the discussion of his delusional explanations, recognises the starting-point of these delusions, and seems to renounce his delusion of persecution. Yet now he comes to make more and more frequent allusions to a very remarkable explanation of his treatment. Although he has never been hypnotised, and although no attempt has ever been made to hypnotise him, he says that he has been subjected to suggestion, has been "possessed" by some one stronger than himself, who unceasingly collaborates with him, and keeps him in the straight road. My assistance, my influence, acts upon him from a distance and through the walls. There is always an occult influence acting upon him; but this time it is a beneficent influence. He fancies that I am continually thinking about him, and that I am sending him this thought by a voice which he hears and recognises as mine. In a word, upon the psychological phenomena of influence he grounds a delusional explanation practically identical with the delusion of persecution from which he previously suffered.

Such transformations of influence into delusion are rare, and I have only come across them in three or four cases; but the before-mentioned disturbances, the manias of guidance, the scruples and the obsessions relating to the director, are fairly common. It was necessary to describe them in some detail, for they greatly complicate the treatment, and it is essential that we should be familiar with them in order that we may know whether the treatment by guidance is dangerous, or whether it ought to be continued.

Explanation of these Disorders. What do these remarkable disorders signify? The psychiatrists of the Freudian persuasion, when they had admitted the accuracy of the description I formerly gave of such phenomena, found it easy to explain them by connecting them, after their customary fashion, with their general theory of pansexualism. The disturbances affecting the patients whom we are trying to guide are, say Freud and his followers, nothing more than the love passion, for in this we perceive the same hesitations, resistances, love of teasing, jealousy, obsessions, delusions. I have already discussed this explanation, and I should like to repeat that such disturbances often occur in patients who have no love sentiment properly so called, and are incapable of any such sentiments. Or they may occur in patients who simultaneously have a love sentiment for another person than the director. But I think that the main objection to the psycho-analytical theory is the typical form assumed by the disorders. No doubt the same form is met with in the love passion, but it is also met with in the case of all the sentiments and all the actions of neuropaths. We are concerned with the reactions of a neuropath, which occur in almost precisely the same way in every kind of situation, and especially in all the different kinds of social relationships.

Whatever the action we are considering, even if it be one which has no connexion with guidance or with the personality of the director, we note hesitations, doubts, imperfect activation of the tendency, a lack of completion, agitations, " attachments," obsessions, delusions. In many cases, as I have just remarked, these disturbances of social action take the form of doubts concerning the worth of persons ; or take the form of teasing, sulking, or jealousy. We had occasion to note many such phenomena when we were studying the influence of the neuropath upon his environment. We are concerned with a general disturbance of his reactions. The craving to tease, to sulk, to be jealous, to torment one's self by scruples, was manifest in the case of a young man of twenty-three, in connexion with his teacher of mathematics, who wanted to make the pupil pay close attention to his work. I saw the same thing in the case of a maidservant of forty in relation to her mistress, who had threatened to discharge the servant. I saw it also in the case of a portress in relation to the owner of the establishment. Are we then to say that all neuropaths are persons in love, and nothing more ? I know that Freud does not hesitate to make this remarkable assertion. For our part, since we are by no means inclined to accept so unduly simplified an explanation of complicated and multiform nervous disorders, we shall not be content to regard the disturbances of influence as nothing more than sexual phenomena. In certain cases, such phenomena may be intermingled with influence without disturbing it in any way. I have referred to cases in which influence was at work between lover and mistress, and yet none of the before-mentioned disturbances occurred ; sexual excitation facilitated guidance and dispelled the patient's symptoms. In other cases, however, such phenomena may complicate and disturb the guidance. But, even then, they are accidental complications. We are not entitled to regard sexual phenomena as the general and sole explanation of these disturbances of guidance.

The disorders we have just been studying depend, in my opinion, upon a more deep-seated cause, upon the essential illness of the subject who is under guidance. The same morbid characteristic is found alike in their reactions to guidance and in all their social activities. What we ask of the patient in the course of this treatment is a social activity of a peculiar and very delicate kind, namely the act of adoption, and the application of a special tendency constructed ad hoc to suit a number of varied circumstances. Many patients, as we have seen, are quite incapable even of beginning such social actions ; but although they clamour for guidance, they will never have it, for they are incapable of adopting a director. Among the others, there are some who have begun this act of adoption, and have developed the corresponding tendency up to a certain point ; they are capable of being commanded and stimulated by the director when circumstances are favourable, but only when the actions to be performed are not very difficult, and when they themselves are not too greatly depressed. As soon as difficulty arises, the activity of the debile tendency is disturbed, and there appear in this connexion disorders identical with those already noted in all the social activities of the same neuropath.

To take only one example, their criticism of the director "who is not an ideal friend" lacks originality, despite all appearances to the contrary. This is a criticism which they have already uttered with regard to every one in their entourage when they were complaining, as they constantly have complained, that they were not "loved for their own sake." We have already studied the significance of this remarkable phrase, and we have learned that it is the expression of a wish to obtain all kinds of services without paying for them, an expression of the desire to find "a cheap slave." Since the director neither will nor can be this ideal person, they naturally recapitulate against him, mutatis mutandis, the criticism they have made against every one else with whom they have come into contact. They say that the director is "a stranger and aloof"; they are troubled by the differences which separate them from him, as they were troubled by the sense of detachment from objects, and by all kinds of social differences. Just when they seem inclined to give themselves up to his guidance, they are inspired by an impulse to despise the director, to dread him, to disobey him, to run away from him, much as they were wont to have impulses conflicting with all their other desires. There is invariably at work the same mechanism of repression, which is applied to this particular kind of social action as to all others. The scruples, the obsessions, and the delusions that ensue, have already been manifested in exactly the same way under other conditions.

Many intelligent patients know well enough that their troubles with the director are identical with those they have had in connexion with other persons.—Nadia admitted it frankly when she said: " I want you to interest yourself exclusively in me. It is just as it was in former days when I was unhappy if mother was interested in one of my sisters."—" The reason why I cannot accept guidance," said Ig. (f., 27), " is the same reason that makes it impossible for me to give myself up trustingly to the will of God and to the hope in a future life ; and it is the same thing which prevents my answering a letter. There are always two beings within me, one who wishes and the other who does not wish. It is the same in this case as in every other case."—" All my doubts are transferred to you," said Fh. (m., 28).—René's phrase was even more striking : " Don't be surprised at my attitude. What happens in your case has happened in every other case. As soon as I have to do with a real sentiment, a check takes place and I cannot go to the end. If I am so much disturbed where you are concerned, and if I have such strange fears and notions in connexion with you, this is because I am trying hard to obey you, and to transform myself. In me, the obsessions return directly anything that I am doing becomes serious."—If we translate these remarks into our own psychological terminology, we shall say that as soon as the patient's psychological condition is characterised by a rising tension, and as soon as a fairly complete activation is in prospect, impotence sets in, and all kinds of derivations are again manifest. This general law of the psychasthenic state applies to all acts of influence, to the activation of the tendency created by adoption, just as to other actions and to the activation of other tendencies.

A last observation will enable us to confirm this explanation. Let us enquire at what moment these disturbances of influence are most conspicuous and most serious. If the disturbances depended upon the influence itself, they would be more marked when this influence was at its maximum, that is to say at the close of successful sittings, and during the happy period which follows them, during the so-called period of influence. But it is precisely at these times that no such disturbances are noticeable, for then the subject feels very well, is delighted with the influence which has transformed him, makes no complaints about its efficacy, and does not dread it in any way. The disturbances are at their climax in the second period, during the latter part of the intervals between the sittings and in the early stage of each sitting. It is when the subject has the greatest need of the director, when he most urgently desires to see the director again, that he is filled with doubts and obsessions antagonistic to guidance. We see in this once more a phenomenon of repression and of antagonism. The disturbances which are the outcome of an increase in the depression are concentrated upon the personality of the director because, at this particular time, the act which circumstances demand is an act which relates to the director. This fact confirms our explanation. We have to do with general disturbances of action brought about by the mental condition of the psychasthenic.

The Treatment of the Disturbances of Influence. The foregoing remarks will help to guide the doctor's behaviour in relation to such disturbances. If he were to regard them as unexpected accidents, as a manifestation of more or less ill-directed amorous passion, he would be surprised at their occurrence, and would dread their onset. He must learn to regard them as natural phenomena depending upon the previous disposition of the persons with whom he is dealing, and he must be prepared to fight against them.

No doubt in certain cases these troubles may become so serious as to be disquieting, and to necessitate the suspension of this kind of treatment. If the delusion of influence or some similar delusion becomes grave, if the conviction grows, and culminates in hallucinations, the doctor must realise that he has to do with a new form of the delusion of persecution from which the patient has already suffered, and that little good is likely to result from the treatment. No doubt a delusion of a beneficent influence is less tormenting to the patient, at first at least, than a delusion of a maleficent influence, but the former is readily transformed into the latter ; the functions of belief and of reasoning will undergo very little improvement ; and often, in cases of this kind, the treatment must be discontinued as useless.

We may have to take the same course when there arise serious crises of doubts and obsessions relating to the director. When the prolongation of the treatment does not dispel them, it may become plain, in exceptional cases, that the harm done to the patient by the treatment exceeds the good. Still, it is our business to recognise that what is amiss here is not that the influence is too strong (as the patient tells us), but that it is too weak. There is a check in the organisation of the direction, a check which usually depends upon the fact that the patient's depression is too great to allow of a correct act of adoption.

Apart from these failures, that occur when the disturbance is too severe, we must not attach much importance to difficulties which are almost unavoidable. I am by no means inclined to regard scruples concerning direction as a sign that the patient is intolerant of the treatment, and that its continuance is contraindicated. To me, rather, it seems to be a favourable sign, an indication of the first stage of adoption, a manifestation of the faltering efforts made by the subject to adopt the director. Patients who show no sign of such disturbances are apt to be those in whom no advance towards adoption has been made, and those in whom adoption is unlikely to occur. On the other hand, the patients who manifest such troubles are often those who will benefit most by the treatment.

Nevertheless, when such disturbances assume an obsessive and distressing form, we must try to reduce them. We shall often succeed in doing this, by our advice and our explanations, for some of the scruples can be lessened by suitable admonitions. No doubt the director is not the " ideal friend," first of all because the ideal friend does not exist, and secondly because if he did exist, the patients would be incapable of making any use of him. Obviously, the director is, to some extent, an artificial parent or an artificial friend. There are drawbacks attached to this fact, and it would be futile to deny them, for they are the direct outcome of the nature of the illness ; but there are advantages accruing thereform likewise. It is precisely because the director is artificial, because he makes things go easily, because he himself effects three-quarters of the journey, that the patient can succeed in making in relation to the director the act of adoption which he has never before succeeded in making in relation to any one else. It is for the very reason that the relationship is artificial that it is comparatively free from risk. In social relationships of a kind which the patient regards as more natural, he will exhibit the same weaknesses, the same lack of control ; but he will not be safeguarded by any kind of pledge, and he will be exposed to all sorts of exploitation. Here his weakness is recognised in advance, and the director's professional obligations prevent his taking advantage of this weakness. The influence which is to be turned to account is based upon the laws of suggestion, education, and excitation. There is nothing mysterious or terrible about these laws ; and, to some extent at least, they can be explained to the patient in order to reassure him. If the artificial character of the relationship is too repugnant to the patient, he may look forward to its subsequent transformation into a more natural relationship. But his first business is to get better, in order to become capable of this.

It is likewise true that the director may be mistaken, and may, despite his best endeavours, contradict himself more or less. He is not a genius, and does not pretend to be one ; but he is sufficiently sincere, and he is competent to direct a poor disordered mind, competent to steer the patient through all the shoals and difficulties. No doubt the director, by imposing direction, would reduce the will power and the freedom of the patient, if the latter had any will power or any freedom. But, in actual fact, he is dealing with some one who has lost will power and freedom ; the only freedom he annuls is the freedom of self-delusion. The only efforts he demands of the patient are efforts which may restore the lost powers of the will. Let the patient postpone his dreams of

independence,, for the best way of realising them at some
future date will be to accept dependence for the time being.
Explanations of this kind, and many others which the director
can think out for himself, will help, in quite a number of
cases, to remove the patient's apprehensions and scruples.

The essence of the treatment, however, is not to be found
in such matters as this. Often we shall do better to avoid
attacking the symptoms directly, and to devote ourselves to
striving against the illness itself, against the lowering of the
psychological tension, which we must try to raise by all the
means at our disposal. The disorders of the influence will
vanish spontaneously when the other disturbances connected
with the disease have been reduced, and when the depression
grows less marked. We can easily perceive that disturbances
which are conspicuous in the phase of need, are absent or
minimised at the close of a successful sitting and during
the happy period which follows it. Lise, like many others,
is greatly obsessed concerning me when she has not seen me
for a long time, but is comparatively free from these troubles
when she sees me frequently and at regular intervals. The
excitation resulting from the visit dispels the depression which
is the main cause of the scruples.

The reader may be surprised to learn that the influence
can continue to make itself felt, and may often do good
notwithstanding the appearance of these manias and obsessions
which seem to annul its action. It is true that in ordinary
life, which is not organised to meet the needs of sick persons,
such disorders rapidly impair social relationships, and even
make social relationships impossible. Fits of bad temper,
attacks of the sulks, agitated resistances, fits of hysterics, hesitations, all kinds of doubts, inertias, a long-continued chilliness
of disposition—such manifestations astonish and discourage the
associates, and speedily put an end to conversation, advice,
or signs of affection. But it is precisely in order that he
may forefend these difficulties, that the doctor must behave
artificially. He does his utmost to avoid an injudicious
provocation of hesitations or doubts, partly by being careful
not to ask certain ticklish questions, but above all by assuming
an affirmative and steadfast mien which would be inadmissible
in ordinary conversation. When alone with his patient,
he will allow himself to utter violent reproaches, to indulge

in sentimental adjurations in an exaggerated tone which would be ridiculous in ordinary life, but which are very wholesome for these persons suffering from moral anaesthesia. When there are signs of bad temper, agitation, or resistance, he knows that in relationship with himself they cannot last long; he knows that the lowness of the patient's tension renders prolonged action impossible; he knows how to overcome the patient's obstinacy by a gentle and continued pressure, like that by which the surgeon overcomes the spasmodic contraction of a sphincter muscle. He watches for the moments of relaxation of tension, which are certain to appear soon, and he seizes his opportunity. He knows how to mask the fact that the patient is obeying orders, for he is aware that all these patients say: " I must be driven with a tight rein, but I do not want to know that this is being done." He must begin the action, and asks nothing more of the patient than the continuance of the action; that is to say, all he asks for is the performance of easy efforts, efforts the patients can make without suffering from the checks which are a part of these invalids' customary experience. Above all, the doctor will display incredible patience, so that the sufferer will be able to act with that extreme slowness which is indispensable to the psychasthenic, as we have previously explained. In a word, the artificial attitude adopted by the doctor is one precisely suited to the disorders from which these patients suffer, and is calculated to enable them to act notwithstanding their malady.

Many of the patients come, in the end, to recognise the nature of the part played by the director. " When I am with you, I can at any rate indulge in these great scenes which seem so quaint to me, and which reduce my relatives to despair, for you, at least, do not take them seriously."—" It does not matter how often I tell you that I detest you, for you understand very well that it is not true, and you know that I am always your big baby."—" I have to be rude for about half an hour before I can become civil and pleasant. Other people, who cannot stand me for more than quarter of an hour, and then go away, are convinced that I am a beast. You know that you must wait half an hour before coming to an opinion."

We have here one more instance of the treatment by

action which we described in the foregoing chapter. When
the doctor pays little attention to reproaches and scruples,
when he gently tries to change the patient's attitude towards
himself, and to make the patient accept the necessary guidance, he is, substantially, exercising a particular kind of
social action upon the subject; he is inducing the subject to
make an act of adoption, and to effect the applications of
this action. He brings about the disappearance of the disorders by means of the correct performance of the action.
The essential factor is always the treatment of the malady
itself, and the preparation for action.

8. The Goal of therapeutic Guidance.

When we study the development of these remarkable
relationships between the patient and the doctor to which
the illness gives rise, we must also study their termination.
How do they end? What is the outcome of these alternations
between satisfaction and uneasy passion? Has guidance an
end? Can it have an end? Ribot wrote an interesting
essay upon the topic, entitled *Comment les passions finissent.*[1]
He could have found very remarkable, almost experimental
data anent this question in the history of our patients and
in the evolution of the somnambulist passion.

In a first category we may class the terminations or the
interruptions of treatment by guidance which supervene for
various reasons before the cure of the patient, although the
illness for whose relief the treatment was begun continues to
run its course. Of course, such interruptions may occur quite
accidentally through the departure of the doctor, through a
change of residence on the part of the patient, through various
changes in situation. In our study of the difficulties of
guidance we saw that such interruptions may sometimes
(though rarely, in my opinion) become necessary because of
the way in which the patient reacts to the treatment, because
the patient has crises of doubt concerning the director, or
becomes affected with obsessions and even delusions bearing
upon the influence. These are familiar causes of the interruption of treatment.

Such terminations are exceptional, and are not of much

[1] The fourth chapter of Essai sur les passions, Alcan, Paris, 1907.

importance. As a rule, when treatment by guidance is broken off before the cure of the disease, the reason is an important one, and one which has a serious bearing upon prognosis. I speak of the *exhaustion of the influence.* We are concerned, here, with a gradual diminution of the therapeutic power of guidance as applied to a particular invalid. This diminution may manifest itself in various ways. One of the simplest, and at the outset one of the most striking, is a reduction in the duration of the period of influence, and the more or less rapid onset of the period of somnambulist passion, or of need. In consequence of this, the sittings have to be held more and more frequently, until the increase of frequency makes the treatment impracticable. Numerous references have been made to remarkable instances of hysterical patients suffering from mutism or other symptoms, who seemed to have been marvellously cured after a hypnotic sitting, but in whom a relapse occurred a few hours later, and who then clamoured for a new sitting. "Dr. Charcot, please help me to get rid of my patient," said a young doctor who was worried several times a day by such a patient.—In connexion with the study of these phenomena I referred elsewhere to the case of Dy. (f., 25). She was suffering from major hysteria. By working hard for two hours or more, I could dispel all her symptoms, and could transform her into a person who appeared perfectly normal. But a few hours later the symptoms infallibly recurred, and to keep her in good health she would have had to be treated several times a day.—The same thing could be noted in other patients. In Bri. (f., 22), the influence only lasted for half a day, in El. (f., 30), it lasted no more than a few hours, and when the benefit of the sitting had passed off the patient pestered the doctor for further treatment.—Irène, in her bad phases, was unable to keep the promises which she had made in all sincerity during the sittings of complete somnambulism. She promised, she swore " upon her mother's portrait," that she would rest. Half an hour later she had forgotten her promise. Meeting a poor woman who had just been evicted, she gave up her bed to this unfortunate, and spent the night in a chair watching her guest asleep. The next day she was more exhausted and depressed than ever, and complained that the sitting had done her no good.—We see the same phenomenon in obsessed persons; in doubters, who are reassured for no more than an instant, who hasten back to the doctor to demand a fresh demonstration, and to torment him with questions. " I leave you with excellent resolutions, which I keep for a quarter of an hour. Then something goes crack in my head and all is lost. You must begin over again."

In favourable cases, we can sometimes train such patients to wait a little longer, and the effort they are thus induced to make gives rise to a favourable excitation. Rk. (m., 40) congratulates himself on not having returned immediately after having left me. " I gave you my word of honour that I would not come back too soon, and I succeeded in keeping my promise. But it was a terribly hard struggle, and I wept like a girl. The effort I was making had a strange effect upon me. The idea of matches which has tormented me so much has suddenly disappeared—so suddenly that I was astonished, for never before had a fixed idea disappeared so promptly." We may see the same thing in the case of treatment by direction when, despite all difficulties, it is going on favourably. But, unfortunately, it often happens that in cases of this kind we have to hold the sittings too frequently, so that ere long the treatment becomes impracticable. When the period of influence grows shorter and shorter, we may infer that the influence of the director is inadequate, that it is diminishing, and that it is doing little good.

Concomitantly with the shortening of the period of influence, the mental modifications caused by the influence become more difficult to secure, and are less and less marked. After the sitting, the subject is almost as ill as before. The doctor will be forced to realise that his influence is less personal than it was, and that he can affect the patient no better than another could do. Before, he was easily able to bring about considerable changes; but now, using the same method, he influences the patient very little.

We are apt to try to explain this exhaustion of influence in accordance with well-known psychological laws, such as are known to act in the case of normal persons. We say that habit blunts the sensibilities. The physical and moral impressions induced by the director no longer have the added power of novelty. The things he says and does during the sitting have become, as it were, stereotyped; the actions which the patient is able to do easily, no longer require an effort, and therefore do not raise the tension. The director must continually renew his consolatory phrases or his criticisms ; he must unceasingly change his methods of procedure. But since this is impossible. it is natural that the influence should be gradually exhausted.

The explanation is plausible, but I do not think it furnishes us with the main reason for the exhaustion of influence. Depressed patients, though they are little capable of new adaptations, may seem to desire changes, just as they desire all kinds of things which appear to be stimulating. In reality, however, they bear changes badly, and derive very little advantage from them. Owing to their lethargy, such patients are faithful in their likings ; they hate changes ; and they are as a rule helped more by familiar methods which have already succeeded in their case and which they have adopted, than by new methods. The beneficial effect of a change of method, or of a change of director, will be transient, and relapse will soon follow. The exhaustion of influence is dependent upon causes which are more deep-seated than the laws of habit.

The exhaustion of influence, like all the disorders previously studied, is an outcome of the development of the illness. The patient does not keep his promises because the performance of a promise, like the acting upon resolutions or beliefs, demands at least as much psychological tension as the making of the promise or the forming of the resolution. The rise of tension has been but momentary, and tension has already fallen again when the time comes for performance. Irène, in whom during the sitting the psychological tension has been raised to the level of reflection, promptly relapses to the level of automatic assent and of impulse, so that she obeys every possible suggestion. Temporarily (and sometimes the time may be considerable), the patient has been sustained, and even uplifted, by guidance. But this arrest of the downward movement is brief ; and, under various influences, operating at a deeper level, the illness continues to develop. The exhaustion of an influence which has for a considerable time been helpful, is, as a rule, a bad prognostic sign. It indicates that the patient has become incapable of being uplifted by means which were previously efficacious.

The symptoms of asthenic delusion, or, more frequently, of asthenic dementia, will speedily appear. This is what I have myself noted in thirteen cases in which, sometimes after several years of easy and successful treatment by guidance, the exhaustion of the influence has set in. The dissolution of a tendency which has been a source of excitation is one of the strangest and saddest characteristics of the permanent lowering of tension which occurs when the disease undergoes such an aggravation. In days to come its study will constitute an interesting chapter in the description of asthenic delusions and asthenic dementia.

These reflections anent the terminations of the influence in the course of the disease, furnish indications for the behaviour of the doctor. Interruptions of direction are especially unfavourable for the patient when they have not been brought about by the evolution of the illness, but by some accidental circumstance. Obviously, therefore, we must do our utmost to avoid them. It would be well at the outset of the treatment of a neuropath to warn the patient or his relatives that treatment of this kind has no resemblance to a surgical operation, that it is not sudden in its effects, that it acts like a sort of education, and must be continued for a certain time without any brusque interruption.[1] When interruption has been inevitable, we shall often find that it induces serious symptoms, especially when we have to do with subjects who have already succeeded in making a more or less satisfactory act of adoption, and who are deriving considerable profit from the guidance. When interruption takes place in these cases, we note obsessions of regret closely akin to those we have occasion to study when some one who has acquired influence over the patient dies or goes away. The crisis of depression may be serious and lasting, but it does not present any special features. It develops just like any other crisis of the kind, and demands the same treatment.

Sometimes, especially in cases in which the direction has been accidentally interrupted, and even in cases in which the direction has been intermittent because of serious disturbance localised upon the personality of the director, we may try the continuance of the treatment with no other change than a

---

[1] Cf. Traitement psychologique de l'hystérie, L'état mental des hystériques, second edition, 1910, p. 679.

change in that personality. Perhaps another person will be able to establish an influence under better conditions, a more durable and stronger influence, one which will be able to prevent the appearance of the scruples which are a manifestation of the inadequacy of the influence. But we must not forget that in most cases such a change involves peculiar difficulties to which attention has already been drawn. It makes the subject feel that he has experienced a new check in his attempts at adoption, so that he becomes more depressed and more discouraged in face of the same problem. Very often, the troubles which have led us to make a change will reappear in a yet graver form in relation to the new director. Patients who are continually changing their director owing to doubts and scruples of this kind, will never achieve a satisfactory result. Still, with perseverance and a certain amount of discipline, we shall sometimes be able, as I know from my own experience, to substitute a new direction for the old, so as to secure very satisfactory results.

When the direction is thwarted by the exhaustion of the influence owing to the fact that the patient has become more profoundly depressed, we shall have to recognise that the treatment has become inapplicable. The patient is, if I may use the phrase, too far down for treatment by direction; he is no longer capable of making the reactions which are essential if this treatment is to be of any use. In most instances it will be better to renounce, at least for a time, treatment by direction properly so called, and we shall get better results from going back to treatment by rest, by education, or by physiological medication. Guidance will have to be replaced by ordinary medical care. This, by means of a lower-grade influence, will enable the patient to avoid the disastrous consequences of his ill-considered impulses. It will render possible the application of other kinds of treatment, and will perhaps enable us, at a later stage and under better conditions, to resume treatment by personal influence.

Happily we are able to note that treatment by direction does not always end in this way. Just as the influence declines when the disease increases, so also it declines, but in a different way, when the disease passes off.

When we have to do with exhaustion of influence dependent

upon an increase in the depression, the modifications brought about by the influence of the doctor are induced with greater difficulty and are less extensive. Notwithstanding the treatment, the patient is little better than he was before, and the advance achieved by the treatment persists for a very short time. But in the cases we have now to consider, while in like manner the changes become less and less extensive, this is because the patient is already better, and because a comparatively small lift of his mental level brings him up to the normal. We find, too, that the progress is more easily secured, and that it lasts longer.

These multiform transformations are easily noted in a number of patients, when, after a few oscillations, the mental level progressively rises. The case of Mb. (f., 33) offers a new example of such methods of treatment. She was suffering from a complicated condition, having simultaneously hysterical symptoms and strange hypochondriacal fixed ideas, tantamount to delusions, as a sequel to a series of misfortunes and sufferings. From the first she was extremely susceptible to hypnotism and to moral guidance, but an hour's sitting was requisite to lessen the strength of her delusions and to raise her mental level a little. Although the effect of influence was very distinct, the period of influence lasted only for a day, and was followed by a typical period of somnambulist passion lasting several days. After six months' treatment, Mb., who by now was a great deal better, could be fully restored by a sitting of a few minutes, and remained in a satisfactory condition for a fortnight or three weeks after each sitting.

It is in cases of this kind, and during this phase of the treatment, that we have occasion to note the easy and rapid transformations to which I have already called attention. The doubts and the obsessions of Kl., the delusions of Vz., and the fixed ideas of Justine, yielded to treatment within a few minutes. The scruples of Lise or of Md. (f., 40), which, to begin with, could only be dispelled by hours of struggle, now disappeared rapidly after the commencement of the sitting, and the patients were soon ready to talk of other things. Hysterical symptoms, such as contractures, would pass off after a few slight touches of the affected limb and after the utterance of a few words, as I have seen in the case of No., although at the outset of the treatment the same symptoms could only be removed by an hour's painful massage and by prolonged suggestion. I could quote numerous instances of the kind. Whereas in the case of many neuropaths we have to deplore the occurrence of frequent relapses, these failures are compensated for in other cases by a gradual decline in the intensity of the illness and by an increasing ease of relief.

The reason why the relief becomes easier in the later stages of the treatment is that the symptom, though apparently still the same, is really different. The fall in psychological tension is much less extensive than of yore. The moral transformation which the doctor has to induce by his influence is much less considerable than it was at the commencement of the treatment. This diminution in the transformation is attended by a remarkable consequence which is especially conspicuous in hypnotised hysterics. The difference between the waking state in which the subjects come into our room, and what is called the somnambulist state artificially induced there, becomes less and less extensive. Sensation, memory, and activity, are now almost identical in the two conditions. The natural result of this approximation of the two states is that there is no longer any modification of memory at the moment of transition from one state to another, so that amnesia no longer occurs when the patient wakens from complete somnambulism. Persons who for years have exhibited a typical loss of memory at this stage of awakening, no longer exhibit such amnesia in any regular fashion ; and during the waking state, when the end of the treatment draws near, they will preserve memories of what has happened in the somnambulist state. I pointed out in former days that hysterics who are fully cured, recover during the waking state the memories of their delusions and of their somnambulisms, even those of very old date. There has sometimes been an inclination to accuse them of fraud, on the ground that if to-day they can remember what happened long ago in the somnambulist state, they ought to have been able to remember it just as well in former days after their awakening. This is a gross error. The amnesia of what has happened in the somnambulist state is a symptom of a peculiar morbid condition which exists especially in the waking state. When this disorder of the waking state passes away, the amnesia also disappears. Moreover, in such conditions the somnambulism itself soon disappears. The disappearance of susceptibility to hypnotism is one of the most distinct and one of the most remarkable signs of the cure of neuropathic conditions.[1]

However this may be, the state of influence is more readily induced and lasts longer. Patients who, to begin with, would relapse after two days, will remain from three to six weeks before relapsing. Moreover, the close of the period of restoration is less distinct. When the patient comes to consult us again, it is not under the pressure of need, and he feels that he might have waited longer before coming. The period of the somnambulist passion or of intense need is much less sharply marked than it was. At the outset of the treatment the patient would clamour for the director the instant the influence passed off, just as a morphinomaniac clamours for a hypodermic injection ; but now, in the later stages of treatment, the need for the director does not manifest itself with the same intensity. The patients clamour less for their sittings, they come late and may even forget the date of their appointment, though this would never have happened at the outset of the treatment.

It is interesting to note the change in the sentiments which accompanies this transformation. The persons who were sounding the praises of their director, who were comparing him to God Almighty, who were hanging on to him in a touching and absurd way, and who were overwhelming him with passionate declarations, have completely changed their attitude. Their tone lowers in proportion as their energy rises. Their feeling towards the director is now a tranquil one ; they no longer put him upon a pedestal, and often allow themselves to criticise him. The reason is that they have become animated by desires for independence, which conflict with their need for support. They vacillate between the two, and only retain an affection for the director in proportion as they still feel need for him. Their indifference grows rapidly. The day comes when, spontaneously, they give up seeing the person from whom a little while ago they could not tear themselves away, and the onset of forgetfulness is as rapid as their demonstrations of affections were

[1] Traitement psychologique de l'hystérie, L'état mental des hystériques, second edition, pp. 649 and 676.

pathetic at the outset. Persons who have acted as guide to such patients, and who have taken the passionate expressions at their face value, are somewhat surprised at the terminal cooling off. In reality, however, this last is their work and their reward, for the patient's love was only the expression of his weakness, and his ingratitude is the best token of his recovery.

An especially typical case is that of Nadia, who for seven years, by word of mouth and by almost daily letters of immense length, displayed for her director an attachment so intense that even she herself found it necessary to excuse herself for " sticking to him like a limpet to a rock." When, by slow degrees, she acquired a higher grade of activity, and when she recovered self-confidence, she no longer felt this urge to stick to a rock like a limpet. She gradually gave up writing to me, became more tranquil, and then colder. More and more she detached herself from me. Then, after a few letters with nothing more in them than polite phrases, she ceased to write to me. The same thing happened with Jean, who, after six years of close attachment, broke away completely. I have had other patients who have vanished from my sight after a phrase of somnambulist passion lasting two years. Others have continued on friendly terms with me, but their friendship now is extremely discreet, and contrasts strongly with their former attitude. I find among my notes those of fifty-four patients who, after a year or two of attachment morbid in its intensity, were cured, and thenceforward exhibited a characteristic coldness. Such experiences, which show once more the pathological nature of the feelings in question, may reassure those who are inclined to be alarmed at the development of so exaggerated an affection.

It is true, none the less, that the doctor who is acquainted with and foresees such a development and such a termination of guidance, must pave the way for it, and must hasten it as far as he can. At the outset of the treatment, he tries to increase the intensity of the influence, and turns it to account in order to bring about the disappearance (temporarily, at least) of the symptoms, and in order to raise the patient's tension. But he must be most careful to avoid allowing the development of a mania for hypnotism, of an impulse to seek excitation, beyond the degree to which these are justified by a real need. That is why he must carefully study the evolution of the patient's mental activity, and must watch the development of the patient's initiative. As soon as any advance can be noted, he must try, above all, to secure a prolongation of the period of influence. To this end he must pay much attention to regulating the interval between the sittings. The interval must not be so long that the somnambulist passion or the need becomes too distressing ; and it must not be so long that the influence passes off altogether and has to be reinstituted. On the other hand, the interval must be as long as possible, so that the subject can become accustomed to practising self-support, so that he shall not relapse too quickly as the mere outcome of the passage of time, so that he shall learn, thanks to the director's teaching, to solve for himself the little problems of life. As R. C. Cabot tells us, we must lead the patient to act on his own account without having recourse at every moment to this " spiritual cocktail." [1] A gradual spacing out of the sittings, a reduction in the number of suggestions and in the intensity of the excitation, will ultimately enable the patient to dispense with the doctor, or at least it will do this in the fairly numerous cases in which the restoration of mental energy is possible.[2]

Such cures are not always definitive. Side by side with the patients whom we guide for several years, who gradually become transformed, and whose illness disappears for good, there are others, who are as a rule restored to health more rapidly, but who, after a longer or shorter interval and thanks to various influences, relapse into a condition similar to that from which they first suffered. As a rule, these relapses are easy to understand, and confront us with the same sort of problem as that which we had to face when the patient first consulted us.

It is remarkable to note that, from the beginning of the relapse, the patient returns into the state of mind which was characteristic of his earlier illness, and that he once more and promptly exhibits the same need for guidance. Generally speaking, it is far easier than it was to begin with to reestablish

---

[1] R. C. Cabot, Suggestion, Authority, and Command, Parker's Psychotherapy, II, iii, 26.

[2] Janet, Traitement psychologique de l'hystérie, L'état mental des hystériques, p. 478.

the influence, and the same procedures succeed as before. Let me recall once more the typical case of Kl. The first time she came under treatment, when she was thirty years of age, I had her under my care for nearly three years, the sittings being held at very brief intervals to begin with, but at long intervals towards the close of this period. The result was that I was able to dispel her very remarkable and obstinate obsessions, and to rid her of a number of neuropathic symptoms which had troubled her since the age of twelve. Thereafter, being now in excellent health, she came to look me up once or twice a year during the next three years. Then I saw and heard nothing more of her for seven years. Throughout this later period there remained no trace of the strong influence I had established over her when she first came to consult me. When she was forty-three, family troubles, a law suit, and a divorce, led to a renewed and severe depression of the mental level, and all her old troubles recurred, so that the clinical picture was identical with that of thirteen years earlier. The obsessive over-scrupulousness, the interminable questionings whether her child's birthmark was really a proof that her husband was the father—all these symptoms were identical with the old ones, although now, since she was separated from her husband, there seemed no reason why such questions should trouble her. Furthermore, her susceptibility to hypnosis, her suggestibility, the signs of an exaggerated attachment to and dependence upon the director, all the phenomena which had disappeared eight years ago, were again exhibited in the old form. The treatment was much briefer, for a few months now sufficed to dispel the symptoms. For four years I have heard nothing more of her, which I take as a sign that she is quite well.

Zoé's case is similar. She first came under my care when she was nineteen, suffering from a grave crisis of doubt and of obsessions arising in connexion with her engagement to marry. At this time she manifested a passionate attachment to me as her director. When the crisis was over, the attachment disappeared, and for seven years she completely forgot me. She returned to consult me at the age of twenty-seven in a state of depression brought on because her mother had died and her husband had gone away. She now exhibited the old symptoms, and the old need for guidance. She spoke to me as if the last sitting had been only the day before, and it was surprising that she had not felt the slightest need to see me or to write to me for seven years. The cure on this occasion was quicker than before, and thereafter she passed out of my ken for an idefinite period. Many of my other cases, especially that of Emma, who was under my observation for seventeen years (though with lengthy interruptions), are of the same kind. This sequence of events is common, and the influence varies in accordance with the evolution of the disease.

Finally there is a remarkable form of influence which confronts us with strange problems. I refer to *continuous influence*, to an influence which lasts for many years. Some of the patients under our care get no worse; the disease does not grow more severe; they never suffer from delusions, and never exhibit any typical signs of dementia. Nevertheless they do not get well, for if their sittings are spaced out too much, a serious relapse ensues. Furthermore, we never note in them a disappearance of the need for guidance or a cessation of the influence.

Here are some cases of the kind.—Ky. has been under guidance in the aforesaid manner for fifteen years. Not until recently, after the patient had passed the age of forty, were the sittings held irregularly and at long intervals. Before that I had had to see her frequently and regularly.—Marceline, whose remarkable history I have given at considerable length, was under my care uninterruptedly for seventeen years until her death. Throughout this period, there was no change in her symptoms. She suffered from a peculiar form of hysterical depression, with marked anorexia, contractures, retrograde amnesia, susceptibility to hypnotism, and susceptibility to a peculiar aesthesiogenic action which could restore activity and memory for a definite time.—Things have gone on in the same way with Irène for sixteen years. Although there is obvious improvement, she invariably relapses if left to herself for a time.—Among the psychasthenics, Lox. has been under regular direction for fourteen years. Not until she had passed the age of fifty did she make a little progress in the way of independence. Even now she cannot get on without being " bucked up " from time to time.—Noémi has been under guidance for ten years.—Lydia has been under guidance for twelve years.—Lise has been subject to influence unintermittently for eighteen years. Only for the last two years, since the menopause occurred, has it been possible to intermit the influence a little.—To sum up, I find in my case-books the reports of fifteen cases in which guidance was continued for from four to five years; twenty-one cases in which guidance was continued for a time ranging from five to ten years; and fourteen cases in which guidance has been continued for more than ten years.

Manifestly we have here to do with a morbid habit. The need for continued guidance is part of the illness. We must point out in this connexion that systematised habits play a great part in disorders of the mind, and that the majority of patients suffering from chronic mental affections exhibit types of disease whose monotony is deplorable. This morbid habit arises because the disease is in itself chronic, because it is kept up by permanent conditions which we cannot get rid of. I showed, for instance, that Marceline's circumstances condemned her to excessive labour, far beyond the measure of her powers, and that this helped to keep up her illness. In many cases the exact causes are beyond our ken, but we think of hereditary conditions, organic insufficiencies, intoxications, social circumstances, which keep up the illness despite our best endeavours, and are the cause of the patient's perpetual inadequacy.

We have, then, to ask what part direction, when it has thus become a morbid habit, can play in the course of these chronic illnesses. I am convinced that it has a very important part to play. It sustains the patient at a higher level, rendering possible a degree of social activity which the sufferer could not have manifested had he been left entirely to himself. The patient is a weakling, obviously; the direction plays the part of a crutch. No doubt it is unfortunate to have to use a crutch, but we must not forget that without this crutch our patient could not walk at all. Marceline was bedridden, inert, dying of starvation, when she was partially restored by aesthesiogenism. If its use had been discontinued, she would have relapsed into her former condition, and would have speedily succumbed. Thanks to the regular use of this influence, she has lived seventeen years longer, has been able to work well enough to gain her livelihood and to help in the upkeep of her family. Of course, this is not a cure, and our powerlessness is the measure of our ignorance. Still we have done something for our patient, and we must be thankful for small mercies. I am satisfied that the same remarks apply to other patients who have been sustained for twenty years by psychotherapeutic direction, even though, in these cases, the patient's life was never in danger. The direction has been a crutch which has enabled them to live socially, and has saved them from having to spend these years in a lunatic asylum. If, however, we are to discuss so delicate a question, and if we are to understand how psychotherapeutics can thus be a support to weaklings, we shall have to consider a little more closely the conception of mental disorders which I am about to expound in the general conclusion of the present work.

The form of treatment in which the personal influence of the doctor plays a part is not easy to appraise from the medical standpoint. Its value does, in fact, vary much in accordance with the personality of the director, and in accordance with the amount of harmony which exists between his individuality and that of his patient. When we have to do with suggestion and hypnotism, we can, though with some difficulty, define our terms and verify the utilisation of the method. The matter becomes far more difficult when we have to take into account the personal action of the doctor, and when we have to ascertain the modifications in the condition of a patient who has been exposed to multiform influences. Among the signs of the action we are considering, I include the phenomena of electivity, somnambulist passion, and the need for guidance, while admitting that these signs are extremely vague. Out of the very large number of cases which have come under my notice, I can select only a small number, about 180, of patients who have exhibited the foregoing signs, and upon whom this special form of treatment seems to have exercised an influence. From among the 180, I select 125 in whom the influence seems to me to have been definitely favourable. Manifestly, however, these figures are too low, for in a great number of cases in which the improvement was attributed to rest, to the simplification of life, or to excitation by work, personal influence must have played an important part, although it is difficult to isolate this factor and to produce evidence of its working.

Notwithstanding the difficulty of drawing up statistics, and though we can scarcely judge of the value of this method of treatment in terms of the number of cures or improvements obtained, I think its very great value cannot be denied. The method corresponds to a need of many of these patients, a need evidenced by the good effects of chance guidance, by the obsession of being loved, by the impulses to seek support and guidance, by which these patients are so often animated. It constituted an important part of the older treatment by moralisation and by religious influence. Very likely, a more accurate psychological analysis of the social relationships and of the various influences which human beings necessarily exercise one upon another, will some day endow this treatment with greater importance, will render it more precise, and will make its application more fruitful.

CONCLUSION

WHEN I began to write the present work my intention was to include in the title the word " psychotherapy," but I gradually came to realise that a title containing this word would be far too pretentious. Psychotherapy does not yet exist. We are merely beginning to see what it ought to be, and what in due time it will become.

According to a first group of definitions, psychotherapy or psychotherapeutics is regarded as a means of treating the disorders of the mind. "Any method by which the mind can be altered favourably . . . is properly called psychotherapy." [1] Certainly this is one of the aims of psychotherapeutics; but if we are to define psychotherapeutics in this way, we must first of all extend our conception of the disorders of the mind, and must fully realise that we are not thinking solely of mental alienation properly so called, but of all morbid modifications of behaviour, of whatever kind. Even then, such a definition would be insufficient, for we must not forget that many authors speak of psychotherapeutics in connexion with diseases of the stomach, enteritis, diseases of the bladder, and so on—maladies which may be associated with or related to disorders of the mind. Such definitions apply rather to the term " psychiatry," which must not be confounded with psychotherapy.

In the other definitions, for the most part, the mind is not regarded as the object of psychotherapy, but as the means employed by psychotherapy. Thus psychotherapy is defined by the use it makes of certain determinate phenomena. Grasset puts the matter very well when he writes : " Electrotherapy and hydrotherpay are not treatments of electricity or water, but treatments by electricity or water; in like manner, psychotherapy is not treatment of the mind but treatment by the mind." Some authors, while defining psychotherapy in this way, restrict their notion of psychotherapeutic procedures

[1] Beatrice M; Hinkle, in Parker's Psychotherapy, II, i, 5.

to the application of certain special psychological phenomena. Dejerine, for instance, will make use of little else than conversation, explanatory reasoning, sound moral advice. I think there is no justification for any such restriction. When we speak of psychotherapeutics, we must include within its scope all the psychological phenomena which can exercise a valuable influence.

Most of the best-known definitions of psychotherapy take such a line. Hack Tuke said that this method of treatment utilised the "general influence of the physician upon the patient in exciting those mental states which act beneficially upon the body in disease"; and he defined psychotherapeutics as the "practical application of the influence of the mind on the body to medical practice."[1]—"Psychotherapy," said Grasset, "is the treatment of diseases by psychic means, that is to say, by persuasion, emotion, suggestion, distraction, faith, preaching, in a word by thought."[2]—"Psychotherapy" write Camus and Pagniez, "is the totality of the means by which we act upon the sick mind or the sick body through the intermediation of the mind."[3]—Münsterberg's definition runs as follows: "Psychotherapy is the practice of treating the sick by influencing the mental life."[4] Most of the other definitions that have been put forward are of the same kind.

I should be ready to accept one of these formulas were it not for certain scruples. It seems to me that the definitions are still unduly restricted. They appear to imply that the therapeutic action of the doctor must directly induce psychological phenomena; they appear to exclude physical methods which have an indirect action upon the mind. When speaking of psychophysiological methods of treatment, I referred to the experiments with hashish made by Moreau de Tours, to treatment by alcohol, by opium, or simply by purgation; and I insisted that it would be a great mistake to deny their right to be regarded as part of psychotherapy. The characteristics of a therapeutic method depend upon the reasons which determine our choice of it, and not upon the nature of the process itself. If I give a purgative to a patient simply

[1] Illustrations of the Influence of the Mind upon the Body in Health and Disease, etc., second edition, 1884, vol. ii, p. 231.
[2] "Revue des Deux Mondes," September 15, 1905, p. 351.
[3] Isolement et psychothérapie, 1904, p. 26.
[4] Psychotherapy, 1909, p. 1.

because I want to relieve constipation, I am practising physiological therapy ; if I give the same purgative to a patient
suffering from mental confusion, and give it because extended
studies have shown me that there is a regular relationship
between intoxications and psychical disorders of this kind,
if I give it because I hope that disintoxication will clarify the
patient's thoughts, then I am practising psychotherapy.
Furthermore it seems to me that the foregoing definitions
allude to psychological phenomena as if we were still in the
anecdotal epoch, that in which Hack Tuke's book was written
They make no allusion to psychological laws. But all the
practical applications of science depend upon the study of
laws. These reflections lead me to propose the following
definition :

*Psychotherapy is a totality of therapeutic procedures of all
kinds, both physical and moral, applicable alike to bodily and to
mental disorders, procedures determined by the consideration of
psychological phenomena which have previously been studied,
and above all by the consideration of the laws which regulate the
development of these psychological phenomena and their association, either with one another, or with physiological phenomena.
In a word, psychotherapy is an application of psychological
science to the treatment of disease.*

Does such a psychotherapy exist ? Its primary characteristic must be to provide us with a number of precise methods
of treatment, and to tell us their exact effects, to inform us
concerning the definite moral or physical modifications which
result from their employment. This information is what we
find in formularies of physical therapeutics, where we read of
calmative, soporific, purgative, alterative drugs, and the like.
From such formularies a doctor can choose whatever drugs
he needs to suit the particular case. But as far as psychotherapy is concerned, nothing of the kind exists ; and some
even declare that no such classification is possible in this field,
for they contend that psychotherapeutic methods of treatment are personal, and that they vary according to the
individual who applies them. Such a contention is greatly
exaggerated. The originality of every psychotherapeutist is
in many cases apparent merely, and we must not believe that
his treatment is new simply because he calls it by a new

name   Still, it is true that at present these methods of treatment are imperfectly known, and have been described only in very vague terms, so that it is far from easy to ascertain the relationships between the different methods.

A therapeutic method founded upon definite laws ought, above all, to indicate the conditions in which this or that treatment ought to be employed; in a word, it ought to furnish the indications for each kind of treatment. As far as psychotherapy is concerned, there is an even greater lack of such indications. Every specialist vaunts his own method, declares that it is original, and wants to use it as a cure-all. One specialist will apply moralising treatment to every one, another will hypnotise all who come to consult him, another will subject all his patients to rest and hyperalimentation, and another will psychoanalyse all and sundry. What should we think of a doctor who proposed to administer digitalis to all his patients, and of a colleague whose speciality it was to prescribe arsenic in every case? We have no right to reproach psychotherapeutists for the defects of their method; they are merely applying a science, and the inadequacies of the application are but a demonstration of the inadequacies of the science. The diagnosis and the nomenclature of psychological disorders are extremely vague, and are entirely subject to the arbitrary conventions of the schools. Arnaud, in his address to the Clermont-Ferrand Congress, had good reason for speaking of the anarchy of contemporary psychiatry. But this anarchy, this vagueness in the description of syndromes, is entirely due to the inadequacy of our psychological science. One of the greatest services which we owe to the first beginnings of psychotherapy is the disclosure of the gaps in our pretended science of psychology. Never do we feel this inadequacy more keenly than when we attempt to teach psychology to medical men, and to derive from psychology practical methods of diagnosis and treatment. Practical success is the chief criterion of the worth of a science. When anything that claims to be a science cannot be applied, it is a science up in the air, and detached from its object. For a long time psychology, being then subordinate to religion or metaphysics, had no concern with the realities upon which it ought to act. Then, under pretext of adopting a scientific method, it merged itself with mathematical speculations, or with physiological researches with which it had no true concern, and it has never been in a condition to guide either the diagnosis of the psychiatrists or the practice of the psychotherapeutists.

In these circumstances it would perhaps be wise to draw the simple conclusion that an attempt to make use of psychotherapeutics is premature, and to decide that we shall reconsider the matter a century hence. But suffering humanity cannot wait. Medicine is applied to the relief of human distress by scientific discoveries, however incomplete. Medical practitioners want to turn a natural law to immediate practical use, even if it be a law which science has only just begun to glimpse. Psychotherapeutists wanted to make a practical use of the numberless observations of the moralists, the observations which disclosed the existence of a certain relationship between modifications of physical or mental health and the appearance of certain phenomena in the mind. The first attempts at psychotherapy were extremely general and vague. The first mental healers, availing themselves of observations which were as a rule devoid of precision, tried to relieve any and every kind of physical or mental disorder (very loosely defined) with the aid of psychological phenomena which were equally ill-known and no less loosely defined. Such was the essential character of the first attempts at psychological healing, whether religious, philosophical, or moral. We have studied these in the earlier part of the present work. Their main interest is historical.

A somewhat more precise knowledge of a few psychological phenomena and of certain psychological laws, gave rise to rather more scientific attempts at psychotherapy. A study of tendencies, of psychic reflexes, and of the various psychological automatisms, made it possible to turn to account the different forms of suggestion, which aim at inducing an automatic functioning of this or that tendency. Ideas concerning the fatigue, the exhaustion, the depression, which follow the expenditure occasioned by excessive action, led to the adoption of a therapeutic method designed to economise the energies of the mind. This method assumed two different forms. Sometimes there was an attempt to restrict expenditure, to disinfect the mind, and thus to do away with the expenditure connected with certain unhappy memories or certain undesirable tendencies. Sometimes the attempt to restrict expenditure took the form of a suppression of movements and actions ; or of the isolation of the patient, and the restriction of social life. A study of the transformations induced by education in young children gave rise to various methods of treatment by gymnastics or reeducation. Finally, entering into a far more hypothetical field, psychotherapeutists have endeavoured to explain the changes characteristic of awakening, effort, and attention, and to understand the nature of the immense increase of energy which appears to result from confidence, faith and enthusiasm—these researches leading to the therapeutic methods of aesthesiogenism and excitation. Just as the advance of physiological study diclosed the special disorders of digestion, circulation, and glandular secretion, that occur in the neuroses, and made it possible to replace the old adage " mens sana in corpore sano " by more precise indications for treatment, so, in like manner, the advance of psychological study has led to the formulation of more and more precise psychotherapeutic methods.

Have these new psychotherapeutic methods become practical and useful ? Do they enable us to cure neuropathic disorders with the same certainty, or even with the same probability, as a cure can be obtained in many other diseases by medical or surgical methods ? We have, unfortunately, to answer this question in the negative. Far too often, psychotherapeutic treatment is utterly fruitless. A very large number of our patients pass on into incurable dementia, or remain mentally disordered for an indefinite period. In many cases, psychotherapeutic treatment, though it seems to do good for a time, has but a temporary effect, so that we are continually obliged to begin the work anew. Finally, even in the most successful cases, such methods of treatment are unduly tedious ; and we always have to ask ourselves whether the natural evolution of the disease during the long period in which the treatment has been applied might not have spontaneously brought about just as much improvement in the absence of any treatment at all.

Thus a good many doctors are inclined to look upon psychotherapeutic methods as useless. They say that some of our patients will get well spontaneously, and that others will inevitably fall a prey to dementia praecox ; they declare that medical skill can make very little difference here. Gilbert Ballet has gone so far as to write : " I am very doubtful whether psychotherapy, of whatever kind, or whatever methods may be employed, has ever curtailed by a single hour the duration of the most trifling periodic attack, any more than it has curtailed the duration of a very grave attack of circular insanity." [1] Thus many doctors speedily succumb to the " monstrous prejudice " against which Magnan used indignantly to protest, " that we can do nothing for our patients." [2]

Such affirmations anent the regular and immutable evolution of the neuropsychoses, such classifications of mental disorders into fixed categories, such assertions concerning the inevitable development of these diseases, seem to me even rasher than the most enthusiastic dreams of the psychotherapeutists. Except in the case of a few terminal phases, in which a certain regularity does seem to be manifested, the clinical observation of the disorders of the mind shows that these have an amazing variability and a disconcerting irregularity. Physiological and psychological disorders are constantly undergoing change thanks to the effect of all kinds of physical and moral influences, and it would be hard to enumerate all the phenomena which make the mental level of our patients oscillate like a Cartesian devil.[3] But if this be so, what right have we to assert apriori that only chance happenings can exert a favourable influence, and that our voluntary and deliberate procedures can never do any good to the patient ? This would be tantamount to denying the value of human inventions, of all the practical application of science.

To me, at any rate, there seems no good ground for attributing to pure chance all the improvements, all the cures, which have been so excellently described in numberless psychotherapeutic studies. I have myself set forth at great length a number of cases in which the favourable effect of this or that therapeutic method seemed indisputable. Psychotherapy, in the wider sense of the term, including within its scope

---

[1] Ballet," Bulletin Médical," 1906, p. 983.
[2] P. Sérieux, V. Magnan, sa vie et ses oeuvres, " Annales Médico-Psychologiques," October 1917, p. 497.
[3] " Ludion " in the original. It is a hydrostatic toy, also called " Cartesian diver," and sometimes spoken of as the " bottle imp."—TRANSLATOR'S NOTE.

all the methods of treatment based upon a knowledge of psychological or physiopsychological laws, has unquestionably done good service in a very large number of cases. The reason why, in the present work, I have given so much space to the reports of cases, is precisely that I wished to supply evidence of the good effects of psychotherapy.

These first attempts at psychotherapy, however premature they may be, have an additional value. They have reawakened psychology, and have forcibly compelled it to attend to its own subject matter. The evolution of human knowledge rarely pursues a logical course. The applications of science ought to follow in the footsteps of theory ; but, in actual fact, practice often precedes and guides theory. It is the necessities of therapeutic application which are to-day compelling psychology to devote its attention to its own proper topic, which is the description and the scientific explanation of human behaviour. Accurate study of the details of behaviour, of the need to love and be loved, of jealousy, of timidity, etc., which in former days were regarded as minor accessories, as literary adjuncts of true psychology, have now come to be regarded as the very core of a truly practical and useful psychology. The searching out of the laws that regulate changes of temper, degrees of activity, and forms of emotion, must not be left to the novelists, but must be the main concern of psychologists, for the whole of our psychotherapy must be based upon a knowledge of these laws. Medical practitioners have suddenly turned to psychology, and have demanded of this science a service which the psychologists were far from being prepared to render. Psychology has not proved equal to the occasion, and the failure of the science has thrown discredit upon psychotherapy itself. But this very failure has necessitated entirely new psychological studies, whereby the science of psychology has been regenerated.

My recognition of the gaps in the science of psychology has led me in the present work to lay great stress upon the explanation of certain psychological notions, which are of especial importance from the therapeutic point of view. I have done my best to explain the precise significance of certain terms in common use ; I have tried, by means of psychological analysis, to throw light upon the phenomena which play a leading part in mental depression and its treatment. Rightly or wrongly, I believe that both psychological science, and psychotherapy which has to make a practical application of psychology, can derive great benefit from the study of those characteristics of behaviour which may be termed the grades of psychological energy and psychological tension, and also from the study of the various oscillations of mental activity. That is why I have devoted several chapters of the present work to such matters.

In a word, this book, however incomplete it is perforce to-day, attempts to deal with a problem which is still very obscure, the problem of the economical administration of the energies of the mind. Some day we may hope that there will be enough knowledge to make it possible to budget the income and expenditure of a mind, just as to-day we budget the income and expenditure of a commercial concern. When that day arrives, the psychiatrist, the mind healer, will be able to help his patients to turn their poor resources to good account by avoiding needless expenditure and by directing their efforts to the precise point where these efforts can best be utilised. He will be able to do more than this; he will be able to teach his patients how to increase their resources, how to enrich their minds. I am not without hope that my labours will prove of some use to those who, in days to come, will discover the laws of this good administration of our psychological fortune.

BIBLIOGRAPHY

ACHER, Rudolph, Recent Freudian Literature, " American Journal of Psychology," vol. xxii (1911), pp. 408–443.

ADKIN, Thomas F., Vitaeopathy.

AGRELO, J. Antonio, Psicoterapia y reeducacion psiquica, " Archivos de Psiquiatria de M. J. Ingegnieros," 1908.

AIMÉ, H., Etude clinique sur le dynamisme psychique, Nancy, 1897.

ANGELL, J. R., see PARKER's Psychotherapy.

ANTOINE LE GUÉRISSEUR, Le couronnement de la révélation d'Antoine le Guérisseur, l'oréole de la conscience, 1907–1909.

ASCHAFFENBURG, G., Die Beziehungen des Sexuellenlebens zur Entstehung von Nerven- und Geisteskrankheiten, " Münchener Medizinische Wochenschrift," September 2, 1906.

ATKINSON, William Walker, Thought Force in Business and Everyday Life, The Psychic Research Co., Chicago, 1901.

BAIR, J. H., The Development of Voluntary Control, " Psychological Review," 1901, p. 474.

BAÏSSAS, Jérome, Les trésors du Château de Crèvecoeur. Episode de l'affaire Frigard, Paris, 1867.

BALDWIN, James Mark, Dictionary of Philosophy and Psychology, Edited by J. M. B., vol. iii, Bibliography compiled by Benjamin Rand, Macmillan, London and New York, 1905. (Pp. 1059–1067 deal with Hypnotism and Suggestion.)

BARAGNON, Etude du magnétisme animal sous le point de vue d'une exacte pratique, 1853.

BARKER, Lewellys Franklin, On the psychic Treatment of some of the functional Neuroses, 1906.

BARKER, Lewellys Franklin, Some Experiences with the Simple Methods of Psychotherapy and Reeducation, " American Journal of the Medical Sciences," October 1906.

BARRAS, Jean Pierre Tobie, Traité sur les gastralgies et les entéralgies on maladies nerveuses de l'estomac et des intestins, Paris, 1823.

BARTH, J. E. Henri, Du sommeil non naturel, ses diverses formes, Paris, 1886.

BEAUCHÈNE, Edme Pierre Chauvot de, De l'influence des affections de l'âme dans les maladies nerveuses des femmes, etc., Montpellier and Paris, 1781.

BEAUNIS, Henri Etienne, Le somnambulisme provoqué, études physiologiques et psychologiques, Paris, 1886.

BEEDE, see CLAPARÈDE and BEEDE.

BERNHEIM, Hippolyte, De la suggestion dans l'état hypnotique et dans l'état de veille, Doin, Paris, 1884.

BERNHEIM, Hippolyte, De la suggestion et de ses applications à la thérapeutique, Paris, 1886 ; English translation by C. A. Herter, Suggestive Therapeutics, second edition, Pentland, London, 1890.

BERNHEIM, Hippolyte, De la peur en thérapeutique, " Bulletin Générale de Thérapeutique Médicale et Chirurgicale," Sept. 30, 1886.

BERNHEIM, Hippolyte, Définition et valeur de l'hypnotisme, " Journal für Psychologie und Neurologie," Leipzig, 1911, p. 471.

BERNHEIM, Hippolyte, L'hypnotisme et la suggestion dans leurs rapports avec la médicine legale, Nancy, 1897.

BERNHEIM, Hippolyte, Hypnotisme, suggestion, psychothérapie, études nouvelles, Doin, Paris, 1891.

BERTRAND, Alexandre Jacques François, De l'exstase, 1820. [The translators cannot verify the existence of this work. Perhaps it is reissued as part of Du magnétisme animal, 1826, q.v. infra.]

BERTRAND, Alexandre Jacques François, Du magnétisme animal en France, etc., Paris, 1826.

BERTRAND, Alexandre Jacques François, Traité du somnambulisme et des différentes modifications qu'il présente, Paris, 1823.

BERTRIN, Georges, Lourdes, apparitions et guérisons, Lourdes, 1905. [New and enlarged edition (37th thousand), Lourdes and Paris, 1912.]—English translation by Mrs. Philips Gibbs, Lourdes, a History of its Apparitions and Cures, Kegan Paul, London, 1908.

BESANT, Annie, Thought Power, its Control and Culture, Theosophical Publishing Society, London and Benares, 1901.

BINET, Alfred, La suggestibilité, Schleicher, Paris, 1900.

BINET, Alfred, and FÉRÉ, Charles, Le magnétisme animal, Alcan, Paris, 1887; English translation, Animal Magnetism, Kegan Paul, London, 1888.

BIRAN, see MAINE DE BIRAN.

BLEULER, Eugen, Affektivität, Suggestivität und Paranoia, Marhold, Halle, 1906.

BLISS, M. A., The Influence of Mind on Digestion, see PARKER's Psychotherapy.

BOISSARIE, Prosper Gustave, Les grandes guérisons de Lourdes, Téqui, Paris, 1900.

BONJOUR, J., Emploi du sommeil prolongé dans un cas de somnambulisme hystéro-épileptique. " Revue de l'Hypnotisme," 1895.

BONJOUR, J., Psychothérapie et Hypnotisme, " Revue de l'Hypnotisme," June 1906, p. 357.

BONJOUR, J., La suggestion hypnotique, " Revue de l'Hypnotisme," 1908.

BONJOUR, J., La suggestion hypnotique et la psychothérapie actuelle, Sack, Lausaune, and Baillière, Paris, 1908.

BOOTH, Emmons Rutledge, History of Osteopathy and Twentieth Century Medical Practice, Cincinnati, 1907.

BOUCHÉ-LECLERCQ, Auguste, Histoire de la divination dans l'antiquité, 4 vols., Leroux, Paris, 1879–1882.

BOURDEAU, Jean, La philosophie affective, Alcan, 1912.

BOURDIN, Victor, De l'impulsion et spécialement de son rapport sur le crime, 1894.

BRAID, James, Neurypnology, or the Rationale of Nervous Sleep, considered in relation to Animal Magnetism, illustrated by numerous cases of successful application in the Relief and Cure of Disease, 1843. See also WAITE.

BRAMWELL, John Milne, Hypnotism, its History, Practice, and Theory, first edition, 1903 ; second edition, 1906 ; third edition Rider, London, 1913.

BRAMWELL, John Milne, The Evolution of Hypnotic Theory, " Brain," 1896.

BRAMWELL, John Milne, James Braid, his Work and his Writings, Proc. Soc. Psych. Res., xii, 1896, pp. 176–203.

BRAMWELL, John Milne, Obsessions and their Treatment by Suggestion, see PARKER's Psychotherapy.

BRAMWELL, John Milne, What is Hypnotism ? Proc. Soc. Psych. Res., xii, 1896–7, pp. 204–258.

BRÉMOND, Félix, Les passions et la santé, Baillière, Paris, 1893.

BRILL, A. A., Freud's Method of Psychoanalysis, see PARKER's Psychotherapy.

BRIQUET, Pierre, Traité clinique et thérapeutique de l'hystérie, Paris, 1859.

BRISSAUD, Edouard, Le mal du roi, " Journal du Magnétisme," viii, 493.

BRISSAUD, Edouard, Les suggestions hypnotiques au point de vue médico-legale, Paris, 1889.

BUCKLEY, James Monro, Faith-healing, Christian Science, and Kindred Phenomena, Fisher Unwin, London, 1892.

BURQ, Victor, Métallothérapie, traitement des maladies nerveuses par les applications métalliques, Paris, 1853.

BURQ, Victor, Des origines de la metallothérapie ; part qui doit être faite au magnétisme animal dans sa découverte ; le Burquisme et le Perkininisme, Paris, 1883.

CABOT, Richard C., The American Type of Psychotherapy, see PARKER's Psychotherapy.

CABOT, Richard C., Analysis and Modification of the Environment, see PARKER's Psychotherapy.

CABOT, Richard C., Suggestion, Authority, and Command, see PARKER's Psychotherapy.

CABOT, Richard C., The Use and Abuse of Rest in the Treatment of Disease, see PARKER's Psychotherapy.

CABOT, Richard C., Veracity and Psychotherapy, see PARKER's Psychotherapy.

CABOT, Richard C., Whose Business is Psychotherapy ? see PARKER's Psychotherapy.

CABOT, Richard C., Work Cure, see PARKER's Psychotherapy.

CADÉAC, Célestin, and MEUNIER, Albin, Recherches expérimentales sur les essences, contribution à l'étude de l'alcoolisme ; étude physiologique de l'eau d'arquebuse ou vulnéraire, " Annales de la Société d'Agriculture," Baillière, Paris, 1892.

CALMET, Augustin, Traité sur les apparitions des esprits et sur les vampires ou les revenants de Hongrie, de Moravie, etc., 2 vols., Paris, 1751.

CAMUS, Jean, and PAGNIEZ, Philippe, Isolement et psychothérapie, etc., Alcan, Paris, 1904, with a preface by J. Dejerine.

CANFIELD, Practical Considerations in the treatment of neurasthenia, " Boston Medical and Surgical Journal," 1907.

CANTONNET, La rééducation de la vision dans le strabisme, " Presse Médicale," May 15, 1919.

CARRÉ DE MONTGERON, Louis Basile, La vérité des miracles opérés par l'intercession de M. de Pâris, Utrecht, 1737.

CHARCOT, Jean Martin, The Faith-Cure, " New Review," January 1893 ; La foi qui guérit, " Archives de Neurologie," January 1893.

CHARCOT, Jean Martin, Oeuvres complètes, in nine volumes, Paris, 1885–1890 ; vol. ix, Hémorrhagie et ramollissement du cerveau, métallothérapie et hypnotisme, électrothérapie.

CHARCOT, Jean Martin, and RICHER, Paul, Contribution à l'étude de l'hypnotisme chez les hystériques, du phénomène de l'hyperexcitabilité neuro-musculaire, " Archives de Neurologie," 1881, ii.

CHARMA, Antoine, Du sommeil, Hachette, Paris, 1851.

CHARPIGNON, Louis Joseph Jules, Physiologie, médecine et métaphysique du magnétisme, Paris, 1848.

CHARPIGNON, Louis Joseph Jules, Rapports du magnétisme avec la jurisprudence et la médicine légale, Paris, 1860.

CHASLIN, P., La confusion mentale primitive, Asselin and Houzeau, Paris, 1895.

CHERVIN, Arthur, Comment on guérit les bègues, 1882.

CHERVIN, Arthur, Du bégaiement et de son traitement, 1879.

CHERVIN, Claudius (dit l'ainé), Du bégaiement considéré comme vice de prononciation, Paris, 1867.

CLAPARÈDE, Edouard, L'association des idées, Doin, Paris, 1903.

CLAPARÈDE, Edouard, and BEEDE, W., Recherches expérimentales sur quelques phénomènes simples dans un cas d'hypnose, " Archives de Psychologie," July 1909.

CLEMENS, Samuel Langhorne, see TWAIN.

CONANT, Albert F., Complete Concordance to Science and Health with Key to the Scriptures, Stewart, Boston, 1916.

Concordance to Science and Health, see CONANT.

CORIAT, Isador H., A Contribution to the Psychopathology of Hysteria, " Journal of Abnormal Psychology," 1911.

CORIAT, Isador H., Discussion of the Symposium, " Journal of Abnormal Psychology," July 1917.

COULEVAIN, Pierre de (pen-name of Mademoiselle Favre de Coulevain), Sur la branche, Paris, 1910 ; English translation by Alys Hallard, On the Branch, Nash, London, 1909.

COURBON, P., see LAVASTINE.

CROTHERS, Samuel McChord, A literary Clinic, " Atlantic Monthly," September 1916.

DAMAGE, Henri, Les affections mentales curables et leur traitement, " Journal de Neurologie," April 20, 1911, p. 141.

DEJERINE, Jules, and GAUCKLER, E., Les manifestations fonctionnelles des psychonévroses, leur traitement par la psychothérapie, Masson, Paris, 1911.

DELBOEUF, Joseph Rémi Léopold, De l'origine des effets curatifs de l'hypnotisme, " Bulletin de l'Académie Royale de la Belgique," 1887.

DELEUZE, Joseph Philippe François, Histoire critique du magnétisme animal, 2 vols., 1813.

DELEUZE, Joseph Philippe François, Instruction pratique sur le magnétisme animal, Paris, 1825.

DEMANGEON, Jean Baptiste, De l'imagination considérée dans ses effets directs sur l'homme et les animaux et de ses effets indirects sur les produits de la gestation, avec une notice sur la génération et les causes les plus probables des difformités de naissance, Paris, 1829.

DEMARQUAY, Jean Nicolas, and TEULON, Giraud, Recherches sur l'hypnotisme on sommeil nerveux, etc., Baillière, Paris, 1860.

DESCHAMPS, Albert, Les maladie de l'énergie, thérapeutique générale, etc., Alcan, Paris, 1908.

DESCHAMPS, Albert, Le rapport psycho-moteur, " Paris Medical," June 1912.

DESLON, Charles, Observations sur le magnétisme animal, London, 1780.

DESPINÉ, Charles Humbert Antoine, De l'emploi du magnétisme animal et des eaux minérales dans le traitement des maladies nerveuses, etc., Paris, 1840. [The same book as Observations pratiques, Anneci, 1838, the only difference being in the title-page.]

DESPINE, Charles Humbert Antoine, Observations de médecine pratique faites aux bains d'Aix-en-Savoie, Anneci, 1838. [See also De l'emploi du magnétisme animal, etc., supra.]

DESPINE, Prosper, Etude scientifique sur le somnambulisme, sur les phénomènes qu'il présente et sur son action thérapeutique dans certains maladies nerveuses, Paris, 1880.

DESPINE, Prosper, Psychologie naturelle, étude sur les facultés intellectuelles et morales dans leur état normal et dans leurs manifestations anormales chez les aliénés et chez les criminels, 5 vols., Savy, Paris, 1868.

DESSOIR, Max, Bibliographie des modernen Hypnotismus, Duncker, Berlin, 1888–1890.

DODS, John Bovee, The Philosophy of Mesmerism and Electrical Psychology, comprised in two courses of lectures, edited by J. Burns, London, 1876.

DODS, John Bovee, Electrical Psychology : or the electrical philosophy of mental impressions, including a new philosophy of sleep and of consciousness, from the works of Rev. J. B. Dods and Prof. J. S. Grimes, revised and edited by H. G. Darling, London and Glasgow, 1851.

DODS, John Bovee, Six Lectures on the Philosophy of Mesmerism, Boston, 1843.

DONLEY, J. E., Freud's Anxiety Neurosis, " Journal of Abnormal Psychology," 1911.

DONLEY, J. E., Psychotherapy and Reeducation, " Journal of Abnormal Psychology," April 1911.

DRESSER, Annetta Gertrude, The Philosophy of P. P. Quimby, with Selections from his Manuscripts and a Sketch of his Life, Ellis, Boston, 1895.

DRESSER, Horatio W., The Quimby Manuscripts, second edition, Werner Laurie, London, 1922.

DRESSER, Horatio W., A History of the New Thought Movement, Harrap, London, 1920.

DRESSER, Horatio W., Health and the Inner Life, with an Account of the Life and Teachings of P. P. Quimby, Putnam, New York, 1906.

DRESSER, Julius A., The true History of mental Science, Boston, 1887 ; new edition, 1899.

DUBOIS, Paul, Un cas de phobie guéri par la psychothérapie, Société Suisse de Neurologie, Berne, March, 1909.

DUBOIS, Paul, L'éducation de soi-même, 1909 ; English translation by Edward G. Richards, The Education of Self, Funk and Wagnalls Co., New York and London, 1911.

DUBOIS, Paul, The Method of Persuasion, see PARKER'S Psychotherapy.

DUBOIS, Paul, La pathogénie des états neurasthéniques, Rapport au dixième congrès de médecine, Geneva, September 1908.

DUBOIS, Paul, Les psychonévroses et leur traitement moral (with a preface by Jules Dejerine), Masson, Paris, 1904 ; English translation by Smith Ely Jelliffe and William A. White, The Psychic Treatment of Nervous Disorders ; the Psychoneuroses and their Moral Treatment, Funk and Wagnalls, New York and London, 1908.

DUMAS Alexandre (the elder), Urbain Grandier.

DUMAS, Georges, La tristesse et la joie, Alcan, Paris, 1900.

DUMAS, Georges, Troubles mentaux et troubles nerveux de guerre, Alcan, Paris, 1919.

DUMONTPALLIER, Amédée, Etude expérimentale sur la métalloscopie et la métallothérapie du docteur Burq, Delahaye, Paris, 1879.

DUPAU, J. Amédée, Lettres physiologiques et morales sur le magnétisme animal, etc., Paris, 1826.

DUPOTET DE SENNEVOY, J., Editor of " Journal du Magnétisme," vols. i to xx, Paris, 1845–1869 ; author of numerous works on magnetism, spiritualism, occultism, etc.

DUPOTET DE SENNEVOY, J., Manuel de l'étudiant magnétiseur ou nouvelle instruction pratique sur le magnétisme, etc., Baillière, Paris, 1846 ; second edition, 1850 ; fifth edition, 1887.

DUPUIS, L., Le moindre effort en psychologie, " Revue Philosophique," 1911, vol. ii, p. 164.

DUPUIS, L., Les stigmates fondamentaux de la timidité, " Revue Philosophique," 1915.

DURAND, Joseph Pierre (dit DURAND DE GROS, having been born at Gros, near Rodez, Aveyron ; wrote also under the pseudonym of J. P. PHILIPS), Cours de braidisme, ou hypnotisme nerveux, Baillière, Paris, 1860.

DURAND, Joseph Pierre, Electrodynamisme vitale, etc., Baillière, Paris, 1855.

DURAND, Joseph Pierre, Essais de physiologie philosophique, Baillière, Paris, 1866.

EASTMAN, Max, The new Art of Healing, " The Atlantic Monthly," 1908, i, p. 645.

EDDY, Mary Baker, Christian Healing, 1888.

EDDY, Mary Baker, Christian Science, No and Yes, 1888.

EDDY, Mary Baker, Mind Healing, an historical Sketch, 1888.

EDDY, Mary Baker, People's Idea of God, 1888.

EDDY, Mary Baker, Science and Health, Boston, 1875. (This was the first edition, which has been considerably modified in later official issues. There is an unauthorised reprint of the 1875 edition, published by Winifred W. Gatling, Jerusalem, 1924.)

EDDY, Mary Baker, Science and Health with Key to the Scriptures, Boston, 1890. Authorised Literature of the First Church of Christ, Scientist. (The official French and German translations bear a similar imprimatur.)

EDDY, Mary Baker, Unity of Good, 1888.

ELLIS, William Charles, Traite de l'aliénation mentale, etc., Paris, 1840 ; the French translation of A Treatise on the Nature, Symptoms, Causes, and Treatment of Insanity, etc., London, 1838.

ESPINAS, A., Du sommeil provoqué chez les hystériques, Bordeaux, 1884.

ESQUIROL, Jean Etienne Dominique, Des maladies mentales, etc., 2 vols., Paris, 1838 ; English translation by E. K. Hunt, Mental Maladies, Philadelphia, 1845.

ESQUIROL, Jean Etienne Dominique, Des établissements des aliénés en France et des moyens d'améliorer le sort de ces infortunés, mémoire présenté . . . en 1818, Hugard, Paris, 1819.

EVANS, Warren Felt, The divine Law of Cure, 1881.

EVANS, Warren Felt, Esoteric Christianity, 1886.

EVANS, Warren Felt, The Mental Cure, 1869.

EVANS, Warren Felt, Mental Medicine, 1872.

EVANS, Warren Felt, The primitive Mind Cure, 1885.

EVANS, Warren Felt, Soul and Body, 1875.

EYMIEU, Antoine, Le gouvernement de soi-même, essai de psychologie pratique, 2 vols., Perrin, 1906, 1910.

FAREZ, Paul, La dormeuse d'Alençon, " Revue de Psychothérapie," August and September, 1910.

FARIA, José Custodio de, De la cause du sommeil lucide, Paris, 1819 ; reprint, with a preface by D. G. Dalgado, Jouve, Paris, 1906.

FAURE, Maurice, La rééducation motrice, " Revue Scientifique," 1902, vol. ii, p. 73.

FEINDEL, E., see MEIGE, Henry.

FELLOWS, Samuel, Insomnia, its Nature, and its Treatment, in PARKER's Psychotherapy.

FÉRÉ, Charles, Sensation et mouvement, Alcan, Paris, 1887.

FÉRÉ, Charles, see also BINET.

FERENCZI, S., Die Introjektion in der Neurose und die Rolle der Uebertragung bei der Hypnose und Suggestion, " Journal für psychoanalytische Forschung," 1910, vol. i, p. 1.

FISCHER, Lorenz, Le magnétisme animal, 1883.

FISCHER, Lorenz, Der sogenannte Lebensmagnetismus oder Hypnotismus, Mainz, 1883.

FLEURY, Maurice de, Introduction à la médecine de l'esprit, Alcan, Paris, 1897 ; English translation by S. B. Collins, Medicine and the Mind, Downey, London, 1900.

FLOURNOY, Théodore, Des Indes à la planète Mars, étude sur un cas de somnambulisme avec glossolalie, Alcan, Paris, 1900.

FLOWER, Sydney, Hypnotism or Psychotherapy, " Pacific Medical Journal," San Francisco, 1898.

FONTAN, Jules Antoine Emile, and SÉGARD, Charles, Elements de médecine suggestive : hypnotisme et suggestion, faits cliniques, Doin, Paris, 1887.

FOREL, Auguste, L'âme et le système nerveux, hygiène et pathologie, Steinheil, Paris, 1906.

FOREL, Auguste, Hygiene der Nerven und des Geistes im gesunden und kranken Zustande, Zurich, 1905 ; French version 1906, L'âme et le système nerveux, hygiène et pathologie ; English translation by A. Aikins, Hygiene of Mind and Nerves in Health and Disease, Murray, London, 1907.

FOREL, Auguste, Der Hypnotismus, seine psycho-physiologische, medicinische, strafrechtliche Bedeutung und seine Handhabung, second edition, Stuttgart, 1891 ; English translation by H. W. Armit, from fifth German edition, Hypnotism, or Suggestion and Psychotherapy, Rebman, London, 1906.

FOREL, Auguste, Die sexuelle Frage, eine naturwissenschaftliche, psychologische, hygienische und soziologische Studie für Gebildete, eighth and ninth edition (36th to 45th thousand), Munich, 1909 ; English adaptation by C. F. Marshall, The Sexual Question, a scientific, psychological, hygienic, and sociological study for the cultured classes, Rebman (now Heinemann), London, 1908.

FOUILLÉE, Alfred, L'enseignement au point de vue national, Paris, 1891 ; English translation by W. J. Greenstreet, Education from a National Standpoint, Arnold, London, 1892.

FOY, Robert, Le bégaiement, nouveaux essais pathogéniques et théra-peutiques, " Bulletins et mémoires de la Société Française d'Oto-Rhino-Laryngologie, Congrès de 1913."

FRANCO, Pierre (dit " de Turriers "), Chirurgie de Pierre Franco, composée en 1561, new edition, Alcan, Paris, 1895.

FREUD, Sigmund, Beiträge zur Psychologie des Liebesleben, " Jahr-buch für psychoanalytischen Forschungen," 1910.

FREUD, Sigmund, Eine Krankheitserinnerung des Lionardo da Vinci, Deuticke, Leipzig and Vienna, 1910 ; 3rd edition, 1923.—English translation by A. A. Brill, Leonardo da Vinci, a psychosexual Study of an infantile Reminiscence, Moffat Yard & Co., New York, 1916, Kegan Paul, London, 1922.

FREUD, Sigmund, Die Traumdeutung, Deuticke, Leipzig and Vienna, 1900, seventh edition, 1922 ; English translation by A. A. Brill from the third German edition, The Interpretation of Dreams, Allen and Unwin, London, 1913.

FREUD, Sigmund, Die psychogene Sehstörung in psychoanalytischer Auffassung, 1910.

FREUD, Sigmund, Ueber wilde Psychoanalyse, " Zentralblatt für Psychoanalyse," 1910, vol. iii, p. 91.

FREUD, Sigmund, Zur Aetiologie der Hysterie, 1896.

GAUCKLER, see DEJERINE and GAUCKLER.

GAUTHIER, Aubin, Histoire du somnambulisme chez tous les peuples, sous les noms' divers d'extases, songes, oracles et visions, etc., 2 vols., Paris, 1842.

GEER, Curtis Manning, Formulary of English Medical Practice in the Eleventh Century, see PARKER's Psychotherapy.

GEER, Curtis Manning, Healing in the Middle Ages, see PARKER's Psychotherapy.

GERRISH, Frederic Henry, The Therapeutic Value of Hypnotic Sug-gestion. See, Psychotherapeutics, a Symposium.

GILLES DE LA TOURETTE, Georges, Les états neurasthéniques, second edition, Baillière, Paris, 1900.

GILLES DE LA TOURETTE, Georges, L'hypnotisme et les états analogues au point de vue médico-legale, Plon, Nourrit, Paris, 1887.

GILLES DE LA TOURETTE, Georges, Traité de l'hysterie d'après l'enseigne-ment de la Salpêtrière, 3 vols., Paris, 1891–1899.

GIRARD, Paul, L'Asclepieion d'Athènes d'après de récentes découvertes, Paris, 1881.

GODDARD, Henry H., The Effects of Mind on Body, as evidenced by Faith Cures, " American Journal of Psychology," vol. x (1899), pp. 431–502.

GOLDSCHEIDER, Alfred, and JACOB, Paul, Handbuch der physikalischen Therapie, 4 vols., Leipzig, 1901–1902.

GRIMES, J. Stanley, see DODS, J. B., Electrical Psychology, etc.

GRAF, Max, Richard Wagner im " Fliegenden Holländer," ein Beitrag zur Psychologie des künstlerischen Schaffens, Leipzig, 1911.

GRASSET, Joseph, La défense sociale contre les maladies nerveuses, " Revue des Idées," 1906.

GRASSET, Joseph, L'hypnotisme et la suggestion, Doin, Paris, 1903.

GRASSET, Joseph, Prophylaxie individuelle, familiale et sociale, " Revue des Idées, 1906.

GROSSMAN, J., Die Bedeutung der hypnotischen Suggestion als Heilmittel, Berlin, 1894.

GUISEZ, J., De l'étiologie et de differentes formes des sténoses inflammatoires de la région cardiaque de l'oesophage, " Presse Médicale," June 4, 1917.

GUYAU, Jean Marie, Education et hérédité, Paris, 1889 ; English translation by W. J. Greenstreet, Education and Heredity, London, 1891.

HABERMAN, Jules Victor, Hypnosis, its psychological Interpretation and its practical Use in the Diagnosis and Treatment of Diseases, " Clinical Lectures in the Department of Neurology at the College of Physicians and Surgeons," New York, March 17, 1910.

HALLOCK, F. K., The Methods of Education and simple Conversation in Psychotherapy, see PARKER'S Psychotherapy.

HART, Ernest Abraham, Hypnotism and Mesmerism and the New Witchcraft, London and New York, 1893, enlarged edition, 1896.

HARTENBERG, Paul, Traitement des neurasthéniques, Alcan, Paris, 1912.

HÉBERT, L. M. (of Garnay), Petit catéchisme magnétique, on notions élémentaire du mesmerisme, Paris, 1852 ; second edition, 1852 ; third edition, 1854.

HEIDENHAIN, Rudolf, Der sogenannte thierische Magnetismus, Leipzig, 1880 ; English translation by L. C. Wooldridge, with a preface by G. J. Romanes, Animal Magnetism, Kegan Paul, London, 1880.

HESNARD, see RÉGIS and HESNARD.

HEUBNER, P. M., Perpetual Health, How to Secure a New Lease of Life by the Exercise of Will Power.

HINKLE, Beatrice M., Methods of Psychotherapy, see PARKER'S Psychotherapy.

HOLMES, Oliver Wendell, Medical Essays, 1842–1882, Houghton Mifflin & Co., Boston, Mass., 1883.

HUBERT, Henri, and MAUSS, Marcel, Esquisse d'une théorie générale de la magie, " Année Sociologique," 1902–3.

HUCHARD, Henri, Maladies du coeur, artériosclérose, Baillière, Paris, 1911.

HULETT, Guy Dudley, Text-book of the Principles of Osteopathy, Cleveland, Ohio.

JACOB, Paul, see GOLDSCHEIDER.

JAMES, William, Automatic Writing, Proceedings of the S.P.R., 1889.

JAMES, William, The Energies of Men, " The Philosophical Review," January 1907.

JAMES, William, The Principles of Psychology, 2 vols., New York and London, 1890.

JAMES, William, Talks to Teachers on Psychology and to Students on some of Life's Ideals, Longmans, London, 1899.

JAMES, William, The Varieties of religious Experience, a Study in human Nature, Longmans, London, 1902.

JANET, Jules, Les troubles psychopathiques de la miction, essai de psycho-physiologie normale et pathologique, Paris, 1890.

JANET, Pierre, Les accidents mentaux des hystériques, 1893.—This work is now incorporated in L'état mental des hystériques, which see.

JANET, Pierre, L'alcoolisme et la dépression mentale, " Séances et Travaux de l'Académie des Sciences Morales," September and October, 1915.

JANET, Pierre, L'amnésie et la dissociation des souvenirs par l'émotion, " Journal de Psychologie Normale et Pathologique," September 1904.

JANET, Pierre, L'automatisme psychologique, essai de psychologie mentale sur les formes inférieures de l'activité mentale, Alcan, Paris, 1889.

JANET, Pierre, Un cas d'aboulie et d'idées fixes, " Revue Philosophique," 1894.

JANET, Pierre, Un cas d'hémianopsie hystérique transitoire, " Presse Médicale," October 23, 1899, p. 241.

JANET, Pierre, Cours sur les degrés de l'activation des tendences, " Annuaire du Collège de France," 1917.

JANET, Pierre, Cours sur les tendences intellectuelles élémentaires, " Annuaire du Collège de France," 1913.

JANET, Pierre, La définition de l'émotion, " Revue Neurologique," December 30, 1909.

JANET, Pierre, Dépersonnalisation et possession chez un psychasthénique, " Journal de Psychologie Normale et Pathologique," 1904.

JANET, Pierre, L'état mental des hystériques, Rueff, Paris, vol i, Les stigmates mentaux, 1893, vol. ii, Les accidents mentaux, 1894 ; second edition in one volume, Alcan, Paris, 1911 ; English translation (from first edition) by Caroline R. Corson, The Mental State of Hystericals, Putnam, New York and London, 1901.

JANET, Pierre, Les états intermédiaires de l'hypnotisme, " Revue Scientifique," 1886.

JANET, Pierre, Une extatique, " Bulletin de l'Institut Général Psychologique," 1900-1901, p. 209.

JANET, Pierre, Une Félida artificielle, " Revue Philosophique," vol. i, p. 329 ; cf. also L'état mental des hystériques, second edition, 1911, p. 567.

JANET, Pierre, Histoire d'une idée fixe, " Revue Philosophique," February 1894.

JANET, Pierre, Les idées fixes de forme hystérique, " Presse Médicale," 1895.

JANET, Pierre, Influence somnambulique et le besoin de direction, in Névroses et idées fixes, which see.

JANET, Pierre, La kleptomanie et la dépression mentale, " Journal de psychologie normal et pathologique," 1911, p. 97.

JANET, Pierre, Les névroses, Flammarion, Paris, 1909.

JANET, Pierre, Névroses et idées fixes, 2 vols., Paris, 1898.

JANET, Pierre, Les obsessions et la psychasthénie, 2 vols., Paris, 1903.

JANET, Pierre, Les problèmes psychologiques de l'émotion, " Revue Neurologique," 1909, p. 1556.

JANET, Pierre, Notes sur quelques spasmes des muscles du tronc chez les hystériques et sur leur traitement, " La France Médicale," December 6, 1895.

JANET, Pierre, On the Pathogenesis of some Impulsions, " Journal of Abnormal Psychology," April 1906, p. 1.

JANET, Pierre, Rapport sur la définition de la suggestion au premier congrès de la Société Internationale de Psychothérapie, 1910, published as Sonderabdruck of the " Journal für Psychologie und Neurologie," Leipzig, 1911.

JANET, Pierre, Rapport sur le problème de la subconscience, Comptes rendus du congrès de Psychologie, Geneva, 1909.

JANET, Pierre, Traitement psychologique de l'hystérie, in Albert Robin's Traité de thérapeutique appliquée, 1898, etc., vol. xv.

JOLY, Henri, L'imagination, étude psychologique, Hachette, Paris, 1877.

JOLY, Henri, Problèmes de science criminelle, Hachette, Paris, 1910.

JONES, ERNEST, The Action of Suggestion in Psychotherapy, " Journal of Abnormal Psychology," vol. v. (This article is reprinted in the same author's Papers on Psychoanalysis.)

Jones, Ernest, Papers on Psychoanalysis, Baillière, London : first edition, pp. 432, 1913 ; second edition, pp. 715, 1918 ; third edition, pp. 731, 1923.

Jones, Ernest, The Pathology of morbid Anxiety, " Journal of Abnormal Psychology," July 1911.

Jones, Ernest, Psychoanalysis in Psychotherapy, see Psychotherapeutics, a Symposium.

Jones, Ernest, Papers on Psychoanalysis, Baillière, London, 1913 ; second edition, 1918 ; third edition, 1923.

Jong, Arie de, Het Hypnotismus als Geneesmiddel, second edition, 's-Gravenhage, 1888.

Jouffroy, Théodore Simon, Mélanges philosophiques, second edition, 1838, fifth edition, 1875 ; English translation by G. Ripley, Philosophical Essays, London, 1838.

Jung, Carl Gustav, Ueber das Verhalten der Reaktionszeit beim Assoziations-experimente, Leipzig, 1905.

Knapp, Philip Coombs, Traumatic Neurasthenia, " Brain," 1897.

Knowles, E. R., The true Christian Science, Providence.

Kouindjy, P., La crampe professionnelle et son traitement par le massage méthodique et par la rééducation, " Nouvelle Iconographie de la Salpêtrière," July 1906.

Ladame, Névroses et sexualité, " L'Encéphale," 1913.

Lafontaine, Charles, L'art de magnétiser, ou le magnétisme animal considéré sous le point de vue théorique, pratique et thérapeutique, third edition, Baillière, Paris, 1860. [First edition, 1847.]

Lagrange, Fernand, Les mouvements méthodiques et la " mécanothérapie," Alcan, Paris, 1899.

Lasègue, Ernest Charles, Catalepsies partielles et passagères, " Archives générales de médecine," 1865.

Lasègue, Ernest Charles, Etudes médicales, 2 vols., Paris, 1884.

Lasserre, Henri, Les épisodes miraculeux de Lourdes, 1883.

Laumonier, J., Traitement de la paresse, " Bulletin Général de Thérapeutique," February 23, 1913.

Laurent, L., Les états seconds, variations pathologiques du champ de la conscience, Doin, Paris, 1893.

Lavastine, Laignel and Courbon, P., Prophylaxie et traitement de l'insincérité chez les accidentés de la guerre, " Paris Médical," November 17, 1917.

Leclercq, see Bouché-Leclercq.

Leroy-Allais, Jeanne, Comment j'ai instruit mes filles des choses de la maternité, Maloine, Paris, 1907.

Leuba, James Henry, A psychological Study of Religion, its origin, function, and future, Macmillan, New York, 1912.

LEURET, François, Essais psychologiques sur la folie, 1848.

LEVILLAIN, Fernand, La neurasthénie, etc., Maloine, Paris, 1891.

LEVILLAIN, Fernand, see also VIGOUROUX, Romain.

LÉVY, Paul Emile, La cure définitive de la neurasthénie par la ré-education, " Archives Générales de la Médecine," February 6, 1906.

LÉVY, Paul Emile, L'éducation rationnel de la volonté, son emploi thérapeutique, Alcan, Paris, 1898 ; English translation by Florence K. Bright, from the ninth French edition, The rational Education of the Will, Rider, London, 1913.

LÉVY, Paul Emile, Les névroses méconnues. Pathogénie psychique et psychothérapie, " Journal des Practiciens," 1906, no. 32.

LÉVY, Paul Emile, Les principes de la psychothérapie, la rééducation, " Bulletin de la Société de l'Internat," November 1904.

LÉVY, Paul Emile, Traitement psychique de l'hystérie, " Presse Médicale," April 29, 1903.

LIÉBEAULT, Ambroise Auguste, Du sommeil et des états analogues considérés surtout au point de vue de l'action moral sur le physique, Nancy and Paris, 1866.

LIÉBEAULT, Ambroise Auguste, Etude sur le zoomagnetisme, Nancy, 1883.

LIÉBEAULT, Ambroise Auguste, Le sommeil provoqué et les etats analogues, Paris, 1889.

LIÉBEAULT, Ambroise Auguste, Thérapeutique suggestive . . . pro-priétés diverses du sommeil provoqué, Paris, 1891.

LIÉGEOIS, Jules, De la suggestion hypnotique dans ses rapports avec le droit civil et le droit criminel, Paris, 1884.

LINDSTRÖM, see TAYLOR, E. W.

LORD, Henrietta Frances, Christian Science Healing, its principles and practice, Redway, London, 1888.

LOURIÉ, Ossip, Le language et la verbomanie, essai de psychologie morbide, Alcan, Paris, 1912.

LOUYER-VILLERMAY, Jean Baptiste de, Traité des maladies nerveuses ou vapeurs, et particulièrement de l'hystérie et de l'hypochondrie, Paris, 1816.

LOWELL, Percival, Occult Japan, or the Way of the Gods, an esoteric Study of Japanese Personality and Possession, Houghton and Mifflin, Boston and New York, 1895.

McDOUGALL, William, The Sensations excited by a single momentary Stimulation of the Eye, " British Journal of Psychology," 1904.

MAEDER, A., Essai d'interprétation de quelques rêves, " Archives de Psychologie," April 1907.

MAEDER, A., Sur le mouvement psychoanalytique, un point de vue nouveau en psychologie, " L'Année Psychologique," 1912.

MAGNAN, Jacques Joseph Valentin, De l'alitement, clinothérapie dans le service central d'admission des aliénés de la ville de Paris, " Bulletin de l'Académie de Médecine," July 23, 1912.

MAINE de BIRAN, Marie François Pierre Gouthier, Oeuvres inédites, three vols., Paris, 1859.

MALEBRANCHE, Nicolas, De la recherche de la vérité, 1674 ; English translation by T. Taylor, Treatise concerning the Search after Truth, Oxford, 1694.

MANACÉINÈ, Marie de, Le sommeil, tiers de notre vie, Paris, 1896 ; this is the French translation by E. Joubert of a Russian work by Mariya M. Manaseina ; English translation, 1897, Sleep, is vol. 34 of the Contemporary Science Series.

MANGIN, Marcel, Les guérisons de Lourdes et les phénomènes métapsychiques, " Annales des Science Psychiques," December 1907.

MANTO, Georges S., Sur le traitement de l'hystérie à l'hôpital par l'isolement, Steinheil, Paris, 1899.

MARK TWAIN, see TWAIN.

MARRO, Antonio, La pubertà studiata nell'uomo e nella donna in rapporto al l'antropologia, alla psichiatria, alla pedagogia ed alla sociologia, second edition, Turin, 1900 ; French translation by J. P. Medici, La puberté chez l'homme et chez la femme, etc., Schleicher, Paris, 1901.

MARTHA, Constant, Les moralistes sous l'empire romain, Hachette, Paris, 1864.

MASON, R. Osgood, Hypnotism and Suggestion in Therapeutic Education and Reform, New York, 1901, Kegan Paul, London, 1901.

MATHIEU, Albert, and ROUX, J. C., Hystérie gastrique, " Gazette des Hôpitaux," February 1, 1906.

MAUDSLEY, Henry, The Pathology of Mind, being the third edition of the second part of " The Physiology and Pathology of Mind " . . . enlarged and rewritten, London, 1879 ; The Pathology of Mind, a Study of its Distempers, Deformities, and Disorders, Macmillan, London, 1895.

MAUSS, see HUBERT and MAUSS.

MAXWELL, William, De medicina magnetica libri iii, Frankfort, 1679.

MEIGE, Henry, Histoire d'un tiqueur, " Journal de Médecine et de Chirurgie," August 25, 1901.

MEIGE, Henry, and FEINDEL, E., Les tics et leur traitement, Masson, Paris, 1902.

MESNER, Friedrich (or Franz) Anton, De planetarum influxu, 1766.

MESNET, Ernest, De l'automatisme du mémoire et du souvenir dans le somnambulisme pathologique, considérations médicolégales, Malteste, Paris, 1874.

MESNET, Ernest, Outrages à la pudeur, violences sur les organes sexuels de la femme dans le somnambulisme provoqué et la fascination, étude médicolégale, Rueff, Paris, 1893.

MIGNARD, M., Les états de satisfaction dans la démence et dans l'idiotie, thèse, 1909.

MILL, John Stuart, Autobiography, Longmans, London, 1873.

MILLER, Dickinson S., What Religion has to do with Psychotherapy, see PARKER's Psychotherapy.

MILLS, Charles K., The Treatment of Nervous and Mental Diseases by Systematised Active Exercises, The Transactions of the Philadelphia County Medical Society, January 11, 1888.

MILMINE, Georgine, The Life of Mary Baker G. Eddy and the History of Christian Science, reprinted, with additions, from " McClure's Magazine," Doubleday, New York, and Hodder and Stoughton, London, 1909.

MITCHELL, Silas Weir, Mary Reynolds, a Case of Double Consciousness, 1889.

MOLL, Albert, Christian Science, Medicine, and Occultism.

MOLL, Albert, Der Hypnotismus, Berlin, 1889 ; third edition, enlarged, 1895 ; English translation, Hypnotism, Walter Scott, London, 1891.

MONTARANI, A. [A Case of painful Writer's Cramp cured by rational Psychotherapy], " Rivista Sperimentale di Freniatria," December 1909.

MONTGERON, Carré de, see CARRÉ DE MONTGERON.

MOREAU DE TOURS, Jacques Joseph, De haschisch et de l'aliénation mentale, 1845.

MOREL, Bénédict Augustin, Traité des maladies mentales, Paris, 1860.

MORENO, Bravo y, Notas de psicoterapia, " Archivos de psiquiatria de M. J. Ingegnieros," 1908.

MORICOURT, J., Manuel de metallothérapie et de métalloscopie, etc., Paris, 1888.

MÜNSTERBERG, Hugo, Psychotherapy, Moffat, Yard & Co., New York, 1909.

MYERS, A. T., and MYERS, F. W. H., Mind, Faith-cure, and the Miracles of Lourdes, Proceedings of the Society for Psychical Research, 1893-4, pp. 160-209.

NOIZET, François Joseph, Mémoire sur le somnambulisme et le magnétisme animal, adressé en 1820 à l'Academie royale de Berlin, et publié en 1854, Plon, Paris, 1854.

OPPENHEIM, Hermann, Letters on Psychotherapeutics, translated by Alexander Bruce, Schulze & Co., Edinburgh, and Stechert, New York, 1907.

OPPENHEIM, Hermann, Psychotherapy in Child Training, see PARKER'S Psychotherapy.

PAGET, Stephen, The Case against Christian Science, Cassell, London, 1909.

PAGNIEZ, Philippe, see CAMUS.

PARKER, William Belmont, Psychotherapy, a Course of Reading in sound Psychology, sound Medicine, and sound Religion, 3 vols., New York, 1909.

PAUCHET, V., Gastroptose, traitement, " Presse Médicale," April 11, 1918.

PAUCHET, V., Traitement de l'ulcère chronique de l'estomac, " Presse Médicale," October 9, 1916.

PAUL, Eden, Pathological and prolonged Sleep, " Journal of Mental Science," July 1911.

PAULHAN, Frédéric, L'activité mentale et les éléments de l'esprit, Alcan, Paris, 1889.

PAYOT, Jules, L'éducation de la volonté, Alcan, Paris, 1894.

PETERSON, Fred, The Effects of Emotion on the Body, see PARKER'S Psychotherapy.

PETETIN, Jacques Henri Désiré, Mémoire sur la découverte des phénomènes que présentent la catalepsie et le somnambulisme, Lyons, 1787.

PHILIPPON, Emmanuel, La médication mentale dans la doctrine de la Christian Science.

PRINCE, Morton, see Psychotherapeutics, a Symposium.

PHILIPS, Joseph Pierre, see DURAND.

PIGEAIRE, Jules, Puissance de l'électricité animale, etc., Paris, 1839.

PINEL, Philippe, Traité medico-philosophique sur l'aliénation mentale, ou la manie, Paris, an ix (1801), second edition, Paris, 1809.

PITRES, A., Leçons cliniques sur l'hystérie et l'hypnotisme, 2 vols., Paris, 1891.

PITRES, A., Tics convulsifs géneralisés, traités par le gymnastique respiratoire, " Journal de Médecine de Bordeaux," February 17, 1901.

PITRES, A., and RÉGIS, Emmanuel, Rapport sur les obsessions au Congrès de Médecine de Moscow, 1897, p. 54.

PLANQUES, J., De l'isolement dans le traitement de l'hystérie et de quelques autres maladies, Paris, 1895.

PLAYFAIR, William Smoult, The Systematic Treatment of Nerve Prostration and Hysteria, Smith, Elder & Co., London, 1883.

PLICQUE, A. F., Maladie par insuffisance d'alimentation, " Journal de médecine et de chirurgie," November 10, 1917.

PRINCE, Morton, Association Neuroses, "Journal of Nervous and Mental Diseases," May 1891.

PRINCE, Morton, Discussion of the Symposium, "Journal of Abnormal Psychology," January 1911.

PRINCE, Morton, The Educational Treatment of Neurasthenia and Certain Hysterical States, "Boston Medical and Surgical Journal," October 6, 1898.

PRINCE, Morton, Fear Neurosis, "Boston Medical and Surgical Journal," September 1898.

PRINCE, Morton, The Mechanism of Recurrent Nervous States, "Journal of Abnormal Psychology," 1911, p. 135.

PRINCE, Morton, The Psychological Principles and Field of Psychotherapy, see Psychotherapeutics, a Symposium.

PRINCE, Morton, The Mechanism of Recurrent Psychopathic States, "Journal of Abnormal Psychology," July 1911.

Psychotherapeutics, a Symposium, by Morton Prince, Ernest Jones, and others, Fisher Unwin, London, 1910, and Boston, Mass., 1910.

PUEL, Edmond, De la catalepsie, Baillière, Paris, 1856.

PUTNAM, James Jackson, Considerations on Mental Therapeutics, Harvard Medical School, Department of Neurology, 1906, p. 14.

PUTNAM, James Jackson, The Nervous Breakdown, see PARKER'S Psychotherapy.

PUTNAM, James Jackson, The Psychology of Health, see PARKER'S Psychotherapy.

PUYSÉGUR, Armand Marie Jacques de Chastenet, Lettres de Puységur, May 8, 1784.

PUYSÉGUR, Armand Marie Jacques de Chastenet, Rapport des cures opérées à Baïonne par le magnétisme animal, adressé a M. l'abbé de Poulanzet, conseiller-clerc au parlement de Bordeaux, 1784.

RAND, Benjamin, see BALDWIN, James Mark.

RAULIN, Joseph, the Elder, Traités des affections vaporeuses du sexe, etc., Paris, 1758.

RAYMOND, Fulgence, Leçons sur les maladies du système nerveux (année 1895–1896), 2nd series, Doin, Paris, 1897.

RÉGIS, Emmanuel, see PITRES, A.

RÉGIS, Emmanuel, and HESNARD, A., La doctrine de Freud et de son école, "L'Encéphale," April 10, 1913, May 10, 1913.

RÉGIS, Emmanuel, and HESNARD, E., La psychoanalyse des névroses et des psychoses, ses applications médicales et extra médicales, Alcan, Paris, 1914.

REGNARD, Paul, Les maladies épidémiques de l'esprit : sorcellerie, magnétisme, morphinisme, délire des grandeurs, Plon Nourrit, Paris, 1887.

Ribot, Théodule Armand, Essai sur les passions, Alcan, Paris, 1907.

Ribot, Théodule Armand, Problèmes de psychologie affective, Alcan, 1909.

Ricard, Jean Joseph Adolphe, Traité théorique et pratique du magnetisme animal, ou méthode facile pour apprendre à magnetiser, Paris, 1841.

Richer, Paul, see also Charcot and Richer.

Richer, Paul, Etudes cliniques sur l'hystéro-épilepsie, ou grande hystérie (with preface by J. M. Charcot), Paris, 1881 ; second edition, enlarged, 1885.

Richet, Charles, L'homme et l'intelligence, fragments de physiologie et de psychologie, Alcan, Paris, 1884.

Riley, Woodbridge, Mental Healing in America, " American Journal of Insanity," January 1910.

Riley, Woodbridge, The personal Sources of Christian Science, " Psychological Review," November 1903.

Robin, Albert, Traité de thérapeutique appliquée, 20 vols., Rueff, Paris, 1895–1898.

Rostan, Article in " Hermès."

Roux, see Mathieu, Albert.

Sadger, Isidor, Aus dem Liebesleben Nicolaus Lenau, " Schriften zur angewandten Seelenkunde," 1909.

Sage, X. Lamotte, Personal Magnetism, an advanced Course of Suggestive Therapeutics, New York, 1902.

Salverte, Eusèbe Baconnière, Des sciences occultes, essai sur la magie, les prodiges et les miracles, third edition, Paris, 1856. (First edition 1829 ; second edition, 1843.)

Savill, Thomas Dixon, Clinical Lectures on Neurasthenia, Glaisher, London, 1899, second edition, 1902, third edition, 1906, fourth edition, 1908.

Schneider, J. P. F., L'hypnotisme, Paris, 1894.

Schneider, J. P. F., Die psychologische Ursache der hypnotischen Erscheinungen, 1880.

Schofield, Alfred Taylor, Faith Healing, Religious Tract Society, London, 1892.

Schofield, Alfred Taylor, Nervousness, a brief and popular Review of the moral Treatment of disordered Nerves, Rider, London, 1910.

Ségard, Charles, see Fontan.

Séglas, Jules, Traitement des paralysies par l'exercice musculaire, " Annales médico-psychologiques," March, 1887.

Seguin, Edward Constant, Lectures on some Points in the Treatment and Management of Neuroses, Appleton, New York, 1890 ; French version by the author, Leçons sur le traitement des névroses, Doin, Paris, 1893.

SEMELAIGNE, René, Les grands aliénistes français, Steinheil, Paris, 1894.

SÉRIEUX, Paul, V. Magnan sa vie et ses oeuvres, " Annales Médico-Psychologiques," 1917 ; reprinted, Paris, 1921.

SIDIS, Boris, Fear, Anxiety, and psychopathic Maladies, " Journal of Abnormal Psychology," July 1911.

SIDIS, Boris, The psychotherapeutic Value of the hypnoidal State, see Psychotherapeutics, a Symposium.

SIMON, Paul, Max, Le monde des rêves, Paris, 1882.

SIMPSON, Frederick T., Alcoholism and Drug Addictions, see PARKER'S Psychotherapy.

SIMPSON, Frederick T., Hysteria its Nature and Treatment, see PARKER'S Psychotherapy.

SMITH, R. K., " Massachusetts Journal of Osteopathy," November and December, 1905.

SOLLIER, Paul A., " Archives des Conférences de l'Internat," 1905, p. 5.

SOLLIER, Paul A., Coenesthésie cérébrale et mémoire, " Revue Philosophique," July 1899.

SOLLIER, Paul A., De la localisation cérébrale des troubles hystériques, " Revue Neurologique," 1900, p. 102.

SOLLIER, Paul A., Genèse et nature de l'hystérie, recherches cliniques et expérimentales de psycho-physiologie, 2 vols., Paris, 1897.

SOLLIER, Paul A., L'hystérie et son traitement, Alcan, Paris, 1901.

STORER, Maria Longworth, The Story of a Miracle at Lourdes, New York, 1908.

STURGIS, Russell, The Use of Hypnotism in the First Degree as a Means of Modifying or Eliminating a Fixed Idea, " Boston Medical and Surgical Journal," 1894.

TAYLOR, E. W., Simple Explanation and Re-education as a Therapeutic Method, see Psychotherapeutics, a Symposium.

TAYLOR, E. W., and LINDSTRÖM, E. A., Experiences in the Treatment of Tabes by Coordinate Exercises, " Boston Medical and Surgical Journal," December 13, 1906.

TAYLOR, J. Madison, The Amelioration of Paralysis Agitans and other forms of Tremor by Systematic Exercises, " Journal of Nervous and Mental Diseases," 1901, pp. 28 and 133.

TESTE, Alphonse, Le magnétisme animal expliqué, Paris, 1845.

TESTE, Alphonse, Manuel pratique de magnétisme animale, Paris, 1840 ; English translation by D. Spillan, A Practical Manual of Animal Magnetism, Baillière, London, 1843.

TEULON, see DEMARQUAY.

THAYER, W. Sydney, On the Importance of simple physical and psychical Methods of Treatment, " The Johns Hopkins Medical Bulletin," November 1907.

THIJSSEN, E. H. M., Contribution à l'étude de l'hystérie traumatique, Paris, 1888.

THORNDIKE, Edward Lee, Animal Intelligence, New York, 1898 ; Animal Intelligence, Experimental Studies, New York, 1911.

TÖPFFER, Rodolphe, Voyages en zigzag, etc., Paris, 1844 ; new edition, 1885.

TOURETTE, see GILLES DE LA TOURETTE.

TRACKER, D. L., The Principles of Osteopathy, Los Angeles.

TRÉNEL, Traitement de l'agitation et de l'insomnie dans les maladies mentales et nerveuses, Congrès de Bruxelles, 1903.

TUCKEY, Charles Lloyd, How Suggestion Works, see PARKER's Psychotherapy.

TUCKEY, Charles Lloyd, Treatment by Hypnotism and Suggestion, Psychotherapeutics, fourth edition, London, 1900.

TUKE, Daniel Hack, Illustrations of the Influence of the Mind upon the Body in Health and Disease, designed to elucidate the Action of the Imagination ; Churchill, London, 1872 ; second edition, 1884.

TUKE, Daniel Hack, Metalloscopy and expectant Attention, Lewes, London, 1879.

TUKE, Daniel Hack, History of the Insane in the British Isles, London, 1882.

TUKE, Daniel Hack, Sleepwalking and Hypnotism, Churchill, London, 1884.

TUKE, Samuel, Description of the Retreat near York, 1813.

TURNBULL, W., Course of Personal Magnetism.

TWAIN, Mark (pen-name of CLEMENS, Samuel Langhorne), Christian Science, Harper, New York and London, 1907.

VIGOUROUX, Romain, Métalloscopie, Métallothérapie, Aesthésiogénie, " Archives de Neurologie," 1880–1881, p. 257 ; see also " Progrès Medical," 1878.

VIGOUROUX, Romain, Neurasthénie et arthritisme, urologie, régime alimentaire, traitement, introduction par le docteur Levillain, Malsine, Paris, 1893.

VILLERMAY, see LOUYER-VILLERMAY.

VINCENT, Ralph Harry, The Elements of Hypnotism, . . . its Danger and Value, London, 1895.

VIRES, J., L'hypnotisme et la suggestion hypnotique, Coulier, Montpellier, 1901.

VITTOZ, Roger, Traitement des psychonévroses par le rééducation du contrôle cérébral, Baillière, Paris, 1911.

WAITE, Arthur Edward, Braid on Hypnotism, a reissue of James Braid's Neurypnology (see BRAID), edited, with a biographical introduction, by A. E. Waite, Redway, London, 1899.

WALTON, Deafness in Hysterical Anaesthesia, " Brain," 1883.

WARREN, S., Autohypnotism, " Medical News," 1898.

WATERMAN, George A., The Treatment of Fatigue States, see Psycho-therapeutics, a Symposium.

WELLS, Frederick Lyman, Critique of impure Reason, " Journal of Abnormal Psychology," June and July, 1912.

WETTERSTRAND, Otto Georg, Hypnotism and its Application to Practical Medicine, Putnam, New York, 1897. (Translation by H. G. Petersen, from the German edition of 1891, which was translated from the Swedish original of 1888, with additions.)

WETTERSTRAND, Otto Georg, Ueber den künstlich verlängerten Schlaf besonders bei der Behandlung der Hysterie, " Zeitschrift für Hypnotismus," 1892.

WHIPPLE, Leander Edmund, The Philosophy of Mental Healing, 1893

WHIPPLE, Leander Edmund, Practical Health, 1907,

WILBUR, Sibyl, The Life of Mary Baker Eddy, Concord Pub. Co., New York, 1908, Harrap, London, 1908.

WILLIAMS, T. A., A few Hints from personal Experience in Psycho-therapy inculcated by physiological Analogies, " Monthly Cyclo-paedia and Medical Bulletin," July 1908.

WOOD, Henry, New Thought Simplified, Lothrop, New York, 1903.

WOODWORTH, Robert Sessions, The Accuracy of Voluntary Movement, New York, 1899.

WOODWORTH, Robert Sessions, Dynamic Psychology, Columbia University Press, New York, 1918.

WUNDT, Wilhelm, Hypnotismus und Suggestion, Engelmann, Leipzig, 1892 (part of the author's Pilosophische Studien) ; French trans-lation by A. Keller, Hypnotisme et suggestion, Alcan, Paris, 1893.

YUNG, Emile, Le sommeil normal et le sommeil pathologique, mag-nétisme animal, etc., Paris, 1883.

ZOLA, Emile, Lourdes, Fasquelle, Paris, 1903.

INDEX

Classics in Psychiatry

An Arno Press Collection

Feuchtersleben, Ernst [Freiherr] von. **The Principles Of Medical Psychology.** 1847

Georget, [Etienne-Jean]. **De La Folie: Considérations Sur Cette Maladie.** 1820

Haslam, John. **Observations On Madness And Melancholy.** 1809

Hill, Robert Gardiner. **Total Abolition Of Personal Restraint In The Treatment Of The Insane.** 1839

Janet, Pierre [Marie-Felix] and F. Raymond. **Les Obsessions Et La Psychasthénie.** 1903. Two volumes

Janet, Pierre [Marie-Felix]. **Psychological Healing.** 1925. Two volumes

Kempf, Edward J. **Psychopathology.** 1920

Kraepelin, Emil. **Manic-Depressive Insanity And Paranoia.** 1921

Kraepelin, Emil. **Psychiatrie:** Ein Lehrbuch Für Studirende Und Aerzte. 1896

Laycock, Thomas. **Mind And Brain.** 1860. Two volumes in one

Liébeault, A[mbroise]-A[uguste]. **Le Sommeil Provoqué Et Les États Analogues.** 1889

Mandeville, B[ernard] De. **A Treatise Of The Hypochondriack And Hysterick Passions.** 1711

Morel, B[enedict] A[ugustin]. **Traité Des Degénérescences Physiques, Intellectuelles Et Morales De L'Espèce Humaine.** 1857. Two volumes in one

Morison, Alexander. **The Physiognomy Of Mental Diseases.** 1843

Myerson, Abraham. **The Inheritance Of Mental Diseases.** 1925

Perfect, William. **Annals Of Insanity.** [1808]

Pinel, Ph[ilippe]. **Traité Médico-Philosophique Sur L'Aliénation Mentale.** 1809

Prince, Morton, et al. **Psychotherapeutics.** 1910

Psychiatry In Russia And Spain. 1975

Ray, I[saac]. **A Treatise On The Medical Jurisprudence Of Insanity.** 1871

Semelaigne, René. **Philippe Pinel Et Son Oeuvre Au Point De Vue De La Médecine Mentale.** 1888

Thurnam, John. **Observations And Essays On The Statistics Of Insanity.** 1845

Trotter, Thomas. **A View Of The Nervous Temperament.** 1807

Tuke, D[aniel] Hack, editor. **A Dictionary Of Psychological Medicine.** 1892. Two volumes

Wier, Jean. **Histoires, Disputes Et Discours Des Illusions Et Impostures Des Diables, Des Magiciens Infames, Sorcieres Et Empoisonneurs.** 1885. Two volumes

Winslow, Forbes. **On Obscure Diseases Of The Brain And Disorders Of The Mind.** 1860

Burdett, Henry C. **Hospitals And Asylums Of The World.** 1891-93. Five volumes. 2,740 pages on NMA standard 24x-98 page microfiche only